Nursing: A Human Needs Approach

NURSING
A Human Needs Approach

Janice Rider Ellis

R.N., B.S.N., University of Iowa
M.N., University of Washington
Professor of Nursing, Shoreline Community College, Seattle, Washington

Elizabeth Ann Nowlis

R.N., B.S.N., University of Cincinnati
M.N., University of Washington
Professor of Nursing, Shoreline Community College, Seattle, Washington

Houghton Mifflin Company   Boston

Atlanta   Dallas   Geneva, Illinois   Hopewell, New Jersey   Palo Alto   London

Cover photo: Elizabeth Wilcox

Illustrations by Kenneth Dewey / Daniele Deverin

Printed in the U.S.A.
Library of Congress Catalog Card Number: 76-12023
ISBN: 0-395-24067-0

Contents

Part One   Becoming a Nurse   1

1 Introduction to Nursing   2

2 Participating in the Health Care Team   16

10 Dependent Nursing Functions 146

11 Infection 174

12 Hygiene 194

Part Three Physiological Needs of the Patient 213

13 Basic Vital Functions 214

14   Nutrition and Fluids   238

15 Elimination 264

16 Activity and Rest 282

Preface

We have written this textbook for the beginning student on the basis of our own experience as practicing nurses and as instructors in a two-year nursing program. The topics and approaches presented in *Nursing: A Human Needs Approach* are those we are using and have found helpful to nursing students.

We believe that nurses are crucial members of the health care team and that nursing practice demands a sound base in theory as well as technical skills. This book presents the theory and rationales that underlie nursing practices, but does not attempt to teach how to perform skilled nursing tasks. Such skills are more appropriately taught in independent study modules, in practice laboratories, and in clinical situations.

The book is divided into four parts. Part One, "Becoming a Nurse," introduces the student to the health care setting. Those students with prior backgrounds in health care may be able to cover some of this material rapidly. But many entering nursing students have had no health-related experience. It is our belief that on the very first contact with a patient, students must see themselves in the role of nurse. Furthermore, we believe the patient has a right to expect the practitioner, whatever his or her role, to fit into the total plan for care in a meaningful way. To do this, the student needs an understanding of the total health care situation.

Part Two, "The Theory and Practice of Nursing," focuses on nursing as a problem-solving process in which communication and interpersonal relationships are central elements. Awareness of the physical, psychological, and spiritual needs common to all human beings, and of differences among patients of different ages, greatly enhances the nurse's ability to help patients cope with illness. And a thorough understanding of the goals of the nursing process enables the nurse to function more effectively and to communicate with the patient in a more meaningful way.

Part Three examines the physiological needs of the patient. Because of differing science backgrounds, students will vary in their familiarity with the subjects discussed in this part. We have, therefore, taken pains to define terms and to explain basic processes wherever necessary. We have not tried, however, to present material on general anatomy and physiology. Textbooks on those subjects are an excellent source of such information.

Part Four, "Major Challenges in Patient Care," discusses matters that concern nurses in every setting—pain, death, sensory disturbance, disturbances of body image integrity, and aging. Though this material is often reserved for a more advanced level of study, these problems are confronted by beginning students as well as by advanced practitioners. We consider it important to provide students with the essential information they will need to recognize and respond to such problems.

Each chapter begins with a set of objectives intended to guide students in their study. The nature of the objectives varies with the subject under consideration: some are presented in very specific behavioral terms, while others are more general. A list of study terms to aid students in review and a list of references suitable for beginning students are provided at the end of each chapter. Certain more advanced references that have become classic in nursing are included, but we have tried to avoid listing publications that are not available in the usual nursing library.

We view the instructor as the facilitator of the learning process, and recognize that learning can take place only if the student is actively involved. Students will need opportunities to test the concepts presented in this book before accepting them; it is a challenge to the instructor to provide this kind of meaningful experience.

We recognize that students begin their nursing practice in a wide variety of settings, and that patients do not conveniently present only those problems that students have already studied. Therefore, while we have organized the material in what seems to us a logical order, we have also tried to make each section sufficiently independent to allow study out of sequence of those chapters that are relevant to a given situation. The instructor may thus choose to assign the material in a different order, to conform to a particular curriculum or an individual course outline. Chapter 5, on the nursing process, is a prerequisite to most of the subsequent chapters, however, and we recommend that it be studied as early as possible.

Instructors who wish to supplement the material in this book with a basic skills manual will find our *Modules for Basic Nursing Skills*, written with Patricia M. Bentz, a helpful student guide. The modules, perforated and punched for insertion in a looseleaf binder, provide step-by-step instruction in specific nursing skills. Learning objectives, performance checklists, and review quizzes are included in each module. The modules are self-contained for easy rearrangement to suit individual course outlines.

JANICE RIDER ELLIS
ELIZABETH ANN NOWLIS

Acknowledgments

Our first thanks go to our families, who have supported us in difficulties and rejoiced with us when things went well. For the time they have sacrificed in deference to "The Book," we shall always be grateful.

We also wish to thank Frances H. Zaleski, R.N., M.N., Professor Emeritus at Shoreline Community College, who encouraged us to begin this project and believed that we could do it well.

Additional thanks go to all the members of the nursing faculty at Shoreline Community College, who have provided a climate in which we could grow and have shared their considerable experience and expertise with us.

Throughout the preparation of this manuscript, we have been aided by the thoughtful responses of nurse educators across the country, whose comments have helped us in numberless ways to bring this project to completion. They are: Lois Bodinski, Carol Connolly, Mary Delaney, Mary Gradishar, Judith Holdcraft, Carol Mutzebaugh, Marian O'Laughlin, Sue Petrovich, Isabel Shannon, and Roberta Windle.

Nursing: A Human Needs Approach

Part One
Becoming a Nurse

1 Introduction to Nursing

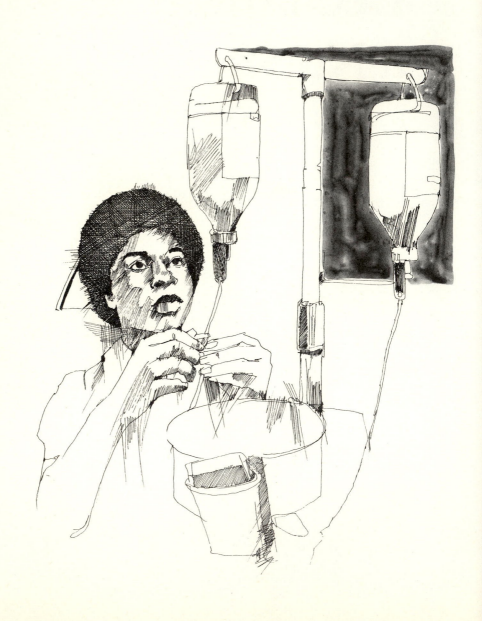

Objectives

After completing this chapter, you should be able to:

1 Discuss the definition of nursing.
2 Identify the three pathways to becoming a registered nurse.
3 Discuss the difference between ethical and legal issues.
4 List some common legal concerns for nurses.
5 Discuss the rule of the reasonably prudent nurse.
6 Identify a resource to consult on ethical issues.
7 Discuss consumer rights as a component of health care.

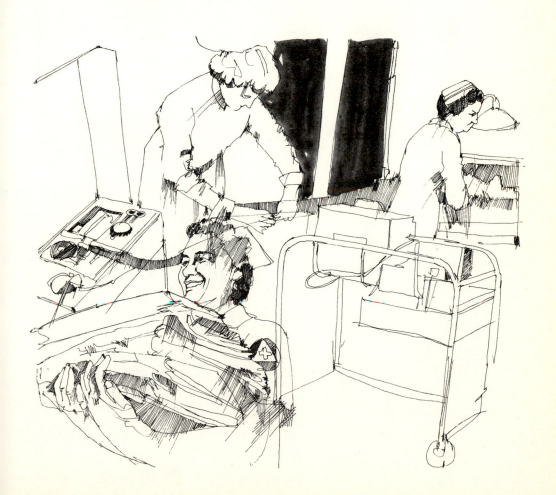

AS YOU BEGIN the new venture of preparing to become a registered nurse, you will find that nursing students today are a highly varied group. Among you are recent high-school graduates and persons in their forties embarking on new careers. Your educational attainments may vary from a general equivalency diploma (G.E.D.) gained through independent study to a baccalaureate degree in another discipline. And your employment experience is also widely varied, some of you having had no previous health-related employment and others having worked for years as licensed practical nurses or members of medical corps.

This rich variety of backgrounds is adding depth and breadth to nursing education. As an individual, you can contribute to the education of others by sharing your background, knowledge, and experiences with them; and you can learn from those around you.

Definitions of nursing

The views of nursing held by beginning nursing students are undoubtedly as divergent as their experiences. Many still think of a

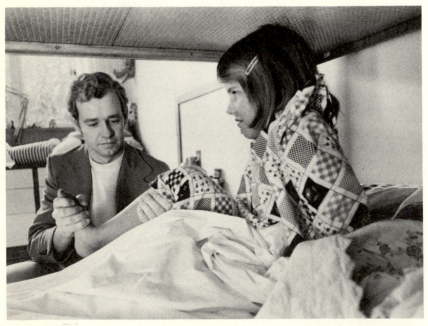

"Nurses today are extraordinarily diverse in their work settings": a visiting nurse and patient
Chris Maynard

nurse as a woman in a white uniform who works in a hospital. But nurses today are extraordinarily diverse in their backgrounds, work settings, and roles. Nurses may be found working in industry, in storefront clinics, in rural homes, and in research laboratories. And the number of men in nursing is growing. What then unites such various people? We find that the excerpt from *The Nature of Nursing*, written by Virginia Henderson, most clearly articulates what we believe nursing to be (see page 6).

You will note that Henderson's definition focuses not on curing patients of illness but rather on caring for them in such a way as to facilitate their own life patterns. In other words, it deals with health, not just with illness. Above all, this definition emphasizes the independence and autonomy of the patient. As you progress in your nursing education, you will gradually develop a working definition of what nursing is for you. And this definition will continue to change and expand as you acquire experience as a registered nurse.

Pathways to nursing careers

The goal of becoming a registered nurse can be reached by three routes. Each one has a slightly different focus, but all prepare the graduate to take the state board licensing examination. Every school of nursing must be approved by its own state's board of nursing, or the equivalent, and some are accredited by such organizations as the National League for Nursing.

Diploma programs

Diploma programs conducted by hospitals' schools of nursing are the oldest type of program, and still produce the majority of registered nurses. Although students may be offered some experience at other facilities, most of their clinical experience takes place in the sponsoring hospital. Relative to other programs, greater amount of time is spent in clinical practice, and graduates are generally expected to have acquired more proficiency in clinical performance. Many such programs arrange for all science and social science subjects to be taught at a nearby college or university. The graduate receives a diploma on completion of the program, which lasts two and one-half or three years. A few programs are structured so that a student receives an Associate Degree in Nursing from an affiliating college as well as a diploma from the hospital school.

The Nature of Nursing

The unique function of the nurse is to assist the individual, sick or well, in the performance of those activities contributing to health or its recovery (or to peaceful death) that he would perform unaided if he had the necessary strength, will, or knowledge. And to do this in such a way as to help him gain independence as rapidly as possible.

. . . . The nurse is the authority on basic nursing care—by basic nursing care I mean helping the patient with the following activities or providing conditions under which he can perform them unaided:

1 Breathe normally.
2 Eat and drink adequately.
3 Eliminate body wastes.
4 Move and maintain desirable postures.
5 Sleep and rest.
6 Select suitable clothes—dress and undress.
7 Maintain body temperature within normal range by adjusting clothing and modifying the environment.
8 Keep the body clean and well groomed and protect the integument.
9 Avoid dangers in the environment and avoid injuring others.
10 Communicate with others in expressing emotions, needs, fears, or opinions.
11 Worship according to one's faith.
12 Work in such a way that there is a sense of accomplishment.
13 Play or participate in various forms of recreation.

From Virginia Henderson, The Nature of Nursing (New York: Macmillan, 1966), pp. 15–16. Revised 1969, International Council of Nurses, Geneva. Reprinted with permission.

Associate degree programs

The newest type of preparation for nursing, associate degree programs, are conducted by community or junior colleges. Some have evolved as a result of cooperation between a college and a hospital that formerly had its own nursing school. Clinical facilities are obtained by contract with hospitals and other health care providers in the community. The general goal of these programs, which last two years, is to prepare students for entry-level positions in direct care. Because clinical experience is limited in such a program, the graduate will need time to increase proficiency and competence when first employed. The graduate receives an Associate Degree in Nursing from the college.

Baccalaureate programs

Four-year baccalaureate programs in nursing are offered by some colleges and universities. Baccalaureate students receive more training in background sciences and social sciences than do students in other types of programs, and nursing theory is taught in greater depth. Nursing in community health, some leadership skills, and beginning research procedures are also taught, to prepare the student for further education and for roles requiring these skills. The baccalaureate graduate acquires sufficient clinical skills to fill entry-level staff positions.

Graduates of all three types of programs take the same licensing examination to become registered nurses. Employment opportunities for graduates of the various programs differ widely, depending on such factors as local nursing needs, the type of experiences a given program provides, and individual ability. Graduates of all types of programs are prepared for entry-level staff positions in hospitals, nursing homes, and ambulatory care settings.

The ladder concept

Many practicing nurses find that they want further education or more advanced degrees. Getting it is not an easy task; in some locales previous education is not credited, and the student is required to enroll at the beginning level of a program. Increasing efforts are being made to provide for career mobility and progression from one degree level to another. The steps in such a progression may be seen as a ladder, as illustrated in Figure 1.1. The nurse who wishes to obtain a

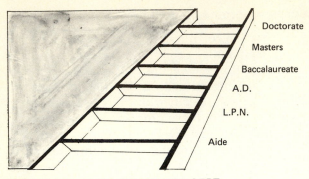

FIGURE 1.1   THE LADDER CONCEPT

higher degree will need to inquire about the program and policies of the college of choice. Some colleges and universities allow credit for previous experience if the applicant passes an examination. Others will allow the student to construct an independent study program to meet his or her own needs. As education becomes more flexible to allow for the individuality of students, nursing education is also changing.

Legal and ethical concerns in nursing

Legal concerns

The legal definition of nursing practice is determined by the legislature of each state, and regulated by the state board of nursing in accordance with the law. Further interpretation of the law is also provided by the courts through litigation on specific issues. Although the specifics of such laws differ in different states, they share certain features. Only persons who have complied with all the requirements of the state licensing law are entitled to call themselves registered nurses. Nursing is seen by the law as entailing a specific body of actions and expertise. In addition, the law recognizes areas of practice, such as giving medication, that can be undertaken on the direction of a licensed physician, dentist, or osteopathic physician.

Let us examine some legal terms applicable to the practice of nursing and some legal principles to which nurses are subject. *Negligence* is a legal term applied to (a) an act that resulted in harm to another person, or (b) the omission of an act that would have prevented harm to another. To be found negligent, a person must have failed to act as a "reasonably prudent person" would act in a given situation.

Malpractice is a narrower term referring to negligence by a professional person.

The standard of the reasonably prudent person is modified in the case of a nurse or other professional, so that standard for action is held to be the "reasonably prudent nurse." An understanding of this principle is important to the student nurse. Whenever you perform a nursing procedure, you are subject to the standard of the reasonably prudent *registered nurse*. You may be slower or less dextrous, but the outcome for the patient must be the same as would be provided by a registered nurse. This principle insures safety and a high standard of care for the patient. It is not reasonable that a patient should suffer for having received care from a student. Malpractice is a civil wrong, and is punished by a monetary fine rather than a jail sentence. It is assumed that the harm caused by malpractice was not intentional.

Another legal charge of potential concern to medical practitioners is assault and battery. *Assault* is threatening to do bodily harm and *battery* is touching or harming a person without consent. This may seem entirely irrelevant to health care, but medical procedures or surgery of any kind performed without *informed consent* may constitute battery in the eyes of the law. Consent for such procedures as injections, catheterizations, and enemas may be verbal; in some hospitals, patients sign a form giving consent for such general care procedures when admitted. More extensive procedures, such as those that involve anesthesia, cutting into the body, or a measure of risk, require specific written consent. Informed consent requires that the patient not be under the influence of medication that impairs judgment and that he or she be apprised of any risks and of the expected result of the procedure. Such consent must be written and the signature must be witnessed. Informed consent may be given by a parent for a minor child, or by the next of kin for an individual unable to be responsible for himself or herself. Exceptions are made to the rule of informed consent only in true emergencies.

Also of concern in nursing is the legal charge of false imprisonment, or confining a person without consent and without due process. The use of restraints and refusal to allow a person to leave a health facility without due process are defined as *false imprisonment*.

Nurses are always legally responsible for their own actions. Because of their educational background, they are expected to know both their role and the limits of their capability. Under no circumstances can nurses take refuge behind the directions of others. This is a weighty responsibility and must be taken seriously. In order to function appropriately, then, a nurse must keep abreast of current practice through education and constant learning on the job.

Code for Nurses

1 The nurse provides services with respect for the dignity of man, unrestricted by considerations of nationality, race, creed, color, or status.

2 The nurse safeguards the individual's right to privacy by judiciously protecting information of a confidential nature, sharing only that information relevant to his care.

3 The nurse maintains individual competence in nursing practice, recognizing and accepting responsibility for individual actions and judgments.

4 The nurse acts to safeguard the patient when his care and safety are affected by incompetent, unethical, or illegal conduct of any person.

5 The nurse uses individual competence as a criterion in accepting delegated responsibilities and assigning nursing activities to others.

6 The nurse participates in research activities when assured that the rights of individual subjects are protected.

7 The nurse participates in the efforts of the profession to define and upgrade standards of nursing practice and education.

8 The nurse, acting through the professional organization, participates in establishing and maintaining conditions of employment conducive to high-quality nursing care.

9 The nurse works with members of health professions and other citizens in promoting efforts to meet health needs of the public.

10 The nurse refuses to give or imply endorsement to advertising, promotion, or sales for commercial products, services, or enterprises.

By the American Nurses' Association, Committee on Ethical, Legal, and Professional Issues, Elizabeth C. Stobo, Chairman. Revised 1968. Reprinted with permission.

As a student nurse, you have the same legal responsibilities as a nurse. You must know your own abilities and limitations, and should seek supervision and assistance whenever you need it. If you practice beyond your competence and make an error, you could be held legally responsible for any untoward effects of that error.

Most registered nurses and student nurses find it prudent to carry some form of professional liability insurance, which pays attorneys' fees, court costs, and a judgment (if obtained) in case of a lawsuit. Such insurance is available through the American Nurses' Association for registered nurses, through the National Student Nurses' Association for its members, and from private insurance companies.

Ethical issues

Ethical issues are those that have moral dimensions, and an ethical action is one that is morally right. Clearly, there may be a variety of opinions on any ethical issue. This does not mean, however, that there is no accepted standard of ethical conduct. Nurses acting together through the American Nurses' Association have developed a set of ethical principles for registered nurses, known as the A.N.A. Code for Nurses (see page 10). An interpretation of the code is available from the A.N.A. The code is revised periodically to reflect current concerns.

Let us examine some general ethical issues that will concern you as a student.

Confidentiality is protection of the patient's privacy through careful use of both written and oral communication. The patient's problems and condition should be discussed only with those who have a need for such information in order to provide or improve his or her care. The patient has a right to decide what information will be shared. In establishing a relationship with a patient, therefore, you may explain that you will share what you are told with your instructor and/or the nurse in charge of the patient's care. Thus, the patient can decide what he or she wants to share with you and others.

You should judge carefully which portion of the patient's remarks are relevant to his or her care, and thus should be shared, and which should be kept confidential. For instance, a patient might confide that she had a child as an unmarried fourteen-year-old. If the patient were in obstetrics this information could be important to her care and would need to be shared. If the patient were being treated for pneumonia or bronchitis, however, such information would not be helpful. If you are in doubt about the relevance of any information a patient has given you, consult with your instructor or with an experienced nurse before sharing the information more broadly.

Sometimes information about a patient is shared for teaching purposes. In such a case, the identity of the patient is concealed to protect his or her privacy. Thus, if you are writing a paper on the care of a particular patient, you must take care to conceal the patient's identity. In order to maintain privacy and confidentiality, discussions of patients, even when appropriate, should not be conducted in public places where others may overhear. Even when names are not used, personal characteristics may be mentioned, and rumors, either false or true, may result.

Confidentiality of written records is preserved by allowing access only to those who need such information in order to enhance the patient's welfare. In general, the law requires the patient's written permission for the record to be viewed by anyone uninvolved in his or her care. Even within the health care team, however, there may be those who are simply curious. Reading a patient's record simply to satisfy curiosity is considered unethical.

The *behavior* of the nurse or student nurse while at work is also a matter of ethics. What you do as a student nurse reflects not only on yourself but also on all other student nurses. This is an area in which there is considerable difference of opinion as to what constitutes correct and incorrect behavior. A useful guideline is to consider whether certain behavior will enhance or impair your ability to work effectively with the patient. For example, seductive or flirtatious behavior toward a patient may inhibit your ability to function as a nurse with that patient, and is thus considered unethical.

Because nurses and student nurses are responsible for matters of life and death, their behavior must reflect recognition of the importance and seriousness of their tasks. As a nurse you are obliged not to treat serious matters frivolously, to take seriously the patient's request for help, and to put the patient's well-being before your own.

Nonjudgmental attitudes that reflect acceptance of the patient as a person, regardless of your opinion of his or her behavior and life style, are an obligation of health care professionals. The man wounded in a gun battle with the police and the policeman wounded in the same incident deserve the same quality of care. On a less spectacular level, the patient who fails to follow medical directions and is thus the cause of his or her own problems is still entitled to acceptance and care. This means not that nurses are "super people" who have no feelings in such situations, but that they display nonjudgmental attitudes toward the patient and express such feelings elsewhere. If you find this impossible in a particular situation, you have an obligation to withdraw from the patient's care so that you do not increase his or her problems.

Consumers' rights in health care

Attention to the rights of consumers of health care is increasing, in conjunction with the growth of consumer movements in other areas of life.

The first statement of patients' rights was formulated in 1959 by the National League for Nursing but was not widely published or known outside the League. Then, in 1973, the American Hospital Association published a "Patients' Bill of Rights." Because of the A.H.A.'s size and influence, and because the public had become very interested in consumer rights, this document was widely published and became the subject of much discussion.

As a result, other groups began to formulate bills of rights, each with a different focus. State nurses' associations were among those who did so. The Health Consumers' Bill of Rights on page 14, enacted by the Washington State Nurses' Association, was formulated with particular reference to the role of the nurse.

Still more recently, the Michigan legislature has passed a legally binding Patients' Bill of Rights. Its substance is somewhat less specific than private organizations' statements, which have only ethical—not legal—force. The law has not been in effect long enough to determine whether it will bring about changes in health care.

Bioethics is the name of a new field of study that considers the ethics of modern health care technology. In brief, bioethics is concerned with questions of human life. When should maximum life-supportive measures be used? Is it ever ethical to withhold maximum life support or to withdraw it, once begun? If care is only available for a few, how and by whom are those few to be chosen? How is death to be defined? The list of such questions is virtually endless, and none have universally accepted answers. Some, such as the definition of death, have legal aspects as well, and lawyers are working with health professionals to seek satisfactory solutions. At present, the thrust of such work is to encourage recognition of these issues as ethical or moral, not scientific, and to emphasize the need for all citizens—not just the health and legal communities—to become involved in these decisions.

As you work, you will undoubtedly confront bioethical decisions. One such decision involves elective abortion. Some nurses find abortion an ethically defensible alternative, and thus participate in the procedure and in care of the patient. Others who consider the procedure unethical cannot in good conscience participate in any phase of care. Still others decline to participate in the abortion, but consider it ethical to care for the patient after the abortion. All of these are individual ethical decisions, and as such are to be respected and honored by others.

Conclusion

To become a student nurse is to enter a new role in life, a role that involves both learning and providing for patients' needs. Your conduct in this new role is governed by both legal and ethical restraints. The rules governing your behavior as a student nurse are

Health Consumer Bill of Rights

Access to the highest quality of care that can be provided is a pervading right of each citizen of the state unrestricted by any personal circumstances. Consistent with a purpose of WSNA to foster high standards of nursing practice to the end that all people may have better nursing care, the 1972 WSNA House of Delegates hereby adopts the following Bill of Rights for patients:

The patient has a right to:

1 Services which respect the dignity and worth of man, unrestricted by consideration of nationality, race, creed, color, status, age or sex.

2 Maximum self-determination in health care situations, consistent with his well-being or health status. Maximum self-determination includes making informed decisions about such things as:

a Total care planning that is in accord with his value system

b Refusal to accept aspects of his care with which he is not in accord after receiving adequate information or teaching

c Determination of the extent to which his family is involved in his care

d Right to die in dignity consistent with his personal values

3 Information and knowledge about his health status and related care.

4 Be well informed as to what constitutes quality health care and what mechanism may be used for obtaining action, when, in his opinion, quality care is not given.

5 Expect a health care advocate to speak on his behalf when his care and safety are affected by incompetent, unethical or illegal conduct of any person.

6 Individualized care related to his unique needs and life style regardless of nationality, race, creed, color, status, age or sex.

7 Privacy by having information of a confidential nature judiciously protected, sharing only that information relevant to his care.

8 Be taught self-care consistent with his capabilities.

By the Washington State Nurses' Association, House of Delegates, 1972. Reprinted with permission.

the same as those that will eventually govern you as a registered nurse. Your learning cannot and should not take precedence over the well-being of the patient. While legal decisions are made for you by others, you must make ethical decisions for yourself. Nursing is not always an easy road, but it is filled with many rewards.

Study terms

assault

associate degree programs

baccalaureate programs

battery

bioethics

confidentiality

consumer rights

diploma programs

ethics

informed consent

ladder concept

legal issues

malpractice

negligence

patients' rights

reasonably prudent nurse

registered nurse (R.N.)

References

Allen, M. 1974. Ethics of Nursing Practice. *Canadian Nurse* 70:5:22-23.

Bachand, M. 1974. Wanted: A Definition of Nursing Practice. *Canadian Nurse* 70:5:26-29.

Barritt, E. R. 1973. Florence Nightingale's Values and Modern Nursing Education. *Nursing Forum* 12:1:6-47.

Bill of Rights for Patients. 1973. *Nursing Outlook* 21:82 (February 1973).

Creighton, H. 1973. Ten Commandments in Nursing. *Nursing '73* 3:1:7-8.

Facing a Grand Jury. 1976. *American Journal of Nursing* 76:398-400.

Judge, D. 1975. The New Nurse: A Sense of Duty and Destiny. *Nursing Digest* 3:6:20-24.

Kelly, L. Y. 1976. Keeping Up With Your Legal Responsibilities. *Nursing '76* 6:3:81-93.

————. 1974. Nursing Practice Acts. *American Journal of Nursing* 74:1309-1310.

Lowe, G. M. 1974. Let's Have More Human Nursing Care. *Nursing '74* 4:1: 10-11.

Schmiedel, E. G. 1973. One Rung at a Time Up the Career Ladder. *Nursing Outlook* 21:400-403.

Tyrer, L. B., *et al.* 1974. The New Morality, Ethics and Nursing. *Nursing Digest* 2:4:89-91.

Wood, L. 1973. Proposal: A Career Plan for Nursing. *American Journal of Nursing* 73:532-535.

Wozmak, D. 1973. External Degrees in Nursing in New York State. *American Journal of Nursing* 73:1014-1018.

2 Participating in the Health Care Team

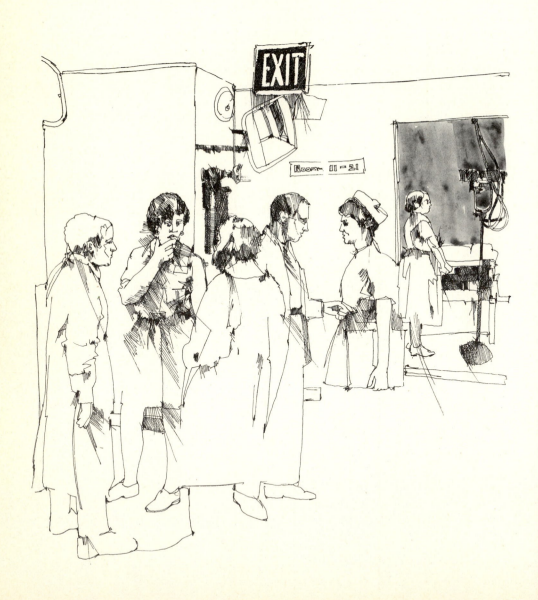

Objectives

After completing this chapter, you should be able to:

1 Define the health care team and discuss its scope.

2 Identify strengths and weaknesses in the team approach to health care.

3 Explain the various ways individuals can function within the health care team: independently, interdependently, and dependently.

4 Apply this knowledge in working cooperatively with others to provide health care.

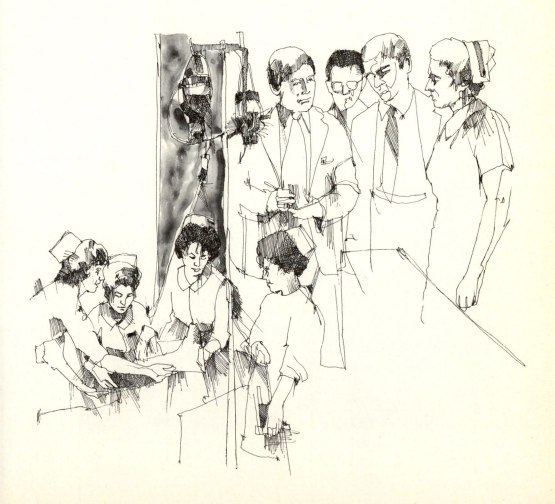

THE INCREASING COMPLEXITY of health care makes it impossible for an individual working independently to provide total health care to a patient. This circumstance has given rise to an ever-growing number of health care occupations, each with a specific area of expertise and responsibility. Any of these individuals who has a direct or indirect impact on the patient's care is considered a member of the health care team in the broadest sense of the term. And the patient too must of necessity, be a central member of this team if it is to accomplish its goal of optimum health care.

Some health care occupations

Some of the occupations that compose the health care team, such as medicine and nursing, are well known. Others such as the orthotics technician, who makes braces and prosthetic appliances, are familiar only to specialists. Many of the newer and less well-known occupations have developed to administer new diagnostic or treatment techniques or to assist more extensively prepared persons.

The chart on the opposite page outlines a variety of health care workers you may encounter. You may find that some of these occu-

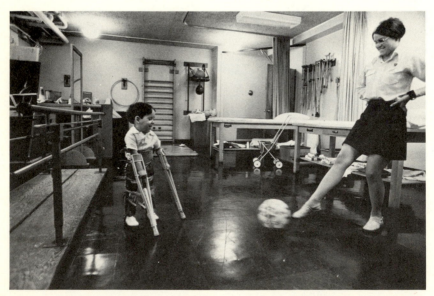

The physical therapist: one member of the health care team
Chris Maynard

18

Some Health Care Occupations

CHILD CARE
Pediatrician
Pediatric Nurse Practitioner

DENTAL CARE
Dentist
Dental Hygienist
Dental Assistant
Dental Laboratory Technician

DRUG THERAPY
Pharmacist
Pharmacy Technician
Pharmacologist

EYE CARE
Ophthalmologist
Optometrist
Oculist

LABORATORY TESTING
Pathologist
Cytologist
Medical Technologist
Medical Laboratory Technician
Certified Laboratory Assistant
EEG (electroencephalographic)
    Technician
ECG (electrocardiographic)
    Technician

NURSING
Registered Nurse
Licensed Practical (Vocational)
    Nurse
Nursing Assistant (Aide or
    Orderly)

MEDICINE
Physician (many specialties, some
    listed in specific categories)
Resident
Intern
Extern
Physician's Assistant

MENTAL HEALTH
Psychiatrist
Psychologist
Psychiatric Social Worker
Mental Health Technician

**PHYSICAL MEDICINE AND REHABILI-
TATION**
Physiatrist
Physical Therapy Technician
Registered Physical Therapist
Registered Occupational
    Therapist
Occupational Therapy Technician

RADIATION AND RADIOLOGY
Radiologist
X-Ray Technician
Radio Isotope Technician

RECORD KEEPING
Medical Records Librarian
Medical Records Technician
Medical Records Secretary

RESPIRATORY CARE
Respiratory Therapist
Inhalation Therapist
Respiratory Technician

SOCIAL WORK
Medical Social Worker
Caseworker
Community Liaison Worker

SPEECH AND HEARING
Otolaryngologist
Audiologist
Speech Therapist

SURGERY
Surgeon
Operating Room Nurse
Operating Room Technician
Anesthesiologist
Nurse Anesthetist

pations are not represented in your locality. Some may have different titles, and certain of these occupations may have overlapping functions. It is important, nevertheless, that you have some understanding of these occupations and their areas of responsibility. If you are unfamiliar with some, look them up in a medical dictionary. As you meet fellow workers in the health care setting, you may want to inquire about their roles in order to gain a greater understanding of the entire health team. It will also be one of your responsibilities as a nurse to interpret to patients the function of those who participate in their care. Thus your own perceptions need to be clear.

Differences in preparation for health care roles

Educational preparation for the various health care careers differs greatly. Perhaps the longest preparation is that of the physician who chooses a specialty or subspecialty. Each move into a more specialized level of practice increases the length of the physician's preparation. In contrast, preparation for some health careers consists entirely of on-the-job training, such as that received by most nurse's aides.

Educational preparation may also vary within a single occupational group. Nursing, as we have seen, provides three pathways to registration: a diploma, associate degree, or baccalaureate degree. However, nursing education programs are subject to approval by state boards of nursing, which tends to have a standardizing effect.

Some health care workers with identical titles may have had vastly different amounts of preparation for their roles, because there are no laws governing their training. One such field is inhalation therapy. Some inhalation therapists have formal educational backgrounds of considerable depth, while others have received only on-the-job training.

Recognition of such differences is important when you are responsible for delegating tasks or sharing them with others. A licensed practical nurse can be expected to observe a patient more knowledgeably than would an orderly. If a patient is in need of close observation, therefore, you would delegate this task to the L.P.N., not the orderly. It is also necessary to know the range and limits of others' expertise. For instance, a respiratory therapist with a thorough background in respiratory physiology might help you to understand a particular patient's problem, while an inhalation therapist with on-the-job training would be unable to give you such assistance.

Credentials for practice

Just as educational preparation differs, so do the credentials necessary for practice. The standards for registration as a nurse are relatively uniform throughout the country and serve to certify minimum ability to practice safely. Registration is *mandatory* in most places. Medicine, dentistry, practical (or vocational) nursing, and other health care occupations have similar standards.

For other categories of workers, registration is not mandatory but *permissive*. This means that you may be licensed but can also practice your occupation without licensure. In some states, registration of practical (vocational) nurses falls into this category.

Some professional organizations provide *certification* for practitioners of their own occupation. Competence is determined by tests and other criteria, and certification is completely controlled by the occupation itself. Physicians are certified as specialists in this fashion. Nurses are being certified in specialized fields by the same kind of mechanism.

In the United States, laws relating to health care occupations are made at the state level. The resulting local variations may affect the mobility of individuals in certain occupations.

All of these variables make it difficult for the beginning nurse to know "who is who." It is, of course, far more difficult for patients, who usually turn to a familiar figure for interpretation and guidance as they move through the modern health care system. The nurse is often that familiar figure, and therefore must be responsible for investigating and understanding the roles of other members of the health care team.

Problems in the delivery of health care

Although the ideal of a coordinated health care team in which each person functions optimally is seldom achieved, it is a goal toward which we are striving. However, many problems currently stand in the way of its realization. We shall discuss some of these problems here, and you may encounter others in your particular work setting.

Certain geographical areas are subject to shortages of persons in some occupational fields. In such situations, less well-prepared persons are often hired, which can result in a lower level of care for the patient and in job dissatisfaction on the part of the inadequately prepared workers.

Another problem is the increase in types of health care workers, which sometimes causes overlapping responsibilities. Such overlap can and does create feelings of competition and occasional antagonism.

Also, as health care has grown more complex, certain occupational groups have had to upgrade their skills and to relinquish tasks requiring less skill. This circumstance has sometimes been perceived as threatening, and those who feel threatened tend to resist change.

One of the most complex problems is communication. As more persons become involved in care, communication among them becomes both more important and more difficult. Communication can and does break down. The result is fragmented care, which causes patients to feel that no one sees them as whole persons and that some of their needs are neither recognized nor met.

In the face of all these problems, what can you do as a nursing student—and later as a registered nurse—to further progress toward the ideal of a functioning, coordinated health care team? You can act effectively both as a nurse and as a concerned citizen.

If insufficiently prepared individuals have been given responsibilities that exceed their competence, you can be active in promoting on-the-job educational opportunities for them and in lobbying the power structure to upgrade its hiring criteria.

If individuals with overlapping areas of responsibility are competing, you can promote and participate in negotiations to establish policies or even laws that protect workers' rights but maintain a high level of care. You can demonstrate your own readiness to compromise with others when appropriate, and can make sure that you remain committed to the goal of optimal patient care.

You can keep abreast of current practice through reading, continuing education, and attention to your patients so that you are able to meet and adapt to change.

You can strive to make your communication with other members of the health care team more complete and more direct. You can ask questions and encourage the establishment of routines and procedures that improve communication. Through such actions, you will be making the health care team more effective.

Functioning within the health care team

An individual member of a health care team may, at any given time, function dependently, independently, or interdependently. Each of these ways of functioning has its place and needs to be understood in relation to the efforts of the team as a whole.

Dependent functioning

On many occasions the person with the most extensive preparation and/or experience in a given area of health care makes decisions to be carried out by others whose backgrounds do not qualify them for such decision making. This practice makes the expertise of one individual available to a large number of patients. Most people are familiar with the practice whereby the physician writes "orders" to be carried out by others. In the past, health team personnel have tended to function dependently only in response to the physician's orders. This is no longer true. Today various persons may make decisions for others to carry out. The nurse in charge of a patient's care may write "nursing orders" to be carried out by other nurses and by aides and orderlies. The physical therapist may write a "prescription" for the patient's exercises, to be carried out by the assistant or by nursing personnel. The person who carries out such orders is functioning in a dependent role.

It must be clearly understood that dependent functioning does not relieve an individual of responsibility for his or her own actions. It does mean that direction or orders must be obtained before acting and that the person who gives the order is responsible for his or her own decision-making process. When acting in a dependent mode, it is your responsibility to make sure you understand the directions clearly, perform the task skillfully, evaluate the results of what you do, and recognize potential contraindications to that action. You also need to be aware of the expected result of a given action, so that it can be discontinued if an unexpected result occurs. You can be held legally liable for damage resulting from lack of skill, performance of an action when clear contraindications are present, or failure to stop when an unexpected or adverse result occurs. As you can see, dependent functioning does not absolve you of responsibility.

Independent functioning

An individual functions independently when working within his or her own area of expertise. Within that area, he or she ascertains what needs to be done and initiates action. Others may or may not be consulted, but the final decision is the individual's. Throughout this text, we will point out areas in which it is appropriate for registered nurses to function independently.

A nursing structure in which independent functioning is the dominant model is *total patient care*. In such a structure, one nurse has complete responsibility for the patient's nursing care—supportive care, hygiene, and all other nursing needs—while he or she is on duty. Of course, the nurse in such a setting works cooperatively with other personnel, and performs some dependent functions related to the physician's medical plan of care, but he or she is fully and exclusively responsible for all nursing functions. This procedure minimizes communication problems, enhances continuity of care, and often makes patients feel that they are being seen as whole persons. The major drawbacks of total patient care are its high cost and the shortage of registered nurses in some areas of the country.

Independent functioning may take a different form for nurses with additional specialized educational preparation. Those with backgrounds in such areas as coronary care and anesthesia function independently in ways unavailable to the general staff nurse. They make judgments that were once considered the physician's responsibility. And nurse practitioners in such fields as pediatrics, obstetrics, and family practice exercise an expanded independence justified by their superior education and skill.

Interdependent functioning

Interdependent functioning means that decisions are made jointly by those involved in the care of a specific patient. One common setting for interdependent functioning is the team approach to certain long-term health problems, such as rehabilitation after spinal cord injury. The physician, the nurse, the occupational and physical therapist,

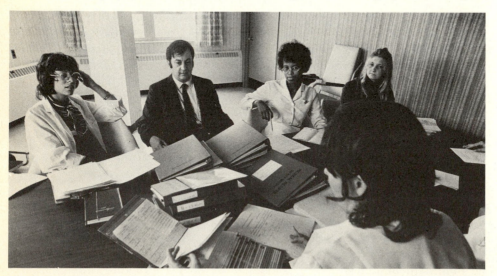

A team conference
Dan Bernstein

and others involved in the patient's care meet to discuss the patient's problems and determine overall priorities and goals. Increasingly, the patient and his or her family participate in such efforts. After the general priorities and goals have been established by the team, its individual members may work together on some problems and independently on others. This method of making decisions is quite time-consuming, but can result in exceptionally high-quality care.

Nurses probably function interdependently most frequently when they engage in *team nursing*. The team nursing concept is an effort to make the most effective use of various types of personnel and to provide the most effective nursing care through joint decision making. The team leader is usually a registered nurse with the background and ability to organize and plan care for a group of patients. Members of the team may be other registered nurses, licensed practical nurses, student nurses, and nursing assistants.

The core of the team nursing concept is team planning of care. At daily *team conference*, care is planned and problems are considered. Of course, some aspects of care are best dealt with by a single individual, for the sake of efficient time use and of the patient's needs, and need not be considered by the entire team. Conferences usually consider difficult problems or overall direction and guidance of the patient's care. Specific aspects of care are then assigned to different team members for implementation. Herein lies one drawback of team nursing. Because different team members perform different tasks, the patient encounters many individuals in the course of his or her care and may not know where to turn with a given question or request. The patient may also feel that no one sees him or her as a whole. Communication is the solution to this problem.

Maintaining continuity of care

As emphasis has shifted from illness care to health care, the need has grown to provide more continuity as the patient moves from outpatient care to acute care to convalescent care to supervised self-care. Changes in setting can occur in a variety of directions and sequences. If care is to proceed smoothly, good communication among those who supply it is essential.

Nurses are active in many settings in promoting this kind of continuity. Some hospitals and public health departments have hired nurses to assume the role of patient care coordinators. Such nurses work with patients and with health care personnel in different settings to assure a smooth transition of care. More and more nurses are also performing the nursing role outside acute care facilities, in health screening, teaching programs, and ambulatory care settings.

Conclusion

The complex modern health care team can be bewildering to patient and worker alike. New occupations seem to emerge every day. Familiarity with the various occupations will make you a more effective nurse, and understanding of their interrelationships will increase your ability to work effectively with them to improve total health care.

Study terms

certification
continuity of care
credential
dependent functioning
health care team
independent functioning
interdependent functioning
levels of preparation
licensure

mandatory licensure
nurse practitioner
orders
patient care coordinator
permissive licensure
prescription
team conference
team nursing
total patient care

References

Arras, B. 1975. Don't Underrate Those Clinical Conferences! *RN* 38:6:41-42.

Cano, P. 1971. Group Efforts Change Care. *Nursing Outlook* 19:61-113.

Deming, E. A. 1971. A Practicing System for Professional Nursing. *Nursing Clinics of North America* 6:311-320.

Epstein, C. 1974. Breaking the Barriers to Communication on the Health Team. *Nursing '74* 4:9:65-68.

Golden, A.S., *et al.* 1974. Non-Physician Family Health Teams. *Nursing Digest* 11:49-54.

Lee, I. M. 1973. Cope with Resistance to Change. *Nursing '73* 3:3:6-7.

Lewis, K. M. 1974. Teamwork: A Key to Better Pre-op Teaching, Part I. *RN* 37:5:61-62.

Menkin, P. 1975. How A Group Can Help You Solve Your Problems. *Nursing '75* 7:67-70.

Ryan, G. C. 1973. The Group Way. *American Journal of Nursing* 73:273-275.

Seiler, K. 1974. The Team Conference. *Supervisor Nurse* 5:9:64-65.

Wilson, A. *et al.* 1973. Team Conferences that Work. *American Journal of Nursing* 73:506-508.

Wilson, C. 1973. The Health Care Team. *Canadian Hospitals* 50:3:27-28.

Zimmerman, D., and Gohrke, C. 1970. The Goal Directed Nursing Approach: It Does Work. *American Journal of Nursing* 70:306+.

Part Two
The Theory and Practice of Nursing

3 Homeostasis and Human Needs

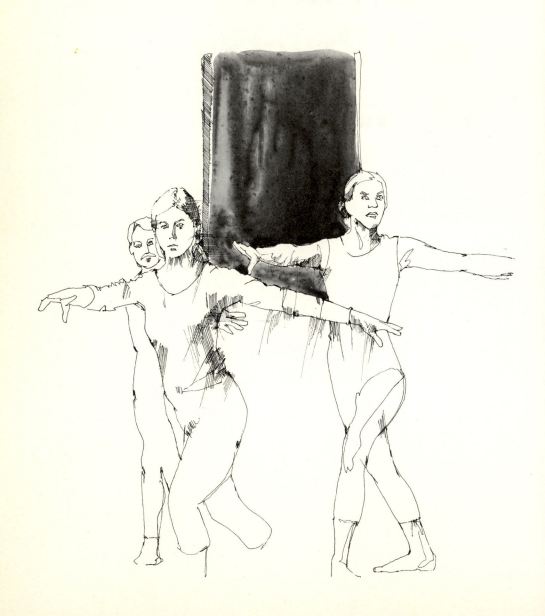

Objectives

After completing this chapter, you should be able to:

1 Define the term *homeostasis*.

2 Explain the relationship of homeostasis to the assessment of the patient's condition and the planning of the patient's care.

3 List, in ascending order, the seven levels of Maslow's hierarchy of needs.

4 Differentiate between a need and a problem.

5 Relate the basic human needs to problems you may encounter in caring for the patient.

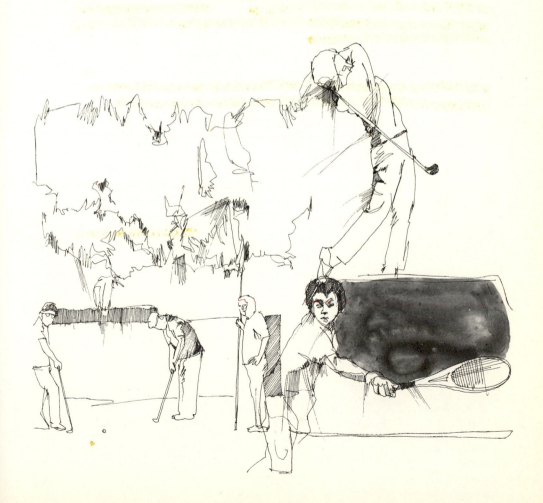

B ASIC TO NURSING PRACTICE is an understanding of homeostasis and human needs. It is on these concepts that we found our judgments of the care needed by individual patients.

Definition of homeostasis

W. B. Cannon, an endocrinologist, originated the term *homeostasis* in 1926. He was describing the ability of primarily physiological processes of the body to maintain a steady state within the organism. Since 1926 the term has been expanded to include the psychological processes as well. For our purposes, homeostasis is the tendency of all living tissue to restore and maintain itself in a condition of balance or equilibrium. The emotional life of the person, evolving from the composition of the brain, is included in the definition "all living tissue."

The word *homeostasis*, however, can be misleading. At first glance you might interpret it to mean "stillness." Far from it, homeostasis is actually a relative state of balance maintained by the constant dynamic shifting and adapting of the body to threat. The process can be compared to the motion of the familiar child's toy (and scientific instrument), the gyroscope. Standing on its slender pedestal on a taut string, the gyroscope appears to be in perfect balance—but only because of its spinning center, which keeps it in an upright position. (See Figure 3.1.) When the movement stops, the balance is lost. So the human being, with the help of the body's internal spinnings, holds to a homeostatic balance.

In his book *Nature and Human Nature*, Lawrence K. Frank

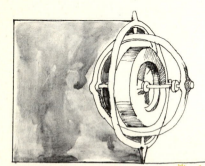

FIGURE 3.1   HOMEOSTATIC BALANCE   Like the balance of a gyroscope, human physiological balance is maintained by the steady functioning of all parts of the body. If any of the physiological processes stops, the balance is lost.

speaks of homeostasis as an orchestra, each organ functioning as a different instrument, sensitively responding to the others to assure stability. "The internal environment is like the external environment—it is continually changing, maintaining a dynamic equilibrium by larger or smaller fluctuations and sometimes by violent alterations as it continues to oscillate between the limits of living existence" (Frank, 1951).

Homeostasis and nursing

The concept of homeostasis gives meaning to patient care. It is not simply an idea that is academically interesting but impractical in day-to-day nursing. On the contrary, it comes into its own when you observe the patient for signs and symptoms of distress—circulatory, respiratory, psychological, and so forth. When you do so, you are actually looking for signs of disequilibrium, or lack of homeostatic balance. Often you will actually see signs that one system in the body is moving to correct an imbalance in another system. For example, the diaphoresis (perspiration) that accompanies a fever occurs to allow evaporation of moisture from the skin, which cools the body. The pallor (paleness) of shock is a compensatory mechanism to bring blood flow to the viscera, where lie the vital life-saving organs.

Good medical management and planning of care revolve around this concept. Much can be done to assist the body's attempts to restore homeostasis. The patient with a fever may be given medications and/or alcohol sponging, which brings about a lowering of body temperature. A patient in shock will probably be given blood preparations that aid vascular distribution and be kept warm and in a flat position to facilitate blood circulation.

With your understanding of homeostasis, you will begin to see that when the patient is in a state of disequilibrium, certain needs are not being met. But do all humans have the same needs? And are some needs more important than others to a given individual?

Basic human needs

Abraham Maslow, a renowned psychologist, developed a conceptual hierarchy of human needs in 1943. In a manner of speaking, it is a layering of needs, the primary or physiological needs at the bottom, and the secondary or nonphysiological needs at the top. (See Figure 3.2.)

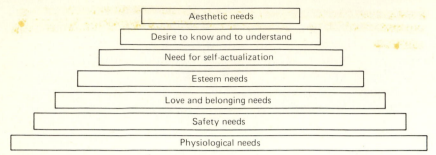

FIGURE 3.2   MASLOW'S HIERARCHY OF NEEDS
Adapted from Abraham H. Maslow, "A Theory of Human Motivation," Psychological Review 50 (1943), pp. 370-396. Copyright 1943 by the American Psychological Association. Reprinted by permission.

Physiological needs

Physiological needs are those needs that are inherent in all humans. If they are not met, homeostasis is seriously threatened. Among these needs are the need for oxygen, food, fluids, sleep, and sexual activity. The physiological needs alone are sometimes referred to as the basic needs, because the effects of their denial are both obvious and measurable. For example, if the body is not receiving oxygen in adequate amounts, a person will hyperventilate (breathe rapidly and deeply) and become pale from the decrease in oxygen in the body's cells. The physiological needs may also serve as channels for other kinds of needs. For example, a person may feel hungry when in fact he or she needs comfort and security (Biehler, 1972).

Safety needs

Maslow places the safety needs just above the level of the physiological needs, although they too may be physical in nature—such as the need for shelter from cold, heat, inclement weather, and attack. But the safety needs are often also psychological. To feel psychologically safe, most of us need some degree of structure, or law; that is, definite social expectations, both of our own behavior and of others. And we need freedom from separation, quarreling, and disorder.

Love and belonging needs

The security we gain from love and belonging enhances the feeling of safety that is so important to us. We learn much about ourselves through the responses of those around us. We learn what in our behavior is acceptable and what unacceptable. Our feeling of structure and security is reinforced when we know where we are in relation to others, and who we are to them. This reflection of ourselves in the eyes of others—as well as our ability to interpret other people's selves to them—is the essence of belongingness. We all need mutually meaningful relationships with other persons.

The love of which Maslow speaks is not, by definition, sexual. It may, to some individuals, be not just the love of another person but the love of or belonging to a group or even a cause. On the other hand, to the infant or the young child, the need for the love of a mother figure is at the more elementary or physiological level. René Spitz's study of two groups of infants and children demonstrates this. Briefly, each group received the same high-quality physical care. But, one group was talked to, fondled and caressed, while the other group received little demonstrativeness. Not only did the children who received little love develop signs and symptoms of lassitude, withdrawal, physical ailments, and delayed development, but their mortality rate was significantly higher (Spitz, 1945).

Adults who are similarly neglected are often able to sublimate

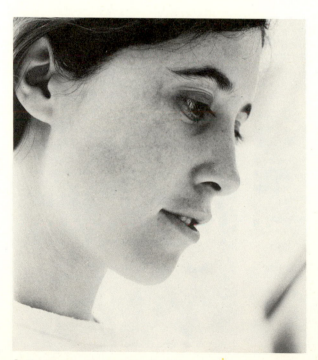

Self-esteem: serving family, job, or profession with competence
John Goodman

or transfer the fulfillment of their love needs to a pet, an artistic endeavor, or a charitable pursuit. Thus, depending on a person's age, the need for love may be considered to exist on more than one level.

Esteem needs

Through belongingness, or being valued, we develop a feeling of self-esteem. We must all justify our existence somehow in order to find meaning in our lives. Self-approval, or liking oneself, is an essential part of satisfying the need for esteem (see Chapter 6). Many of us—parents, teachers, workers, and nurses—gain self-esteem through serving our families, jobs, or professions with competence. But unfortunately, a great many people never rise to this level, spending their lives in self-doubt and sadness. Some people who appear to have achieved great esteem in the eyes of their peers actually lack self-esteem; they push ahead frantically for even more public recognition.

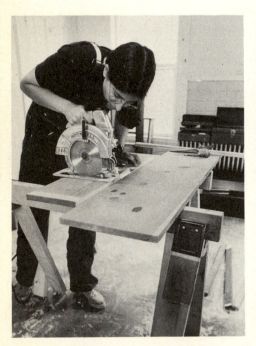 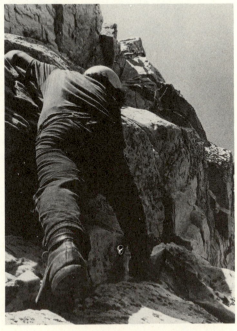

Self-actualization: to do in life, with joy, what one both wants and is suited to do
Left: *Donald C. Dietz / Stock, Boston;* Right: *J. Berndt / Stock, Boston*

The need for self-actualization

Maslow calls self-actualization "being true to oneself." More clearly, it is the attempt to fulfill one's potential; to do in life, with joy, what one both wants and is suited to do. As Maslow writes, "The farmer plants and tends his crops, the nurse nurses." But to be truly self-actualized, a person must grow: the farmer takes increasing pride in his ability to grow plants, and the nurse sharpens his or her skills and deepens the sense of empathy for the patient. This level, then, is not confined to what one chooses to *do* in life, but includes also what one *feels.* Philosophy, morality, and religion, honestly explored, raise the individual to the state of self-actualization.

The need to know and to understand

The striving for knowledge is an extension of self-actualization. Motivated by curiosity, people seek answers to the secrets of their world. Perhaps it is this need that led us to our great advances in

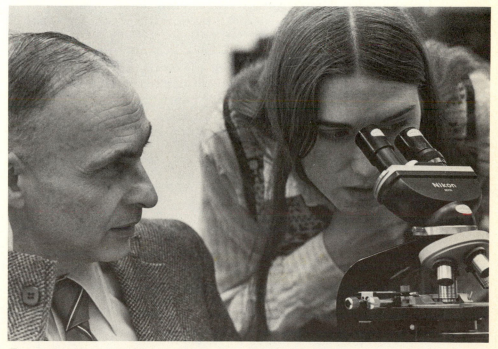

The striving for knowledge—an extension of self-actualization
Chris Maynard

technology and the exploration of outer space. For the need to know and to understand exists solely for its own sake, not for the gratification of immediate goals.

Aesthetic needs

The highest level in the hierarchy of needs, according to Maslow, is the aesthetic level. This level is well developed in the artist, who ardently seeks out beauty and transposes it to paper or canvas for others to enjoy. The fulfillment of the aesthetic need can also be observed in the placement of a single potted yellow rose in a ghetto window.

Maslow wrote of the hierarchy of needs as a motivational force. He hypothesized that as a lower level is satisfied, a person moves on to the next highest level. If, then, a person has the physiological needs fulfilled (and is thus in homeostatic balance), he or she will move upward to the levels of self-actualization and the seeking of knowledge and beauty.

An important qualification must be made to Maslow's theory, however. Although the hierarchy will be useful to you as a nurse, it is at best a relative, not a rigid, series of concepts. People flow, during their lifetimes, up and down, through the various levels, often in response to their external world. It is not uncommon for the secondary needs to dominate the primary or physiological needs. Consider the soldier in battle who chooses to deny his physiological needs as he throws himself on a grenade in order to save the lives of his companions. Or the artist who becomes thin and malnourished, neglecting the need for food in order to continue to fill a canvas with profound beauty.

Needs versus problems

Problems are different from needs. We have just considered, at some length, the basic and secondary needs. If these needs are not met when they are felt, a problem arises. The problem is the situation that develops when a need is not satisfied. Often the water pitcher is inadvertently placed beyond the reach of the debilitated, elderly patient. The patient's *need* is for water or fluid; the *problem* is the situation—that is, the water is not readily available. Lack of water in turn creates such other problems for the patient as dry mouth, flaky skin, and general discomfort. Another example is the nurse who reports to work in the afternoon wearing a sweater, only to find it inadequate because of the falling temperature when leaving work in the evening. The need is for body warmth; the problem is inadequate clothing. When planning care, nurses often confuse needs and problems, causing nursing actions and goals to be poorly defined.

The needs and problems of nurses

In order to assess and respond to the needs and problems of patients effectively, the nurse should have an understanding of his or her own needs and problems. Professional behavior does not allow for your own needs to "spill over" into the process of interaction to the detriment of the patient. For example, if you interpret as personal rejection the patient's refusal to accept some aspect of care, the nurse-patient relationship may be markedly disrupted. Using the patient in any way to fulfill your own needs, except the need for esteem as a result of excellent care, is inappropriate.

Satisfying patient needs

This discussion of needs and problems can prove both relevant and useful to your nursing if you apply it to the process of assessment. Keeping in mind that immediate needs must be met before more mature needs can arise (Peplau, 1952) may give new direction to your care.

You must assist the patient to meet physiological needs first: this is the guiding principle in establishing priorities for care. If the patient is very short of breath and receives oxygen, it is not an appropriate time to discuss the importance of keeping an accurate record of intake and output. And if a patient is in obvious pain, you must delay teaching the patient about a therapeutic diet. Helping the patient fulfill the basic needs first makes it possible for you to assist in the fulfillment of his or her higher needs. In this way, you give real service to the patient. For example, the patient who is pain-free and has recovered almost to the point of homeostasis is ready to be consulted about long-term plans for care and the prevention of recurring disease.

As a nurse, you may also use this knowledge to prevent problems by recognizing when the fulfillment of essential needs may be threatened. For example, recognizing the need for full oxygenation, or lung expansion, after surgery, we teach the patient the technique of deep breathing the evening before scheduled surgery in order to avoid such problems.

Conclusion

An understanding of homeostasis and human needs is a valuable tool for the nurse. No two patients are alike, and no condition remains static. The needs and problems you help define are the challenge you face as a practitioner and the object of the nursing process.

Study terms

compensatory mechanisms   pallor
dynamic balance   primary needs
esteem   problem
hierarchy of needs   secondary needs
homeostasis   self-actualization
hyperventilation   viscera
need

References

Cannon, W. B. 1926. Some General Features of Endocrine Influence on Metabolism. *American Journal of Medical Science* 171.

Biehler, R. F. 1972. *Psychology Applied to Teaching—Selected Readings.* Boston: Houghton Mifflin Company.

Frank, L. K. 1951. *Nature and Human Nature.* New Brunswick, N.J.: Rutgers University Press.

Maslow, A. H. 1943. A Theory of Human Motivation. *Psychological Review* 50.

Peplau, Hildegarde E. 1952. *Interpersonal Relations in Nursing.* New York: G. P. Putnam's Sons.

Spitz, R. 1945. Hospitalism: Inquiry into Genesis of Psychiatric Conditions in Early Childhood. *Psychoanalytic Study of the Child* 1.

4 The Life Cycle

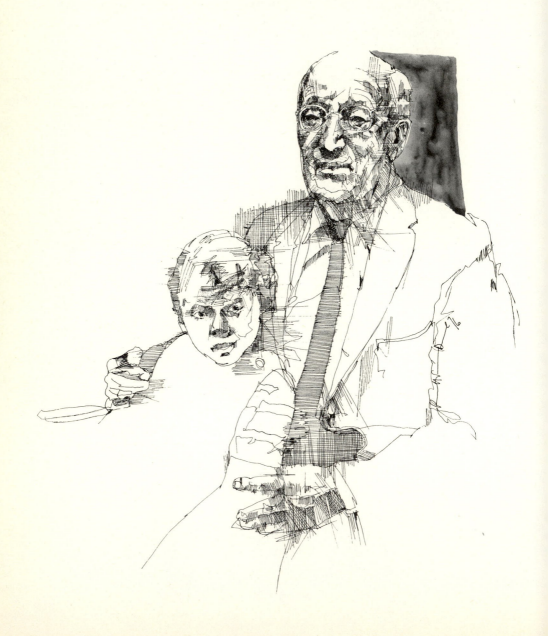

Objectives

After completing this chapter, you should be able to:

1 Name and briefly discuss the eight stages of the life cycle according to Erikson.

2 Outline the main factors in the development of body image throughout the life cycle.

3 Discuss the sexual development of the individual in the context of the life cycle.

4 Describe how the stages of the life cycle affect response to illness.

5 Give four reasons why nurses need a basic knowledge of the life cycle.

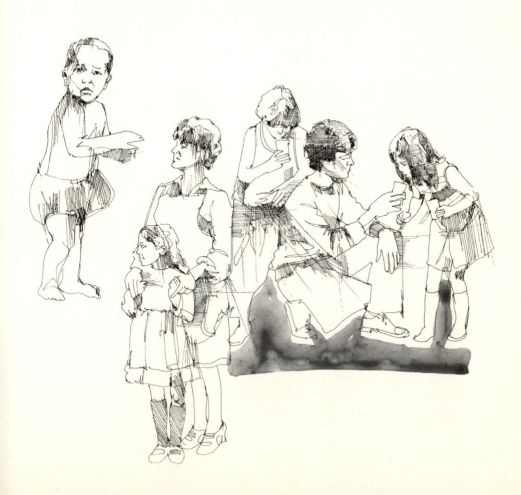

O NE OF THE MOST FASCINATING aspects of nursing is the variety of patients, in terms of age as well as physiological and psychological development. Just as there are no two individuals with identical fingerprints, no two human beings are exactly alike.

The progression through life that is called the "life cycle" is not only a passage of years but also a development of the body and mind. In order to understand the patient fully, the nurse needs basic knowledge of the life cycle—of what is at play physically and emotionally when one reaches a given age. It is perhaps more appropriate in such a discussion to speak of "usual" than of "normal" development, for the term *normal* has come to suggest a standard of sorts. By knowing what is usual for a certain age group, the nurse can identify and assess what is unusual. It is the unusual that may indicate illness.

Theories of the life cycle

In *Childhood and Society*, published in 1963, the psychiatrist Erik H. Erikson divides the life cycle into eight stages. He then defines each in terms of the hoped-for or expected outcome versus the unfavorable outcome that may result if conditions for growth are not present.

Jean Piaget, a zoologist by training and a contemporary of Erikson, views the life cycle primarily from the standpoint of the cognitive or intellectual process. Briefly, he sees the growth of the child as dependent on the intellectual processes that transform experiences into useful concepts, which the child can then apply to new growth experiences.

Erikson's ideas provide a degree of structure to the human responses we see as nurses, and can thus prove helpful in working with patients. The stages of the life cycle are listed and described in Table 4.1. Along with a brief discussion of the conflict characteristic of each of Erikson's eight stages, we will also examine in this chapter the development of body image and sexuality typical of each stage. Though body image and sexuality will be discussed separately for easier learning, you should remember that they are inseparable in the individual.

Body image is one's mental picture of one's body. A three-dimensional view, it encompasses one's appearance from every angle. Appearance is by no means its only component, however. Body image also has a *kinesthetic* aspect, whose source is the response of nerves and muscles to position and spatial relationships.

The sensory component of body image responds to external stimuli, providing the brain with data on objects and air movements the body perceives. Such internal sensations as hunger, thirst, and fullness of the bladder are also incorporated into the body image. In other words, one's body image is the total experience of one's physical self.

Sexual development, which is closely related to body image, may be described as one's sexual image or awareness. Differences in body structure and hormonal determinations, as well as societal conditioning, contribute to the individual's development of sense of womanliness or manliness.

Infancy: birth to one year

It takes only a few minutes for the infant to be propelled from the warm, safe, fluid refuge of the mother's womb into a temporarily hostile world. The maintenance of physiological homeostasis at birth requires profound bodily changes. These changes or, in Frank's words, "violent alterations" (see Chapter 3) result in a new human being who is physically separate from the mother. The infant's first cry expands the countless alveoli, or tiny air sacs, of the lungs, thus initiating a lifelong dependence on the external environment for oxygen. Structural adaptations begin quickly in the heart to complete the formation of the four chambers, and a strong rhythmic pattern of beats begins and persists without interruption for seventy years or more. Peristalsis, the wavelike movements of the intestines, and the flow of gastric juices ensue in preparation for the first feeding. Although almost all newborn systems, and particularly the emotions, are grossly immature, the infant soon becomes responsive to the needs of his or her own body and to certain features of the environment. The newborn stretches, startles easily, listens to his or her own cry, and blinks at bright light.

Although physically separate from the mother and thus in a sense independent, the infant is highly dependent on others for the fulfillment of needs. The newborn is totally dependent for the gratification of all basic needs: sufficient air of a comfortable temperature, fluids and nutrients, a safe crib, and touch that conveys love.

A wet diaper or hunger contractions of the stomach mucosa (lining) signal distress to the infant and elicit a cry for help. The mother hurriedly responds, initiating an emotional as well as a physical dependence that is the most meaningful relationship during the early years of life. Erikson calls this stage *trust vs. mistrust*.

TABLE 4.1 STAGES OF THE LIFE CYCLE ACCORDING TO ERIKSON

	YEARS	CRISES	SIGNIFICANT PERSONS
INFANCY	0–1	Trust vs. Mistrust	Mother or mother substitute
TODDLER	1–3	Autonomy vs. Shame and Doubt	Parents
EARLY CHILDHOOD	3–6	Initiative vs. Guilt	Entire family
MIDDLE CHILDHOOD	6–12	Industry vs. Inferiority	School and neighborhood
ADOLESCENCE	12–18	Identity vs. Role Confusion	Peers, national leadership models
YOUNG ADULTHOOD	18–40	Intimacy vs. Isolation	Intimates, usually of opposite sex
MIDDLE YEARS	40–65	Generativity vs. Stagnation	Expanded family, institutions
LATER YEARS	65–	Integrity vs. Despair	Those who sustain feeling of usefulness

If the parent-infant relationship is one of consistency and genuine affection, the baby perceives the world as trustworthy, safe, and dependable. If, on the other hand, care of the child is inconsistent or neglectful, the infant displays fear, suspicion, and agitation.

The first year is characterized by alternating frustration and pleasure, and by inability to postpone gratification. Infants receive pleasure, give nothing consciously in return, and are unaware of the unique pleasure their existence gives their parents.

Some authorities refer to this period as the oral stage. Indeed, months-old youngsters are orally oriented. They begin early to put their fingers in their mouths and to make sucking movements. The pacifier, once in disrepute, is now accepted as a device to strengthen and fulfill the sucking reflex. At approximately seven months, the twenty tiny teeth lying dormant within the gums begin to push their

TASKS	RESPONSE TO ILLNESS
Expressing frustrations. Dependence upon mother.	Physiological irritation. Fear of environment.
Speech. Walking. Assertion of wishes. Beginning the postponement of pleasure.	Fear of threats to the body and painful procedures. Stress of separation from mother.
Enlargement of vocabulary. Interaction with total family group. Beginning of peer involvement.	Equation of illness with being bad. Guilt.
Increased physical activity. Competitiveness. Dealing with authority in the school environment.	Anger over restrictions due to illness. Guilt over causing family crisis.
Independence from family. Strong influence of peer group. Becoming sexually active. Beginning to choose life goals.	Anger over dependency due to illness.
Carrying out life plans. Choosing a mate. Selecting a life's work.	Fear of possible change in the intimacy relationship. Depression over the interruption of plans.
Forming ideas and plans for the next generation. Carrying out life goals. Assessment.	Depression over the interruption of work and separation from family.
Life review. Finding satisfactions. Setting new goals for retirement. Sharing knowledge with others.	Feelings of no longer being useful. Threat to life. Despair.

way, often painfully, through the surface. Now chewing movements take place in preparation for the firm foods that will soon be introduced into the diet.

Body image

The infant is born without a body image. In the womb the infant and the environment are one, and the self is not perceived as a separate entity. At birth, the processes that lead to the development of the adult self-image begin.

The infant responds to the internal stimuli of pain and hunger, and does not at first distinguish between them. Gradually the infant begins to identify those feelings of discomfort that are relieved by food and to distinguish them from other feelings. The same process occurs with all internal stimuli, and as a result the infant learns to trust his or her body and to develop an understanding of its signals.

External stimuli also assist infants to identify their own bodies. Little babies may even cause themselves pain by biting their own toes, because they do not know their own boundaries. The touch of those who care for the infant also helps to differentiate self from nonself.

Sexual development

Although not pronounced, differences in behavior between the sexes have been noted very early in life. Females appear to be more vocal as infants, and in later life prove somewhat more adept at verbal skills and less prone to speech difficulties than males. Male infants are superior in motor skills, although fine muscle coordination advances earlier in girls. Thus sexual differences, although subtle, are evident even in the first few months of life.

The toddler: one to three years

Between the ages of one and three or so, the child achieves some freedom from total dependence on the parents. Physical freedom results largely from mastery of the art of walking. Everyone knows the wonderful game in which the toddler runs from the pursuing parent amid laughter and squeals of delight. If not pursued, the youngster stops, forlorn, only to find reassurance in the welcoming arms of the waiting parent.

At this age the youngster also gains psychological independence. "The battle of the pottychair" can become a confrontation of wills; the mother imposes conformity and the child discovers a new power to manipulate or control. If rewards exceed punishments, the child gains pleasure from the parents' approval (love) of the new behavior and from a sense of the reality of the environment. The child begins to know what is expected of him or her. A new awareness unfolds of being a distinct individual with the ability to affect the surroundings. The child sees, for the first time, that pleasure postponed can be pleasure gained.

If allowed to do what he or she is capable of, according to Erikson, the child will develop a lasting sense of confidence and autonomy. If thwarted, however, the child may develop an unhealthy doubt of his or her own capabilities and, in turn, of others and the environment.

Body image

The toddler can distinguish self from nonself, has learned to trust feelings (one hopes), and begins to ascribe value to body parts. Some parts are seen as important, some as pretty, some as bad, and some perhaps as unmentionable. These values are acquired from the persons who are significant to the child. Body limits may be seen as more encompassing than by the adult. For example, feces, urine, fingernails, and hair are considered parts of the body, and their removal may be upsetting.

Sexual development

The toddler does not yet have a firm grasp of differences between boys and girls. Young children derive pleasure from touching themselves and from cuddling and fondling by the parents. In fact, many psychiatrists believe that early childhood is the most crucial period in sexual development, because the child receives open love from the mother and learns—or fails to learn—to love and give to another. Some unfortunate children are punished for touching their genitals and are made to believe that all sexual matters are taboo. Other children become confused about the contradictory reactions of the adults around them.

Early childhood: three to six years

Early childhood is an age of intense activity, both physically and mentally. The acquisition of speech, which has both physical and mental components, is an outstanding feature of this stage and affords even more independence. A vocabulary of five thousand or more words is acquired by the age of six. One has only to observe the extreme depression and frustration of the stroke patient suffering aphasia (loss of the ability to speak) to realize how inherently essential is the power of speech. To the four- or five-year-old, the word "No!" is very popular as a response to a decision made by the parent, and allows the child at least verbal initiative in decision making.

The initiative of which Erikson speaks gives the youngster a feeling of accomplishment, and thus diminishes rebelliousness. Children of this age tend toward orderliness, and willingly perform such tasks as balancing blocks, putting away toys, and washing and dressing themselves.

Physical stature is changing from the round "babyfat" appearance of the toddler to the lean, tall body build of the preschooler or first-grader. By age four, the child's weight is double what it was at one year. Temporary teeth begin to be shed in deference to the more solidly rooted permanent teeth. Groups become important, and meals are rushed through in order to play with friends.

Parental attitudes are crucial at this period. If the parents treat the child's activities and questions as significant, the child is encouraged to grow in response to such positive reinforcement. On the contrary, if the child's questions and explorations are treated flippantly or ridiculed, a sense of guilt may delay or undermine further emotional growth.

Body image

Along with physical stature, the body image is also changing. The child no longer feels like a baby and may ascribe this term to a younger sibling. Children of this age may see themselves as "little adults," the boy pretending to go to work "like Daddy" and the girl imitating the activities of her mother.

Sexual development

At this age the child discovers that boys and girls are differently constructed. The three- to six-year-old has a natural curiosity about his or her body. The proximity of the genitals to the organs of elimination, as well as the attitudes of others, may cause the child to think of the sexual organs as "dirty." Learning at this age that nudity is not generally accepted in our culture may mystify the child more about sex.

Parents tend to encourage children to adopt sexual identities very early. For example, a football may be given to a little boy and a soft doll to a little girl. Boys are often dressed in very masculine clothing, and girls in dresses, long before apparel has much meaning to youngsters.

Middle childhood: six to twelve years

Many educators regard the years from six to twelve as the most important formative period for learning. These are the "doing" years. Teachers share responsibility for the child's development, since the youngster in this age group substitutes the teacher's authority for much of the parents'. The encouragement of a sensitive teacher can, as you may have experienced, have a lasting impact. The school-age child has a normal attachment to the parent of the opposite sex commonly referred to as "Oedipal." For both boys and girls, friends and other peers also assume great importance. Boys form groups for team sports, channeling the aggression that is common at this age into competitive agility. Fighting and wrestling dissipate energy. Girls' groups are usually less aggressively oriented. They do, however, form basketball, soccer, and baseball teams which are highly competitive.

If the child's industry is praised and he or she is allowed to undertake and complete tasks, the resolution of this stage will be healthy. However, a child whose efforts are made fun of and criticized becomes discouraged and feels unworthy and inferior.

Body image

By the time children have reached school age, they have become highly aware of others' bodies and have begun to make close comparisons between themselves and others. The child may be acutely aware of differences that are not even noted by the adult. Although the child of this age has begun to learn about the body's functioning, real understanding does not arrive until the age of nine or more. Before then, the child's ideas are often inaccurate and may be very confused. Both boys and girls of this age group may seek out magazines and books that include pictures of the human body.

Sexual development

The early school years have been termed the period of "sexual latency." This may appear to be the case, for a distinct separation of the sexes occurs: boys form groups with exclusively male membership and girls socialize only with girls. In spite of such voluntary separation, boys often perform feats of limited daring and bravery to gain admiration not only from their male peers but from girls. Girls, in turn, are not unaware of the boys' antics, and may demonstrate the beginning of role identification by experimenting with lipstick or wanting to learn homemaking skills from the mother.

Adolescence: twelve to eighteen years

The period of adolescence is usually an exciting but unsettling time for the individual. Today's adolescent is taller, healthier, and more independent than ever before, but a changing society in which wars are commonplace and drugs accessible on the school grounds often forces teenagers to make choices far beyond the wisdom of their years. Rising divorce rates place additional stress on the adolescent. The rise in teenage suicide is of grave concern to social workers.

The sense of identity that evolves during these years, and that sets the stage for adulthood, is largely a matter of reconciling one's self-image ("Who am I?" "What kind of a person am I?") with the image presented to family and friends ("How do other people see me?"). The strengthening of identity is accompanied by a need to separate oneself psychologically from the family group. Family outings become less popular, and peer-group activities increasingly important. Such other signs of independence from the family as the choice of a religion or political affiliation different than that of the parents may also occur. Unfortunately, such acts can increase the emotional distance between the adolescent and the parents. Heterosexual interest and consideration of a life partner and vocation begin. Although the teenager at times appears noncaring and rebellious in the eyes of the parents, their solid support remains essential. Limit setting does become more difficult, but must not be abandoned. Using the reactions of both parents and peers as measurements, the teenager can gradually achieve the security of a valid role identity—that is, his or her self-image becomes congruent with others' views. If this delicate balance cannot be attained, Erikson tells us, role confusion results. Adolescents need acceptable role models on whom to pattern their ideas about life. Parents who exercise too much control cannot function as role models, and as a result the confused young person may grasp at any ready-made identity, such as drug use, sexual precocity, or defiance of authority. Such desperate efforts to be "somebody" may lead to serious problems.

Body image

Many physical changes, both outward and inward, are occurring in the adolescent. Growth is initially very rapid, but ceases altogether in later adolescence, when dreams of what might be must be reconciled with reality. This growth pattern can create awkwardness and a sense of unfamiliarity with one's body. Heads are bumped because they are higher than expected; furniture is a stumbling-block to large feet and uncoordinated legs. Opportunities for physical activity and exercise can help teenagers overcome these difficulties.

Sexual development

Sexual development in adolescence involves both external body changes and new feelings. Adolescents tend to be preoccupied with "normality," and constantly compare their rates of development and the size of their significant body parts, such as breasts and penis, with others'. Facial features take on adult conformation, and adolescents are commonly unhappy with their features. Attitudes and values pertaining to appearance are derived from the peer group rather than the family. The adolescent seeks security in handling the responsibilities of intimacy: the desire for sexual activity may be accompanied by fear of the results. As H. S. Sullivan puts it, an adolescent's task is to learn to handle sex without anxiety (Sullivan, 1953).

Young adulthood: eighteen to forty years

Although the intimacy desired by the young adult is usually a relationship with someone of the opposite sex that has meaning and a sexual component, this is not exclusively the case. The basic need is for closeness and real relatedness to another. The young adult is a competitive, productive, creative person who sees the results—and, one hopes, the rewards—of decision making. He or she enters a vo-

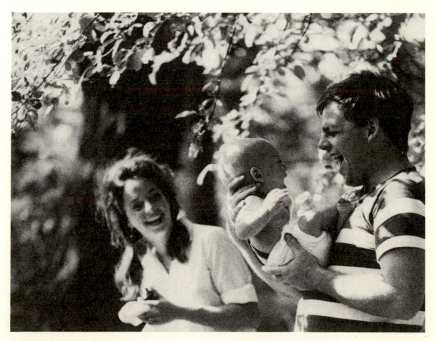

Young adulthood
Elizabeth Wilcox

cation and may establish a family. Physical growth is complete. The attainment of intimacy further enhances the identity first established in the teenage years, though Erikson warns that isolation can occur if "intimacy, competitive and combative relations are experienced with and against the selfsame people." If the person cannot "fuse" his or her identity with others', there occurs self-imposed isolation.

Body image

The body image of the young adult is deeply influenced by prevailing standards of beauty and value judgments about the body. Efforts to discern character on the basis of appearance have a dubious but very long history: the belief that people with beady eyes are untrustworthy, for example, originated centuries ago. More recently, psychological studies of body types have been undertaken in an effort to make such "folk wisdom" legitimate. Stereotyping is thus very common. (Health care workers who try not to respond to patients stereotypically sometimes forget that patients may respond to them, in turn, on the basis of stereotypes. Ideally, any health care worker would be equally acceptable to the patient, but reassignments must be made if the patient's response to care is affected by his or her attitude to the provider of that care.)

In Western cultures, and especially in the United States, the young, beautiful body is idealized. For women, the standard is a very slim figure and conformity to a rather narrow definition of beauty. For men, the range of what is considered handsome is wider: for example the older man with a slightly portly figure and graying hair may be seen as "distinguished." However, height is often equated with leadership ability in men, and the short man may be handicapped in job advancement by his appearance.

Women seem to have clearer and more accurate images of their bodies than do men. They are more acutely aware of physical changes, especially those that affect the face, than men. Women also tend more to equate body with self. Men tend to be less specific in their views of their own bodies and to relate self more to accomplishment and position in life than to body. The women's movement and related phenomena may bring about a convergence of men's and women's attitudes toward their bodies.

Sexual development

Young adulthood should be characterized by sexual fulfillment in long-term relationships of satisfying intimacy. However, it has been

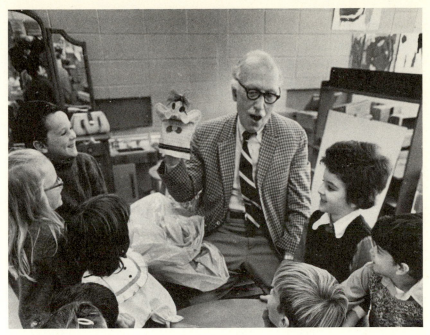

The middle years: a "parenting" of all youth
Dan Bernstein

suggested that many young adults have unrealistic expectations of romantic love and intimacy, and find long-term sexual involvement dull and disappointing. Nevertheless, the young adult typically embraces the sexual role and looks for security in a love relationship.

The middle years: forty to sixty-five

Erikson calls the middle years a period of generativity, in which the individual reviews past accomplishments and assesses what remains to be done. It can, then, be a period of satisfaction or of disappointment. One may make the desirable psychological adjustment of considering one's capacities and past accomplishments in light of their value to the younger generation. The development of such a sense of generativity does not require that one have children of one's own; it is more a matter of "parenting" all youth. Through productivity and political and social responsibility in the middle years, the individual strives to help young people grow.

Physiological changes are also taking place. The hair grays, body fat is redistributed and may increase, and a deficit in visual or hearing acuity may occur. The climacteric, or cessation of reproductive ability, occurs in both sexes. Women stop menstruating, and men somewhat later experience hormonal and psychological changes. Depression is not uncommon in the middle years, perhaps due to the realization that one is not going to achieve all the goals of one's youth. Some degree of depression may also be a result of hormonal alterations.

If, in the middle of life, one can assess oneself realistically and at the same time look toward the younger members of society and their concerns, a state of generativity has been reached that can give rise to a feeling of contentment. If this encompassing view of life is lacking, self-pity, self-interest, and sadness result.

Body image

The decreased hormone production that characterizes the middle years brings about changes in body and feelings. Because of the extreme emphasis on youth in Western culture, some individuals have difficulty facing these changes and make massive efforts to continue looking young. Such a person may dress in a youthful manner, use cosmetics to cover signs of aging, and even undergo plastic surgery. These activities are not harmful in themselves, but may indicate that the person has difficulty accepting body changes.

Occasional individuals react in the opposite way, simply "giving up" at the first signs of aging. They may refer to themselves as old, wear clothing characteristic of elderly people, and withdraw from physical activity. This only accelerates the aging process.

Sexual development

During middle age, sexual activity can be highly gratifying. For example, a woman who is self-assured and contented, and who sees her children, if any, reaching adulthood, may find new joy in her sexuality. But if she feels unfulfilled and has lost the formerly close relationship with her partner, further sexual development can be interfered with.

The middle-aged man commonly experiences brief periods of impotence, usually psychological in origin. The realization that he may not accomplish all that he intended can cause him to feel sexually inadequate. If his sexual partner is understanding and supportive, these problems can be temporary. If they persist, however, professional counseling may be needed.

In spite of the potential problems of middle age, sexual development may be more satisfying than at any other time in life. When the responsibility of childrearing is past, one has more time to appreciate one's partner.

The later years: over sixty-five

Growing old in Western societies is far from the pleasant experience it appears to be in some Asian countries, where age elicits respect and the young solicit the wisdom of the old. Retirement is often mandatory, and usually unwelcome to the individual. However, retirement communities have gained favor as an antidote to the social isolation that plagues the elderly.

In reviewing achievements and disappointments, the individual can acquire dignity and integrity. And many older persons' perspectives broaden as they undertake new ventures and projects. Even so, depression is not uncommon over the age of sixty. As in adolescence, the reactions of others greatly influence the way elderly people feel about themselves. The older family member who

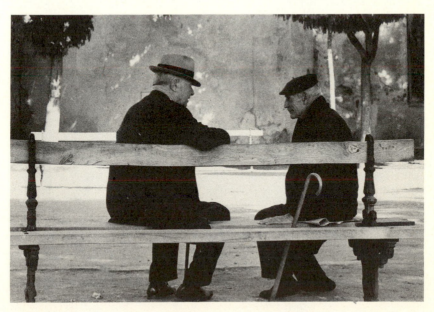

The later years
Ira Gavrin

is looked on as useless feels of no use; and deep despair is the result, according to Erikson. It is prudent to remember that aging, like all other stages of living, is an individual experience (see Chapter 23).

Body image

As old age approaches, the body usually becomes progressively less able to function at previous levels. Eyesight diminishes, hearing may worsen, and muscles are not as strong. These reductions in efficiency occur at different rates to different individuals: there are those who function more slowly, or tire more easily, but who can continue in their normal occupations; for others the aging progresses rapidly to the point of dependence on others.

The changes that occur must be incorporated into the body image, and a realistic adaptation must be made to them if the elderly person is to participate in life optimally. But lack of trust in the body's ability, fear of chronic illness, and anxiety about dependence make this a difficult task.

Sexual development

Perhaps because of changing attitudes toward sexuality, people in their later years now realize that they need not cease their sexual activity. A decrease in hormonal activity does not mean the absence of libido (sexual interest) or the end of intimacy.

Moving through life's stages

Each of the eight stages presents the person two opposing directions toward which to turn. An accepting social environment allows these crises to be resolved in ways that mean the evolution of identity. The individual is thus enabled to move onward to the next stage. Life, then, is a continuing search for an identity appropriate to one's stage of development and the world in which one lives.

Erikson contends that a person cannot move successfully to a later stage until the identity crisis of the present stage has been resolved. The main focus or premise of modern psychotherapy is identity growth. Therapy can bring about the correction or resolution of a crisis not handled well formerly. Thus, an unresolved life stage need not condemn a person to hopelessness; psychotherapy offers an opportunity to relive the developmental past and bring about a new sense of self.

The life cycle and nursing practice

Knowledge of the life cycle is vastly important to nurses for several reasons. First, your assessments of the physical and emotional characteristics of the patient are only valid or meaningful if you can make comparisons to what is usual. Notwithstanding the hazards of "putting people in boxes," knowing the norms of social development will deepen your assessment abilities. For example, if the hospitalized three-year-old cries uncontrollably when the mother must leave the bedside to return home, you can give the child (better) support and assurance if you know that at this age the mother's presence is all-important and that even brief separation is devastating. Second, knowledge of the developmental stages will give you insight into what is important to the patient, and how he or she might respond to care. Knowing this, you can design care that will meet the unique needs of the ill individual.

The nurse can best care for an infant by providing a physically safe environment free of startling noises or bright lights, and by touching, speaking to, and fondling the infant. Nursery-room nurses commonly talk and sing to the infants in their charge. The infant may be irritable, fearful, and anxious. Even without the ability to understand illness, the infant feels systemically unwell and reflects this feeling in behavior. Illness changes the normal "happy" baby into an "unhappy" baby whose responses are expressive. It is important for you to observe and record such behavior; in this way, you directly contribute to an assessment of the infant's physical status.

The toddler who is sick has a special need to know that feeling sick is unrelated to having done something bad. Understanding is very limited at this age, but the child is very sensitive to the surroundings. In addition to guilt for wrongdoing, the primary stress is possible separation from the mother at a time when the child most needs maternal closeness. Hospitals are becoming increasingly aware of the importance of this need, and the mother, unless it becomes too tiring for her, is usually allowed to remain with the child almost continually. Since it relieves some of the anxiety of the child, this kind of arrangement is usually welcome for the child, the mother, and the staff.

As we have said, the body is particularly meaningful to the

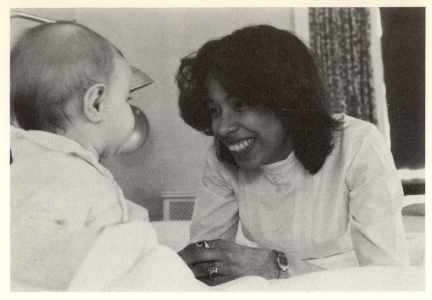

The stage of the life cycle a patient is in affects his or her response to illness.
Chris Maynard

young child. Medical procedures, particularly painful ones, pose a threat to the body in the mind of the child. To the three-year-old, simple explanations can be offered. Lying to any child—or to any patient, for that matter—is inappropriate and not helpful. If the mother cannot or should not be present, a nurse who relates well to the youngster can give needed physical and emotional support during medical procedures. (The parent should be considered, as well as the child: if the procedure is painful or upsetting to watch, the mother may not wish to be present and should not be encouraged to do so.)

Guilt over illness persists in the preschooler, who may readily equate illness to some occurrence that aroused a sense of wrongdoing. Because preschool-age patients are very aware of their bodies, they may relate painful procedures to punishment unless they have been adequately prepared for such experiences.

The ill school-age youngster feels keenly the restrictive atmosphere of the hospital and resents the imposition it places on exploratory activities, a major need of this age group. The less understanding nurse may find the school-age child a demanding patient with behavior problems. You should make time to allow the child to talk about the frustration illness is causing. Such attention and sympathy can help the child become not only less rebellious but also a cooperative participant in his or her management.

Illness is particularly threatening in adolescence since it imposes an ill-timed dependence on an individual who is naturally moving toward and wanting independence. The teenager can be a very unwilling and angry patient. Separation from friends and their activities places considerable stress on the adolescent patient. The inventive nurse can help channel anger into constructive feelings that can aid recovery.

The young adult, when ill, may feel acutely the interruption in productivity. Many also fear change in the quality or character of the intimacy relationship. The nurse's recognition of resulting depression, and acknowledgment of such feelings when they occur, helps the patient work through the experience of illness.

Adulthood is an especially vulnerable time to become ill, for the ideas and plans so essential at this age must be put aside in deference to the illness. Illness may be interpreted as deterioration due to age, and thus cause both depression and fear. Ventilating and sharing these feelings is usually helpful to the patient, and the nurse often facilitates this process.

Illness in an elderly person can undermine the dignity so vital to maturity. Dependence on others may mean to the older patient that he or she is a burden to the family and no longer useful. It is often nursing attitudes that determine whether or not the older patient maintains dignity or gives way to despair.

A third reason why understanding of the life cycle is important is that it will make you more comfortable with the responses described above, which might otherwise appear irrational. Planning care thus becomes both more realistic and more enjoyable and stimulating. It is professionally satisfying to care creatively for the child, the adolescent, or the adult.

Finally, a basic understanding of the life cycle and how it influences human behavior will increase your sensitivity not only to patients but also to others around you.

Conclusion

Erik Erikson has given nurses and others in health care a useful tool for identifying the basic and primary needs of individuals in their care. He does not ignore the fact that each individual is different from every other and that diversity makes people interesting and unique. Erikson identifies the major difficulties each individual confronts at each stage of life, and suggests how others can help promote successful resolution and greater growth.

Study terms

adolescent	isolation
autonomy	kinesthetic
climacteric	life cycle
despair	menses
doubt	mistrust
generativity	Oedipal conflict
guilt	pacifier
identity	role confusion
industry	self-absorption
inferiority	sexual latency
initiative	sibling
integrity	trust
intimacy	

References

American Journal of Nursing 75:10. 1975. Seventy-Fifth Anniversary Issue. (Entire issue devoted to the life cycle.)

Biehler, R. F. 1974. *Psychology Applied to Teaching*, 2nd ed. Boston: Houghton Mifflin Company.

Erikson, E. H. 1963. *Childhood and Society*. New York: W. W. Norton and Company.

Evans, F. 1971. *Psychosocial Nursing*. New York: Macmillan.

Kolb, L. C. 1973. *Modern Clinical Psychiatry*, 8th ed. Philadelphia: W. B. Saunders.

Marlow, D. R. 1973. *Textbook of Pediatric Nursing*, 4th ed. Philadelphia: W. B. Saunders.

Oremland, E. K., *et al.* 1974. How to Care for the "Between-ager." *Nursing '74* 74:11:42-51.

Piaget, Jean. 1963. *Origins of Intelligence in Children*. New York: W. W. Norton.

Smith, D. W., and Bierman, E. L. 1973. *The Biological Ages of Man*. Philadelphia: W. B. Saunders.

Sullivan, H. S. 1953. *The Interpersonal Theory of Psychiatry*. New York: W. W. Norton.

Sutterley, D., and Donnelly, G. 1973. *Perspectives in Human Development*. Philadelphia: J. B. Lippincott.

The Middle Years. 1975. *American Journal of Nursing* 75:6:997-1024 (special supplement). Part I: Emotional Tasks of the Middle Adult. Part II: The Sexually Active Middle Adult. Part III: The Change of Life. Part IV: The Full Life. Part V: Living Sensibly. Part VI: Coping with Chronic Illness. Part VII: The Mid-Stage Woman. Part VIII: A Faculty Member Remembers.

Weiner, I. B., and Elkins, D. 1972. *Child Development: A Core Approach*. New York: John Wiley and Sons.

5 The Nursing Process

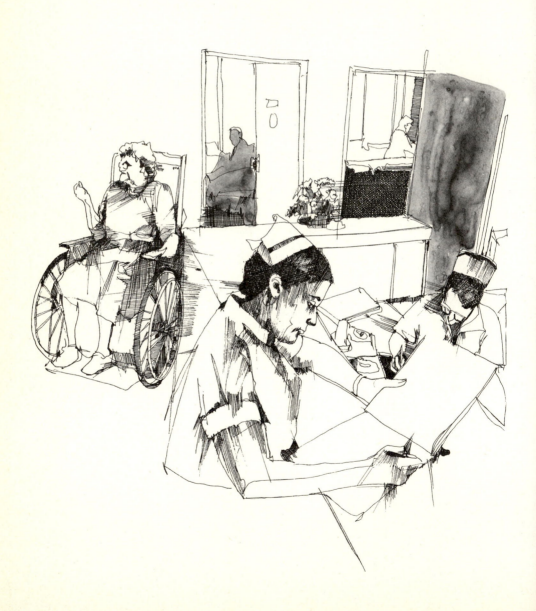

Objectives

After completing this chapter, you should be able to:

1 List the five steps in the nursing process.
2 Discuss the meaning of each step.
3 Apply the problem-solving process to a patient problem.

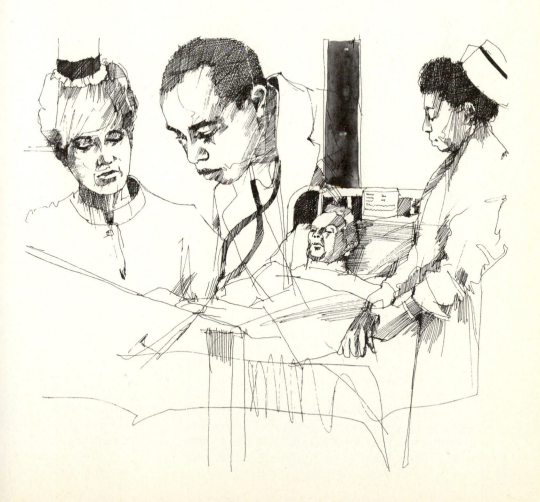

ONLY IN RECENT YEARS have nurses realized that they need a co-ordinated plan for taking care of their patients. Previously, each nurse functioned autonomously. As a result, patient care varied from poor to excellent, was often fragmented, and offered little opportunity for follow-through and evaluation. Since there were few guidelines for planning care, nurses often simply did as they had been taught or used trial-and-error to ascertain what should be done.

Today it is generally accepted that the patient receives the best care when a coordinated approach is planned and the results are evaluated. Nursing education consequently emphasizes the *process* of patient care—that is, the method or manner with which the nurse approaches patient care.

What is this process? What steps insure completeness and can be used reliably in a wide variety of nursing situations? Certainly there are differences of opinion among nurses; however, most agree that a problem-solving approach is basic to the process. You may find that you have been using a similar approach for years without labeling or analyzing it. For example, imagine that you will be taking a final examination in a few days. After taking stock of your performance in the class, you decide you need to do well on the test in order to earn the B you want. You then review testable material, what you already know, what references will be useful, and the previous pattern of testing. When all of this information is in hand, you plan: "I'll review the lecture notes first—that will take an evening. The next day I'll review the text using the lecture outline as a guide. If I have time, I'll review the notes I took on the outside readings." After taking the test, you pat yourself on the back. "I did a great job! I ended up with a B+."

Now reread the above description of your preparation, outlining the steps you took. There are various ways of analyzing the same process, and different people identify different numbers of steps. However, the following analysis of the process has proven helpful to beginning nursing students and to practicing nurses.

First, you assessed the situation, determining that a problem existed by reviewing your previous performance and current knowledge. Information was gathered. Then you clearly defined or stated the problem—in this case, that you needed to do well on the exam.

Second, you stated a concrete and suitable goal, a B in the course. In order to pursue your goal, however, you needed background information.

Third, you collected data—information relating to the course, previous tests, your own strengths and weaknesses, and other matters pertinent to your understanding of the problem and to possible solutions. Then you made a precise plan and timetable.

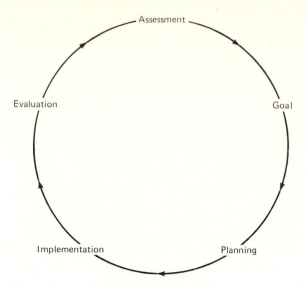

FIGURE 5.1   THE NURSING PROCESS

Fourth, you implemented your plan, doing exactly what you had planned.

Fifth, you evaluated the outcome of your activity, to determine whether your plan resulted in the achievement of your goal.

This, then, is a brief outline of the problem-solving process as it will be described in the next pages (see also Figure 5.1).

1 Assessment
  a Collection of information
  b Statement of the problem
2 Determination of the goal
3 Planning
  a Collection of data
  b Formulation of the plan
4 Implementation of the plan
5 Evaluation

Assessing the problem

Assessment is the process of gathering information and identifying problems. Identification of patients' problems is the foundation of all the nurse does. It is a skill you will begin developing as a student and will never stop expanding.

Many systems and tools have been devised for assessing patients, including Abdellah's "21 Nursing Problems" (Abdellah, 1963), Henderson's "Activities of Daily Living" (Henderson, 1966), and the anatomic systems approach. One of these may work for you, or you may develop your own as you become a more skilled nursing practitioner. All such systems and tools have certain characteristics in common.

The first is *observation*. Observation involves the use of all the senses: sight, hearing, smell, touch, and perhaps even taste. It is the total experience of perceiving and knowing what you have perceived. In a television mystery, for example, a famous astronomer is found dead. The policeman notes nothing unusual about the scene, but the hero, a private detective, recognizes the significance of the fact that the draperies are closed: a telescope is set up by the window, with the apparatus prepared for viewing, and the victim would thus not have closed the draperies himself. The mystery begins to unwind.

In a less spectacular way—but one more significant in real life—the nurse must be alert and recognize the significance of what is seen. A full pitcher of water on the bedside stand is a common sight in the hospital, but the observant nurse relates this observation to the statement heard at morning report that the patient was to be NPO (nothing by mouth). In this way, a potential problem is identified.

However, the nurse must not leap to conclusions. Each bit of information must be considered in the light of others, and a decision must be made as to the additional information necessary. For example, the nurse may need to check the patient's chart to verify the accuracy of the report. Such data is *objective* information—that is, information related to what the nurse sees or hears. Items of information about the patient that can be seen or heard are called *signs*. Some have recently begun using the term *objective symptom* to mean the same thing. The process of gathering objective data about the patient's physical condition is sometimes called a *nursing physical examination*.

The nurse in the situation described above may need to ask the patient questions, such as whether he or she is thirsty. Such *interviewing* is used to collect *subjective* information, or information about what the patient sees, hears, feels, or thinks. Examples are such things as nausea, pain, fear, and dizziness. This information is essential, but should be clearly identified in the nurse's thoughts and in written records as originating with the patient. Traditionally, these subjective facts have simply been called symptoms. However, those who are using the term *objective symptom* as a synomy for *sign* use the term *subjective symptom*, rather than simply *symptom*. For example:

OBJECTIVE SYMPTOMS (SIGNS)	SUBJECTIVE SYMPTOMS (SYMPTOMS)
rapid pulse	heart palpitations
elevated temperature	feeling of warmth
stumbling gait	dizziness
cloudy urine	burning on urination
emesis	nausea
trembling	apprehension
wincing on movement	pain

Many facilities begin nursing contact with a patient (or "client," as the patient is sometimes termed) by collecting a *nursing history*. This is done in a planned interview, by asking questions designed to identify commonly occurring patient problems. As a rule, each facility develops its own form, appropriate to the kinds of patients it receives and the services it offers. (See Figure 5.2.) It is important for the nurse who uses such a form to see it not as an end in itself but as a tool to assist in assessment. Each patient is an individual with unique problems; therefore, the questions you ask may need to vary from those used on the form if you are to discover a given individual's problems.

Sometimes you will perceive cues as to the patient's feelings. These must always be *validated*, or checked with the patient to be certain they are correct. For example, the patient, Miss D., appears to be dizzy. You make an objective observation of her stumbling and irregular gait, and validate your perception by saying, "You are stumbling. Do you feel dizzy?" In this way, you gain subjective information.

As you observe and listen closely to what the patient tells you, you must be constantly relating the resulting information to your knowledge of such basic sciences as anatomy, physiology, pathology, sociology, and psychology. You will also increasingly relate your observations to your knowledge of nursing theory and practice, and will in this way become better able to identify situations in which basic homeostasis is disturbed.

As a beginning practitioner, you may develop your skill at observing more rapidly than your knowledge about your observations. For this reason, you will be communicating your observations and information to other members of the health care team who can determine their significance. But do not lose sight of your objective, which is to be able to interpret the significance of what you observe. As a registered nurse, aides and student nurses will bring their ini-

NURSING CARE HISTORY

Current Health Information

1. Do you have any immediate need? Pain? Excessive fatigue?

   _____
   (Nurse: meet this need before proceeding.)
2. For what problem are you being admitted to the hospital?

   _____
3. Have you been taking any drugs at home? If so, which ones?

   _____
4. Have you been on any special diet at home? If so, what kind?

   _____
5. Do you have any allergies? (Food? Drugs? Other?)

   _____
6. Do you smoke? _____ If others smoke, does it bother you? _____
7. Have you ever had any blood transfusions? _____ When? _____
   Where? _____ How many? _____

Previous Hospital Contacts

1. Have you been hospitalized before? _____
2. If so,
   a. For what condition? _____
   b. Date? _____
   c. Length of stay? _____
   d. Do you recall any nursing actions that were especially helpful to you? If so, please describe
      them. _____
      _____
   e. Do you recall any nursing actions that were not helpful to you or were upsetting to you? If so,
      please describe them. _____
      _____

Activities of Daily Living

1. What are your usual bedtime and wakening hours? _____
2. Are there any things you use to help you sleep? (Number of pillows and covers, food, music,
   medication, etc.) _____
3. Do you have special food likes and dislikes? _____
   _____
4. Do you prefer a tub bath or shower? _____ Time of day? _____
5. Do you have trouble with diarrhea or constipation? _____ Do you take medications for the
   above? _____

Social Background

1. Do you expect to have visitors? _____
2. Do you desire any limitation on visitors? _____ Number? _____ Who visits? _____
   _____Length of Visit? _____
3. Is there someone who will be available to assist you after discharge if you should need help?

   _____

4. What do you prefer in the way of leisure-time activities? _____
_____

Other Information

1. Is there any other information we should know in order to be of better assistance to you? _____
_____
2. Do you have any questions? _____

           Patient's name _____
           Room no. _____ Hospital no. _____
           Adm. date _____ Physician _____

_____
Signature of nurse

FIGURE 5.2   A NURSING CARE HISTORY

tial observations to you, and you will be responsible for determining the significance of such observations.

Stating the problem is so very important that some people treat it as a separate step in problem solving. Some nurses use the term *assessment* to mean only the collection of data, while some writers use it to refer only to the statement of the problem (Weed, 1969). The terms *nursing diagnosis* and *analysis of data* are also used to refer to the statement of the problem. Historically, nursing has used the term *assessment* to encompass both the collection and interpretation of information, and this text will use the term in that way. Terminology is, after all, important only insofar as it enables us to understand one another.

The problem needs to be stated in very clear terms so that it can be understood by all members of the health care team. You will find that your work is more purposeful, and the data you collect more relevant, if you know precisely with what problem you are dealing. Such precision will also enable you to consult with other team members more effectively: not all patient problems are nursing problems, and you must be able to differentiate.

Problems are stated in various ways. For example, the statement "Mr. C. has a decubitus ulcer (bedsore) on the right heel" describes an abnormal condition that is present. In another instance, it might be easier or more appropriate to note what is absent. For example, the statement "Mrs. J. cannot swallow solids" notes the absence of an ability one would expect to be present. The terminology itself is less important than the necessity of making the patient the focus of your statement when you are considering a patient problem. Your concern at this time is Mr. C's bedsore, not the nurse's duty to provide skin care. Finally, if the cause of a problem is known, its inclusion in the statement of the problem will facilitate future planning. For example, "anorexia due to excessive fatigue" would engender different concerns from "anorexia due to odor of wound drainage."

Once stated, a problem must be validated with the patient and other health care team members. Any discrepancy between the patient's and the nurse's perceptions of the problem represents another problem to be solved.

Determining the goal

This step is often omitted because it seems to overlap with the statement of the problem. If you consider the two closely, however, you will see that the problem exists in the present while the goal is the hoped-for future outcome. At first glance, then, a goal may seem to be a statement of what is optimal, since that is what you hope for. However, skill in nursing requires that the goal be realistic and achievable by the patient—neither so low as to underestimate the patient's potential nor so high as to be unobtainable. This is often a fine line to tread.

It is important that patients be involved in setting their own goals and that they see such goals as appropriate. If so, they will participate in their own care to the fullest extent possible. Patients very often come to the health care setting with predetermined goals, which may or may not accord with those of health care personnel. It is the nurse's responsibility to find out what the patient's goals are, to communicate the goals the nurse sees as appropriate, and to negotiate with the patient a set of goals toward which all can work together.

Planning

At this point in the nursing process, you will have collected some data that will be useful as you plan nursing action. But, before acting, it is essential that more data on the specific problem in question be obtained. This data generally falls into two broad classes. The first is objective and subjective data about the patient, acquired from observation, interview, and reading of the patient's record. The second type of information, derived from references, resources, and general knowledge, helps you understand the problem and serves as a basis for planning action. The second type of information forms the rationale, or reason, for your action. Some practitioners use the term *facts and principles* when discussing the rationale for nursing action. A nursing principle is most often defined as two or more facts related by cause and effect that directly suggest a given nursing action. We prefer the term *rationale*, which is somewhat broader and encompasses a wide variety of facts, principles, and other information that can be considered together as a basis for action. The very skilled practitioner may carry much of this knowledge in memory. But for the beginning practitioner and the skilled practitioner faced with new or unusual problems, it will be necessary to consult books and periodicals. Nursing has moved far beyond the era when it was considered necessary only to do, and not to think.

After you have stated the problem, set a goal, and gathered more information, it is time to construct a plan for action. At this point, you will be weighing all your data, deciding what is relevant and what is not. You will be relating the theory, facts, and principles you have gathered to what you know about this particular patient.

All possible actions will have to be judged by a variety of criteria. The first, of course, is "Will it work?" Does this action have the potential for solving this problem? The second is "Are the necessary resources available?" Resources include people and material. If any necessary resource is missing, the proposed action cannot be carried out. For example, if there are not enough people on duty to move a very obese person to a chair, that action is impractical; or if the facility does not have alternating pressure mattresses, you cannot plan to use one. The third criterion is acceptability to the patient. It is necessary to consult the patient on the proposed action, interpreting it if necessary and enlisting cooperation.

The written plan for action is most effective when each part clearly relates in terms of sequence and timing to every other part. (See Figure 5.3.) Steps that are to be taken in sequence or that depend on the completion of a prior task should be listed in the appropriate order. The degree of detail that is specified depends on the person or persons expected to carry out the action, whether you yourself, nursing assistants, registered nurses, or a variety of other persons. However detailed the description, the actions outlined are more likely to be performed consistently if a timetable is also included. For example,

Name __Miller, James_____ Hospital no.000-00-000 Age _60_ Sex _M_ Room _101A_.

NURSING CARE PLAN

Long-Term Goal _Restoration of ability to perform A.D.L. independently_

Current Problems	Nursing Actions
Low fluid intake	Offer fluids (dislikes milk; likes O.J.) q.h. 7:00–3:00 —1000 cc. 3:00–11:00 — 500 cc. 11:00– 7:00 —150 cc.
Does not move self in bed	q.h. — visit and encourage in use of P.T. techniques to turn; give praise when turns with minimum help
Tires easily when trying to converse	Check on pt. when visitors here — ask them to leave before he is too tired
C.V.A.— R. Hemiplegia 3/21/76	M. Jones / J. Scott
Diagnosis Adm. Date	Physician

FIGURE 5.3 TYPICAL FORM FOR RECORDING NURSING CARE PLANS
A.D.L. is short for "activities of daily living"; *o.j.* for "orange juice"; *q.h.* for *"quaque hora"* ("every hour"); *c.c.* for "cubic centimeter"; *P.T.* for "physical therapy"; *pt.* for "patient"; and *C.V.A.* for "cerebral vascular accident."

"good skin care" may be interpreted differently by different people, but "Turn and rub back q2h (every two hours)—even hours" is unlikely to be misinterpreted or ignored. Your plan might also provide checklists or other record-keeping devices to assist those giving care. The Kardex commonly used in many institutions is a practical device for recording a plan for nursing action.

Implementing the plan

In order to achieve the goal, the nurse must next perform or delegate the performance of the actions. Assignment of tasks is not a minor matter, for the nurse must decide on the skills required by the proposed task and by the patient's needs. A task that requires elementary skills, such as feeding a patient, might need to be performed by the registered nurse if knowledgeable attention to the patient's respiratory status and fatigue level is also required during the feeding process.

It is very important for the person who carries out the nursing action to be skillful at it. Skill and confidence in the performance of tasks enhance the patient's sense of trust in the provider of care and can alleviate anxiety and insecurity. By the same token, hesitancy, clumsiness, and carelessness can arouse such feelings where they did not previously exist. Nursing education seeks to enhance the student's skill at common nursing actions.

The actions taken, and the patient's response to them must next be recorded and/or communicated orally so that others on the health care team are aware of them.

Evaluating the results

Evaluation of nursing care is generally regarded as an essential component of nursing practice, but it often receives little time and attention. Evaluation is frequently confined to asking whether or not a given action was taken. The additional questions that ought to be answered involve the result observed in the patient, whether the problem was solved, whether the goal was attained, and whether patient satisfaction was achieved.

If the problem and the goal were originally stated precisely and in detail, evaluation is a relatively easy task. For example, if the problem was that the patient's intake of food was insufficient to provide for healing, and if the goal was for the patient to eat half of what is served on the meal tray, you can simply state "Yes, this was accomplished, the problem is solved, and the plan was a success" or "No, this was not accomplished; therefore the plan was unsuccessful." This is evaluation at its simplest. The criterion—that is, the standard for judging success or failure—is merely success or failure at attaining the goal.

If the problem and the goal were originally stated in general terms, the first step in evaluation is to establish criteria. For example, if the goal in the case described above was simply for the patient to "eat more" or "eat enough," a decision would have to be made about what constitutes "more" or "enough." Only after a criterion is established can one determine whether it has been met.

Written records facilitate the process of evaluation, since care is often provided by different nursing personnel at different times. If actions and results are recorded and if there is a record of the goal and/or criterion being used to measure results, evaluation can be undertaken by someone other than the nurse who made the plan.

More complex evaluation involves subtler questions and determinations. Often the degree of progress made toward the goal must be estimated. If the patient has made progress, the nurse must try to determine whether that progress resulted from the action taken. If so, the nurse must then consider whether the action should be continued or whether the patient would benefit more from a reconsideration of the plan.

So far we have focused exclusively on the nurse's evaluation, but the patient's evaluation of care is equally important. Patients need to be encouraged to examine their goals and their progress. The patient's opinion of care should be actively sought. If care is producing the desired result but is not being delivered in an acceptable manner, the patient can very readily evaluate it.

At its simplest, then, evaluation is simply asking whether the criteria have been met and the goal achieved, and answering "yes" or "no." In its more complex form, evaluation requires that the nurse be able to distinguish degrees of progress toward the goal and to identify the reason or reasons for such progress. The patient ought to be involved in the entire evaluation process, and especially in determining the appropriateness of the method of delivering care.

The purpose of evaluation is to enable you to continue the nursing process. If evaluation reveals that your actions are unsuccessful, you must begin again to examine the problem. Your initial definition of the problem may have been inappropriate, or you may have failed to validate your information with the patient. If you acted before collecting sufficient data, the action may have been inappropriate. If so, you repeat the entire process. If evaluation then shows that you were successful, you may proceed to another problem.

Conclusion

The nursing process outlined in this chapter can be adapted to a wide variety of nursing situations. It may be long and painstaking, or it may be performed quickly in an emergency. Wherever you encounter a patient/client—in the hospital, in the outpatient clinic, in the emergency room, or in the mental health center—the nursing process will enable you to determine his or her problems. Only when problems are clearly defined is it possible to begin solving them. Of course, because the patient seldom has only one problem, the process will be continuous.

CARE STUDY / The problem-solving approach to patient care

Mrs. Sarah Davenport is an eighty-two-year-old widow who was admitted to the hospital because of severe weight loss. The nurse assigned to care for Mrs. Davenport interviews her, using the unit's nursing care history form, and makes careful observations as she assists the patient to bed.

Among the nurse's observations are the following:

1 Mrs. Davenport's skin is thin and transparent and feels dry.

2 All bony prominences are very pronounced, the skin appearing taut (stretched) over them.

3 There is a reddened area over each elbow.

4 Mrs. Davenport stated she "feels tired" and "can scarcely move."

The nurse determines that Mrs. Davenport has beginning skin break-down over the elbows and might easily incur further skin breakdown. On the nursing care plan she writes, "Beginning skin breakdown over both elbows. Potential skin breakdown over all bony prominences."

The nurse reviews what she knows about prevention and treatment of skin breakdown. She reads the patient's chart to learn what activity and diet have been ordered. She spends time talking to Mrs. Davenport about her activity at home, her eating habits, and her concerns about care. She also checks on the equipment currently available to this patient. As the nurse collects all this data, she sorts out its relevance to this patient and this problem. Then the nurse formulates the following plan:

1 Put foam rubber "topper" over mattress.

2 Use cornstarch on sheets at point of contact with elbows to reduce friction. Replace p.r.n. at least q4h (9-1-5 and so on).

3 Assist patient to change position q2h, odd hours (9-11-1 and so on).

4 Visit patient during meals and when nourishment is served to encourage the intake of high-protein, high-calorie foods.

The nurse asks the orderly to get the foam "topper" and, with the assistance of the nurse's aide, to put it on the bed. She gets the cornstarch herself and goes to the patient's bedside to explain what she is going to do and to apply it.

At the end of the fifth day of hospitalization, the nurse reviews all of the patient's current problems. She checks Mrs. Davenport's skin during her morning rounds. Her evaluation is charted: "Redness on elbows gone; skin still appears dry and taut; no skin breakdown apparent on any other bony prominences." Reviewing what has been done, the nurse decides that the plan has been generally successful and should be continued, but that something more needs to be done about the dry skin.

Study terms

assessment   nursing process
criteria   objective data
data collection   observation
evaluation   problem-solving approach
implementation   rationale
interviewing   signs
nursing care plan   subjective data
nursing care history   symptoms
nursing diagnosis   validation

References

Abdellah, Fay G., *et al*. 1960. *Patient Centered Approaches to Nursing*. New York: Macmillan.

Aspinal, M. J. 1975. Development of a Patient Completed Admission Questionnaire and Its Comparison with the Nursing Interview. *Nursing Research* 24:377-381 (Sept.-Oct. 1975).

Bailit, H., *et al*. 1975. Assessing the Quality of Care. *Nursing Outlook* 23:153-159 (March 1975).

Carlson, S. 1972. A Practical Approach to the Nursing Process. *American Journal of Nursing* 72:1589-1591 (Sept. 1972).

DeTornyay, R. Nursing Decisions: Experiences in Clinical Problem-Solving. *RN* 38:9:57-62.

Haffke, E., and Gero, S. 1973. Two Missing Pieces: A New Formula for Solving Nursing Problems. *Nursing '73* 3:3:32-35.

Hefferin, E. A., *et al*. 1975. Nursing Assessment and Care Plan Statements. *Nursing Research* 24:360-366 (Sept.-Oct. 1975).

Henderson, V. 1966. *The Nature of Nursing*. New York: Macmillan, pp. 15-16.

House, M. J. 1975. Devising a Care Plan You Can Really Use. *Nursing '75* 5:7:1214.

Weed, L. L. 1969. *Medical Records: Medical Education and Patient Care*. Cleveland: Case Western Reserve University Press.

Woody, M., *et al*. 1973. The Problem-Oriented System for Patient Centered Care. *American Journal of Nursing* 73:1168-1175.

6 Mental Health

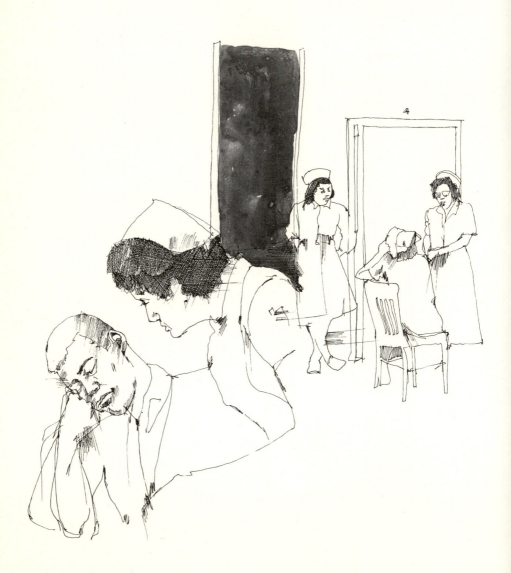

Objectives

After completing this chapter, you should be able to:

1 Discuss the concept of mental health.

2 Review the eleven basic mental health concepts presented and explain how each might be applied to nursing.

3 Discuss how a person's concept of health and illness might affect his or her response to being a patient.

4 List and explain major problems affecting the person who is becoming a patient.

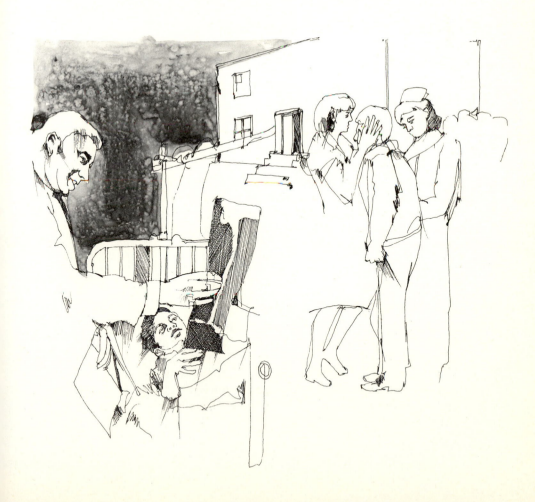

ENTAL HEALTH, which encompasses thoughts, feelings, and responses to life, is closely related to physical, spiritual, and social health. Although many components have been identified, mental health is ultimately a personal matter and must be evaluated by the individual in question.

It is helpful to consider mental health as a continuum, and individuals as occupying different points on that continuum at different times in their lives. Thus mental health is a dynamic state, always changing and always affected by events in one's life.

The degree of mental health an individual possesses at a given time is usually judged by examining his or her ability to function optimally in relationship to the self and to the environment. Let us examine the factors that contribute to one's ability to function optimally (Amis, 1975).

Basic concepts in mental health

Self-understanding

"An understanding of one's self may lead to an understanding of others" (Schmaul, 1966). As a nurse you will be called on to understand others in many situations, and the basis for doing so lies in an understanding of yourself. Self-understanding is not a static state, but a dynamic process in which you strive to know yourself in relation to each new experience and each new person you encounter. As you read about each of the following factors in mental health, consider its application to your own life and the ways it might enhance your self-understanding. Then seek an understanding of its application to your relationships with family, friends, patients, and co-workers.

Human dignity

The concept of human dignity rests on faith in the individual's worth, regardless of race, sex, creed, culture, or behavior (Dunn, 1962). Recognition of the intrinsic worth of each individual is the basis of all supportive, helpful human relationships, and is central to effective nursing. This principle underlies efforts that go unnoticed and supports work toward goals that are not realized. And, when acted upon, it promotes in others a belief in their own dignity and worth.

Basic Mental Health Concepts

1 "An understanding of one's self may lead to an understanding of others" (Schmaul, 1966).

2 The concept of human dignity rests on faith in the individual's worth regardless of race, sex, creed, culture, or behavior (adapted from Dunn, 1961).

3 A human being is made up of interrelated components—physical, mental, emotional, and spiritual—and must be viewed as a whole person (adapted from Amis, 1975).

4 The concept of the self is an important factor in coping with daily life (adapted from Dunn, 1961).

5 Any mutilation or basic change in body structure or function will influence the individual's self-concept and relationships with others and must be understood in terms of the individual's feelings about the change (adapted from Nordmark, 1967).

6 All behavior has meaning and purpose for the individual (adapted from Amis, 1975).

7 Feelings and sentiments are real, and must be treated as such whether or not they appear to be based in fact (adapted from Farnsworth, 1960).

8 Human beings function and experience both as individuals and as members of social groups (adapted from Schmaul, 1966).

9 There is a basic capacity in the individual that continues to seek growth under the proper conditions (adapted from Schmaul, 1966).

10 Psychological balance requires that the individual have adequate means for communication with others and/or for self-expression (adapted from Nordmark, 1967).

11 Anxiety is a subjective experience of apprehension initiated by a threat to oneself, whether physical, mental, emotional, or spiritual (adapted from Peplau, 1963).

The whole person

A human being is made up of interrelated components—physical, mental, emotional, and spiritual—and must be viewed as a whole person (Amis, 1975). The interrelatedness of the individual's components means that physical illness may have a profound effect on psychological well-being, and that psychological status may affect physical well-being in a variety of ways, both positive and negative. The nurse cannot be exclusively concerned with one or the other aspect of the person, but must consistently strive to see the whole person and the relationships among the physical, psychological, mental, and spiritual components.

Self-concept

The concept of the self is an important factor in coping with daily life (Dunn, 1962). One's view of oneself affects one's ability to function. If you see yourself as competent and resourceful, you will tend to behave in ways that support this view. On the other hand, seeing yourself as incompetent may make you reluctant to attempt tasks or even destine you to failure before you begin. An individual's self-concept is based on many factors, one of the most potent of which is the way others see one, or *feedback*.

Body image

Any mutilation or basic change in body structure or function will influence the individual's self-concept and relationships with others, and must be understood in terms of the individual's feelings about the change (Nordmark, 1967). A person's self-concept is closely bound up with the physical self and the body image. If a change occurs in the body, such as the removal of a body part, the person must be reoriented toward the body, reappraise the responses of others, and adjust his or her self-concept. This process may not be difficult, as in the case of an appendectomy that leaves a scar. The loss of a leg, on the other hand, is of maximal concern. The meaning of such a change for the individual is the most significant factor in assessing the seriousness of the difficulty and in deciding whether or not the individual needs assistance in dealing with it (see Chapter 22.)

The meaningfulness of all behavior

All behavior has meaning and purpose for the individual. It can solve problems, relieve anxiety, or help a person to cope with stress

(Amis, 1975). You may not understand certain behavior, or be able to discern its purpose, but a recognition that behavior is not without meaning to the individual can help you be more accepting even when you lack understanding. Some behavior may not even be understood by the individual who engages in it, and your efforts to understand may guide the person to greater self-awareness. When you are attempting to help someone change his or her behavior, it may be essential to search for and understand the meaning or purpose of the behavior you hope to modify.

The validity of feelings

Feelings and sentiments are real, and must be treated as such whether or not they appear to be based on fact (Farnsworth, 1960). It is usually easy to accept feelings—our own or others'—for which we can discern reasons, but when we cannot we frequently label the feeling inappropriate or "wrong." This response can result in a breakdown of the interpersonal relationship. If instead we accept a person's feelings and sentiments without judging them to be right or wrong, we strengthen the relationship and build mutual trust.

Individuality and group identification

Human beings function and experience both as individuals and as members of social groups (Schmaul, 1966). It is important to see others as individuals whose responses are derived from their own experiences, and to abandon expectations of behavior based on stereotyped views of the "good patient," racial and ethnic groups, or males and females. On the other hand, we must not ignore the group to which an individual belongs. A person's family or ethnic group may affect the way he or she responds and functions. Finding an appropriate middle ground between stereotyping and inattention to individual backgrounds is a difficult task, as is distinguishing between behavior based on individual differences and behavior characteristic of the group to which the person belongs. However, a continuing effort to do so will help you deal more effectively with others. For example, some family groups respond to the illness of a member by gathering together and becoming intensely involved in the person's care. An understanding of this practice and its meaning to those involved is necessary if the patient is placed in a unit where the number of visitors and length of visits are very restricted. On the other hand, the patient may prefer that the family not be so intimately involved. As a nurse, your first responsibility in such a situation is to the patient.

The capacity for growth

There is a basic capacity in the individual that continues to seek growth under the proper conditions (Schmaul, 1966). As a person's immediate goals and needs are met, new ones arise to take their place. We expect growth when we ask individuals to adopt new ways of functioning, to learn new skills, and to deal with a variety of complex feelings and problems. If an individual does not appear to be striving for growth, the surrounding conditions need to be examined. Are his or her immediate needs not being met? Is energy available for growth, or is all the patient's available energy being devoted to maintenance? Are you providing a climate suitable for growth?

The need to communicate

Psychological balance requires that the individual have adequate means for communication with others and/or for self-expression (Nordmark, 1967). Some consider communication the most important single factor in mental health. Undeniably, anything that hampers communication with others—whether laryngitis, a language barrier, or a mental attitude—poses a threat to mental health. Inability to communicate significantly affects recovery from any illness, but perhaps most dramatically in the stroke patient. If two patients have equal motor function but differ in speech capacity, the patient who can communicate will invariably be rehabilitated to self-care more easily and rapidly.

It is the nurse's responsibility to provide the patient a means of communication. This task might require seeking the help of another person, such as the speech therapist, or using sign language, pictures, or gestures. For the patient in isolation, it could mean setting aside time to talk together; for the deaf patient, you might provide a "magic slate" for writing. With patients whose mental attitudes block communication, the nurse must work skillfully and patiently at using the nursing process to establish some form of communication.

Anxiety

Anxiety is a subjective experience of apprehension initiated by a threat to oneself, whether physical, mental, emotional, or spiritual (Peplau, 1963). Anxiety may also be described as the generalized energy experienced by the body as it prepares to act in response to a perceived threat. In a mild form, therefore, anxiety is constructive and helps the individual to function effectively. But as it increases in severity, purposeful activity is hampered and anxiety becomes dysfunctional.

Table 6.1 lists some of the physiological responses characteristic of anxiety and some of the behaviors characteristic of the anxious person. You will need to learn the characteristics of anxiety in order to be able to identify it in yourself and in those with whom you work. You must also become highly aware of the effect of anxiety on learning and on perception, since you will be involved in health teaching and in explaining new and strange procedures to patients. Table 6.1 will help you to identify the level of anxiety being experienced. Individuals with mild to moderate anxiety may be functioning very well. However, those suffering from moderate to severe anxiety or panic will benefit from intervention to reduce anxiety to a more manageable level. (See Chapter 7.)

Threats to the patient's mental health

In our daily lives, we all assume a number of different roles. For example, a woman may be a daughter in one setting, an employee in another, and a mother in still another. Each of these roles is characterized by a set of expected behaviors. The term *mother* evokes widely shared expectations, within whose general outlines each person develops a particular way of responding on the basis of life experience and background.

Becoming a patient requires a person to adapt a new role. This role may vary, depending on whether the setting is an outpatient clinic, the home, or an acute care hospital. People's responses to this role also depend on their families and cultural backgrounds which teach them various interpretations of appropriate behavior for the sick person, and on their previous experiences with the patient role.

Individuals differ in their views of health and illness. A person with multiple handicaps who needs ongoing supervision by a health care team may consider himself "healthy" as long as he does not have an acute illness. His response to the patient role will be quite different from that of the person who perceives a sprained ankle as a serious threat to health and assumes a totally dependent role. When the patient's concept of health differs from that of the health care team members, conflict may result. This situation calls for the skillful use of interpersonal communication techniques to resolve the conflict. It may not be possible nor desirable to alter the patient's perception, and health care providers may have to alter their expectations and approaches.

TABLE 6.1 CHARACTERISTICS OF ANXIETY

	NO ANXIETY (−)	MILD ANXIETY (+)
PULSE	Resting rate	Slightly faster
RESPIRATION	Resting rate	Slightly faster
BLOOD PRESSURE	Resting level	Slightly elevated
MUSCLE TONE AND EFFECT ON ACTIVITY	Flaccid, not ready to act; lethargic	Slight tension, ready to act; acts with purpose
MOOD	Calm; may feel lethargic	Alert; feels ambitious and ready to act
EFFECT ON PERCEPTION	Not alert, easily distracted	Alert, sees details well; extraneous material excluded from attention
EFFECT ON LEARNING	Slow	Enhanced, optimal

Whatever the setting, common problems confront the person entering the patient role. You will find the eleven mental health factors to be important guides in helping the patient adjust to role change. A setting that minimizes such problems and provides maximum support to the patient is called a *therapeutic environment*.

Threat to the self-concept

The first problem is the threat to the person's self-concept posed by the patient role. "I'm not a whole person anymore." "I can't fulfill my usual role in life." "What will other people think of me? How will they treat me now?" The answers to these and other questions may require a change in the view of the self. During a temporary illness, such changes may be very minor and easily dealt with by the patient. During a major illness profound changes are frequently required, and the patient may need assistance and support in dealing with his or her feelings.

As we have seen, a threat to self-concept arouses anxiety. Therefore, you can expect most patients to experience some degree of

MODERATE ANXIETY (+ +)	SEVERE ANXIETY (+ + +)	PANIC (+ + + +)
Noticeably faster	Rapid, possibly irregular	Very rapid and irregular
Noticeably faster	Rapid and irregular	Very rapid, possible hyperventilation
Noticeably elevated	High	High; if profound, may suddenly drop and cause fainting
Increased tension; may have headaches and other aches; may act in repetitive manner to release tension; may pace	Extreme tension—may be almost unable to move; no purposeful action; repetitive actions increased in speed and intensity	Extreme tension; either immobilization or eruption into erratic behavior; almost uncontrollable
"Nervous," somewhat upset	Very upset, feels loss of control	Out of control, panicky
Focuses more narrowly; may not perceive whole situation	Focuses on random detail; misses whole situation	Perception distorted
Slow or limited	Greatly diminished or absent	No learning possible

anxiety during their contact with the health care system. Because there is an interrelationship between physical and psychological well-being, this will be true whether the initial problem is physical or psychological. Helping the patient to reduce anxiety to a constructive level is the task of the nurse. It is accomplished through an interpersonal process that provides the patient an opportunity to explore and deal with his or her feelings.

Loss of privacy

A second problem is the loss of privacy. Many different individuals may be asking the patient personal questions. There may be physical examinations that offend modesty. In the hospital, personal belongings are often carefully inspected, inventoried, and stored elsewhere for safekeeping. Elimination may take place while other persons are present or separated only by a curtain. This setting requires the patient to suppress a set of feelings and behaviors related to maintaining personal privacy and modesty.

Belief in human dignity and worth leads you to protect the privacy of the individual in every way possible. It requires that you be sensitive to the patient's feelings and recognize that they may differ from your own. With this principle as your guide, you will provide a full measure of privacy to the individual who is not able to claim it independently: the comatose individual, the child, or the person without speech. Concretely providing privacy means using blankets for draping, pulling curtains, knocking on closed doors, and being discreet when you talk with the patient about personal matters.

Loss of control

A third problem is the feeling of loss of control. Adults in Western society are used to the sense of controlling their own lives. In the health care setting, tests may be ordered, forms filled out, and plans for care made by others; the person may feel as if swept along on the tide. Giving consent does not mean that the patient thoroughly understands all that is happening.

Loss of control may also be a threat to the self-image, and as such may create anxiety. This outcome can be prevented or alleviated by allowing patients to retain control over as much of their lives as possible. Whenever feasible, you can give the patient choices regarding care. For example, does he prefer a bath now or in an hour? In what order does she prefer the tasks of care? Often such decisions are arbitrarily made by nursing personnel even when a choice is feasible. To help the patient feel more control over the situation, you ought to introduce unfamiliar members of the health care team, describe their functions and carefully explain all that is going to happen, including time schedules. You must also explain how beds and call lights work, where the bathroom is, and how the telephone operates. Fear of loss of control over elimination is very prevalent, especially in the elderly. Calm acceptance of such problems and shared planning to solve them can restore dignity and some control to the patient, even when physical control is lost. Control over broader matters also concerns patients. As you review the Health Consumer Bill of Rights in Chapter 1, consider how you can support the patient in the exercise of these rights.

Uncertainty

Patients also experience uncertainty as to the behavior expected of them. "How is a patient supposed to act?" "Is it permissible to ask questions?" "Do I have to ask for pain relief or can I expect it to be provided without asking?" You have faced such uncertainty yourself if you have ever sat in a doctor's examining room wondering what you should do next. "Am I expected to wait in the examining room until the doctor returns or should I get dressed and go to the desk?" Such uncertainty may be multiplied many times over when the entire environment is unfamiliar and one's contact with the health care system has been limited. Anxiety may be especially pronounced among individuals from cultural backgrounds other than those of the health care workers.

You can assist the patient by describing the behavior you expect. The most routine admission to the hospital may be a completely new experience for the patient. "Am I expected to take all my clothes off under that gown?" "Can I leave my underwear on?" "Am I expected to go right to bed?" "Do I ring the buzzer or will you automatically come back?" Explanations of all such matters are necessary, as are any orders regarding activity, policy on leaving the area, and the patient's responsibilities for his or her own care. Be sure to elicit the patient's questions and concerns as well. Hospital admission is not the only time when expected behavior needs to be explained. Explanations are also needed when a new procedure or treatment is to be performed, when the patient is to go to another department for a test, and when changes occur in care. The need for clear statements of expected behavior continues throughout the patient's contact with the health care system.

An unfamiliar pattern of living

In the hospital the patient must adopt an entirely new pattern of living, which can be a further problem. The schedule may be drastically at odds with his or her own. In spite of attempts to individualize care, most institutions find that certain routines and schedules are necessary to function smoothly. As a nurse, you might consider which of the patterns prescribed by the institution are really essential, and whether it is possible to adapt in any way to the needs and desires of the patient. Certain aspects of our routines are indeed based on necessity, but others are unquestionably the result of long-standing traditions that have no rationale and have never been questioned.

Worry over expenses

A major problem facing the consumer of health care in the United States is its cost. For most persons, an extensive illness or hospitalization costs more than insurance pays. Health care costs have been rising much more rapidly than most other sectors of the economy. Even those whose health care plans pay all the costs of illness may be subject to loss of income, expenses for child care, or the cost of home-making services. The nurse is not usually in a position to directly alleviate a patient's financial concerns. However, the nurse can refer the patient to others with the ability and knowledge to do so, such as the social worker. Some hospitals employ individuals to help patients with their financial problems. Sometimes the patient can deal with such problems independently if he or she has access to the business office or insurance carrier.

Fear

In addition to the foregoing problems, the patient may carry a burden of undisclosed fears: of disease, of surgery, and even of death. Such fears can hinder the patient's ability to understand and cope with all that is happening, and as a nurse you can help the patient alleviate them by means of skillful interpersonal communication. This subject is discussed in detail in Chapter 7.

Conclusion

You will find the basic mental health concepts to be useful guidelines to your actions in a wide variety of situations. They can also be of value in dealing with your own feelings and responses within the health care setting.

The role of patient is complex and involves many changes in life style and expected behavior. Supporting the mental health of the patient during stressful experiences of health care is one of the primary functions of the nurse. The nurse is in a position to do a great deal to ease the transition to the role of patient. Understanding of the concerns and problems of the patient is essential if you are to do this effectively.

Study terms

anxiety   dysfunction
apprehension   ethnic group
body image   goal seeking
control   homeostasis
cultural group   human dignity

intrinsic worth   psychological equilibrium
mental health   role
mutilation   self-concept
panic   therapeutic environment
privacy

References

Amis, Dorothy. 1968, 1975. *Basic Mental Health Concepts*. Seattle: Shoreline Community College A.D. Nursing Program.

Azarnoff, P. 1974. Mediating the Trauma of Serious Illness and Hospitalization in Childhood. *Children Today* 5:12-17.

Carstairs, G. M. 1973. Mental Health: What is It? *World Health* 26:4-9.

Carty, R. 1972. Patients Who Cannot Hear. *Nursing Forum* 11:290-299.

Dunn, H. L. 1962. *High Level Wellness*. Arlington, Va.: R. W. Beatty, p. 227.

Elliott, S. 1969. The Day the Students Came. *American Journal of Nursing* 69:551-552.

Farnsworth, D. L. 1960. Mental Health, A Point of View. *American Journal of Nursing* 60:688-691.

Grace, M. J. 1974. The Psychiatric Nurse Specialist and Medical-Surgical Patients. *American Journal of Nursing* 74:481-483.

Issner, N. 1972. The Family of the Hospitalized Child. *Nursing Clinics of North America* 7:5-12.

Meyer, V. R. 1973. The Psychology of the Young Adult. *Nursing Clinics of North America* 8:5-14.

Nordmark, M. T. *et al*. 1967. *Scientific Foundations of Nursing*, 2nd ed. Philadelphia: J. B. Lippincott, p. 276.

Peplau, Hildegarde. 1963. A Working Definition of Anxiety. In *Some Clinical Approaches to Psychiatric Nursing*, ed. S. Burd *et al*., pp. 323-327. New York: Macmillan.

Rickles, Wathan, and Finkle, B. C. 1973. Anxiety: Yours and Your Patients'. *Nursing '73* 3:3:23-26.

Schmaul, J. A. 1966. *Experiment in Change*. New York: Macmillan, p. 30.

Volicer, B. J. 1974. Patients' Perceptions of Stressful Events Associated with Hospitalization. *Nursing Research* 23:235-238.

7 Communication in Nursing

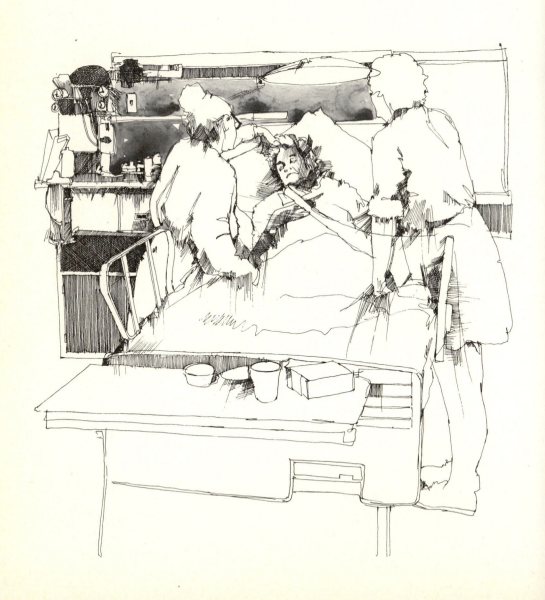

Objectives

After completing this chapter, you should be able to:

1 Define verbal and nonverbal communication and give examples of each.

2 List the four major types of verbal communication and define each.

3 List the categories of facilitating responses.

4 List the categories of blocking responses.

5 Discuss the five guidelines for a nursing care plan.

6 List and define the four kinds of information the nurse must record on the patient's record.

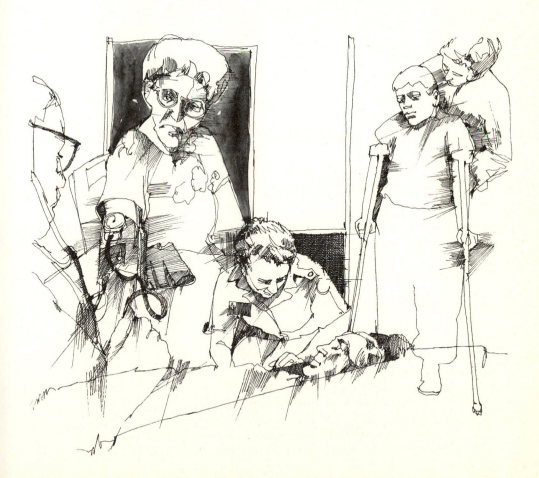

COMMUNICATE: TO MAKE KNOWN. The definition is simple, but the process is one of the most complex in which human beings participate. Transmission of knowledge, experience, and feelings requires the skill and attention of both the sender of a message and its recipient. Meaning is conveyed in a variety of ways, both verbal and nonverbal. Understanding of the ways in which nonverbal and verbal behavior affect interaction is important to you in meeting the needs of patients and working effectively with other members of the health care team.

Communication has various purposes or objectives, and the effectiveness of any given communication can be enhanced by the use of skills and techniques appropriate to its purpose. Thus you need to develop ability to identify patient needs for interaction, to determine the purpose or objective of the interaction, and to interact effectively using the appropriate techniques or skills.

Nonverbal communication

In any human relationship nonverbal behaviors that communicate feelings and attitudes are as important and at times even more important than the words that are exchanged. The infant's first experiences with others are entirely nonverbal. Touch, tone of voice, and facial expressions can communicate caring, anger, indifference, or myriad other feelings even before the child is able to understand the meaning of the spoken word.

We often respond to nonverbal cues without awareness that we are doing so. We may say, for example, "I don't think Mrs. Jones likes me," but be unable to explain why we think so. The reasons may lie in nonverbal cues we have absorbed but not thought about. At other times we may respond only to the spoken words, failing to perceive contradictory nonverbal cues. If, for example, you ask your neighbor, "Would it be all right if I park in front of your driveway temporarily?" and the neighbor answers, "Well, O.K.," you may miss the hesitation and tone of voice that suggest he does indeed mind, responding only to the verbal answer you hoped to hear.

Identification and interpretation of nonverbal communication can be learned. This skill will help you to understand yourself and those with whom you come in contact better, and to respond in the most helpful manner possible. A preoperative patient may state, for example, "Oh, I've had surgery before—it doesn't worry me too much." The patient may indeed have learned to deal very successfully with the entire surgical process; on the other hand,

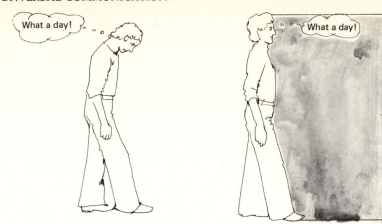

FIGURE 7.1   NONVERBAL COMMUNICATION AND THE PATIENT   What message is the patient communicating?

the patient may be quite anxious but feel he or she "shouldn't be." The nurse may be able to tell the difference by identifying and correctly interpreting nonverbal cues (see Figure 7.1). For example, was the patient pacing restlessly? Did he seem to have difficulty concentrating or was he relaxed? Interpretive skill will help make your response helpful and supportive to the patient and will prevent the emotional isolation of the patient whose verbal and nonverbal messages are inconsistent.

Identifying and interpreting nonverbal behavior

The most common nonverbal cues are tone of voice, facial expression, body position, and gestures. Others are the presence or absence of muscle tenseness, eye movements, and activity. This list is by no means exhaustive, but can serve to suggest the wide variety of factors that need to be observed.

Once nonverbal behavior has been identified, it must be interpreted. In other words, you must ask yourself, "What does this behavior mean?" An entire book, *Body Language* by Julius Fast, has been devoted to the meanings of nonverbal cues; the subject is vast. You might begin by trying to understand the most common nonverbal behavior. Does it communicate a mood or feeling to you? You may want to consult others or psychiatric nursing textbooks. A beginning nurse is not expected to be able to interpret all nonverbal behavior correctly, but a knowledge of behaviors commonly indicative of anxiety or fear is most helpful.

It is also helpful to watch for consistency between nonverbal and verbal communication. Compare patients' facial expression with the verbal messages they are conveying at the same time. Are they congruent or at odds? An angry expression accompanying a positive or bland statement indicates that the patient's feelings may vary from the spoken words.

After interpreting a given behavior, it is often necessary to validate your interpretation. This process simply involves identifying the behavior verbally, giving your interpretation, and asking the person involved if your interpretation is correct. For example, "I have noticed you pacing the room, and it appears to me that you are upset." The other person may confirm your interpretation, elaborate on your comment, or deny that it is correct.

If the person agrees with your interpretation, you may then interact on the basis of that understanding. If the person denies your interpretation, you should first consider that you might be mistaken. Interpreting nonverbal behavior is not simple, and errors are not uncommon. But if further observation and thought reinforces your viewpoint, you might want to seek the opinion of another nurse. If your final interpretation is unchanged, you might try responding to the message of the nonverbal communication as you have interpreted it. This is more often helpful than is responding only to the patient's statement. For example, a patient admitted for diagnostic studies is tossing and turning, unable to sleep. Approaching the patient, the nurse notices that her face looks tense and pale. The nurse says, "I notice that you're having difficulty sleeping and that you look tense. Are you feeling worried?" The patient replies, "Oh, I'm O.K. I'm sure you have lots to do with so many sick patients." The nurse reconsiders the original observation and decides to respond to the nonverbal behavior rather than the verbal statement of well-being. The nurse sits down and talks with the patient, and is able to help relieve her worries. The patient finally falls asleep. In this instance, the patient was helped far more by a response to her nonverbal behavior than she would have been by a response to the verbal message.

Communicating nonverbally

The nurse also conveys meaning to the patient in nonverbal ways (see Figure 7.2). You may say that it is simply routine to change a very malodorous dressing, but the rigidity of your jaw, the distance you maintain, and the speed with which you depart may tell the patient that it is a distasteful task. Such inconsistency between verbal and nonverbal messages may be very upsetting to patients. It is far

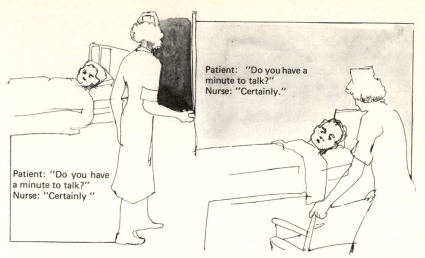

Patient: "Do you have a
minute to talk?"
Nurse: "Certainly."

Patient: "Do you have
a minute to talk?"
Nurse: "Certainly"

FIGURE 7.2 NONVERBAL COMMUNICATION AND THE NURSE   What
message is the patient receiving?

more supportive for the nurse to convey consistent verbal and nonverbal messages. This means that both need to be true expressions of
feeling: most people cannot control nonverbal behavior in the same
way they do verbal behavior, and the attempt may undermine the
patient's trust. Thus it might be more helpful to the patient described
above if you say, "The drainage from your wound is unpleasant.
Therefore I'll change it frequently and place this air freshener in the
room so that it will not trouble you or your visitors so much."

    Touch is a highly significant mode of nonverbal communica-
tion where meaning may vary in different situations and to different
people. Touch may be associated with discipline, rejection, sexual
feelings, or myriad other ideas and attitudes, but the most common
association is probably with mothering and comfort. You may use
this mode of communication to convey your concern, to comfort, or
to reassure. Touch may communicate caring when no other mode of
communication can bridge the barrier between two people.

    Touch may also have value and meaning for the person who
does the touching. It may be a way of expressing feeling, releasing
tension, or making contact. Thus the nurse may touch the dying patient to express grief, or the patient may grasp the nurse's hand for
reassurance. Because touch may be interpreted in various ways, you
need to be alert to what it means to you and to the other person. (It
may sometimes be helpful to clarify verbally what you are trying to
convey with touch: "It's hard to be alone at a time like this. I'll stay

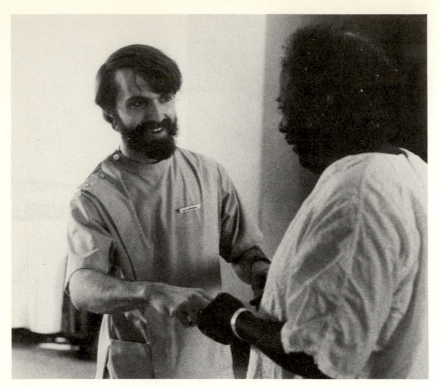

Touch: a nonverbal expression of caring
Elizabeth Wilcox

with you during this test.") When using touch with patients, evaluate it primarily in light of its value and meaning to the patient.

Silence also conveys meaning, and may be used purposefully to enhance communication. Silence at an appropriate moment in a conversation may communicate your willingness to wait for an answer or to allow the other person to think about a reply. Sometimes sitting quietly with someone else, neither talking nor leaving, can communicate your unconditional acceptance. Many people, however, become very anxious during silent moments; if you do, your anxiety may be conveyed by other nonverbal behavior and defeat your purpose. You may be able to overcome such anxiety by initially limiting the time you expect yourself to remain silent to a few minutes, and then gradually increasing its duration as you become more comfortable. If five minutes is the most you can handle without becoming anxious, you might articulate this limit by saying, "I'll stay another five minutes and then I have to leave." You can similarly enhance your abilities to perceive and understand nonverbal behaviors by constant practice.

Verbal communication

Verbal communication is all the words exchanged between people. Words themselves can be a source of considerable confusion: you have probably had the experience of becoming involved in an argument only to discover that you differ only over the use of terms, not over basic ideas. Thus it may be necessary to seek validation of the messages communicated by verbal interaction by asking, "Do you mean. . . ?" or "I understand you to mean . . ."

Verbal communication serves many purposes and may be structured variously to serve those different purposes. We will here discuss socializing, interviewing, and therapeutic interaction as major purposes of interaction with patients. A fourth type of interaction, health teaching, is discussed in Chapter 8. It is valuable to remember that the following principles pertain to interactions with persons, not just patients, and can be used appropriately in interactions with co-workers, teachers, friends, and relatives.

Socializing

Socializing is engaging in ordinary social conversation with someone else. Its subjects may include such impersonal topics as the weather and politics and such personal topics as children, family, and occupation.

A facility in which socializing with patients is rare would be perceived as cold and unfriendly. Socializing contributes to pleasure and relaxation and enhances our knowledge of one another. However, the nurse's social conversation with patients has been a cause of concern for many practitioners. A prime consideration is the physical well-being of the patient—social conversation should not cause fatigue or interfere with needed rest. Another issue is the patient's privacy—social conversation should not pry into personal and family matters. A third concern is the patient's emotional well-being—it may be that the nurse's response to the concerns or feelings the patient expresses should be therapeutic, not social. Finally, social conversation should not become a forum for the nurse's problems and opinions.

As a nurse, you need to assess the situation and the patient's needs and decide what the patient needs. If you decide that socializing is appropriate, it is your responsibility to make sure such conversation does not create a problem where none existed by, for example, causing undue fatigue or probing into personal matters. Socializing is not an opportunity for you to talk about topics of personal interest but a time for patients to discuss topics that interest them.

Conflicting advice has been given nurses on how much of oneself to reveal in social conversation with patients. An important guideline is that socializing must not undermine the possible effectiveness of the professional relationship.

What you reveal of yourself might vary considerably in different situations and with different patients. A student nurse might feel very comfortable sharing personal concerns and thoughts with a patient of the same sex. With a patient of the opposite sex, such talk might be misconstrued as romantic interest and interfere with future therapeutic interaction.

Some nurses feel comfortable revealing their thoughts and feelings to other people, while others are even in their personal lives more private. Individual differences make it necessary for each nurse to make a personal decision on how much and what to share in each situation. What is right for one may not be right for another.

There are those who question whether nurses should establish long-term friendships with patients that will persist outside of the care setting. Again, this is an individual matter. Sometimes such relationships are successful for all concerned. In other instances, the two persons find they have little in common once the professional connection ends. The nurse needs to be aware that a one-sided loss of interest can be painful for the other person. The ex-patient is apt to be in a more dependent position, and thus to be the more hurt when the friendship ceases. Again, recognition of the many possible outcomes, critical self-evaluation, and a well thought-out decision is the best course of action.

Interviewing

An interview is a conversation in which questions are asked by one person and answered by the other. The nurse often interviews the patient or family members as part of nursing assessment. The nursing care history is one type of *structured* interview—that is, an interview in which the questions are planned in advance. Other types of interviews are *unstructured*—that is, the questions are not planned but arise in the course of the interview on the basis of the respondent's answers.

The physical comfort of both participants enhances an interview's effectiveness. Such factors as lighting, heat, drafts, and noise may all affect the patient's response. And recognition of the special physical problems of the ill person—such as pain, fatigue, and shortness of breath—is essential in nursing interviews. Nursing care directed at alleviating such problems may be needed before an interview can be attempted.

The relative physical positions of the two participants may affect the interviewee's feelings about the interview. Positioning yourself on level with the person you are interviewing and making eye contact can facilitate communication. Patients may respond quite unfavorably or reticently to someone who stands over them looking down. Also, sitting down to talk with the patient emphasizes the importance of the interaction and allows the patient to feel that you have time to listen.

Privacy is very important. Some topics may be discussed in the presence of other patients if voice levels are kept low, but others are too private to be discussed where remarks may be overheard. If family members are present, you must decide whether to encourage their participation or ask them to leave. This decision depends on the content of the questions and the physical, mental, and emotional condition of the patient. You may wish to direct some questions to the family (especially if the patient is a child), some to both patient and family, and some to the patient alone. Conducting such an interview requires judgment. The patient may even be embarrassed by the presence of other health care workers. (This is often overlooked.)

The traditional queries of the newspaper reporter—who, what, where, when, and how—are equally valid in a health care setting. *Why* is less useful, since the patient may not know why. Specific questions are needed when specific information is desired. However, if the area of concern is unknown to the interviewer before the interview begins (as in an unstructured interview), questions might initially be general and become more specific as more information is gathered.

You may have to ask questions about an unpleasant or painful matter, such as the circumstances of an accident. At times questions must be very personal, relating to such things as bowel habits and family relationships. People are usually more comfortable in answering such questions if a trust relationship has been established before the interview. One way to elicit trust is to meet the patient's immediate needs—make him or her comfortable—before beginning to ask questions. Another is to explain the purpose of the interview and the use that will be made of the information collected.

During an interview, it is important that you look for nonverbal indications that the questions being asked do not relate to the primary concerns of the patient and cues to other concerns that should be explored. Even in a structured interview, you may find it useful to deviate from the structure in response to cues and responses from the patient. Recognition of questions that arouse anxiety may give you insight into areas where nursing intervention is needed.

Above all, you need to remember that the interview is a purposeful tool for the improvement of patient care. In order to fulfill this purpose, it must remain flexible enough to meet the needs of a wide variety of patients and situations. After the interview is completed, you have an obligation to use the information for the well-being of the patient.

Therapeutic interaction

When a patient experiences unpleasant feelings, such as anxiety, grief, or depression, or has a decision to make or a problem to solve, the nurse can be valuable by helping the individual to minimize anxiety, handle grief, clarify feelings, or work out the problem. Interaction for this purpose is called *therapeutic interaction*.

First, the need for therapeutic interaction must be identified. In the nursing assessment, such things as nonverbal cues indicating anxiety, statements of feelings, and signs of grief must be noted and evaluated. The problem confronting the patient must be identified, if it is known. If you are unsure whether therapeutic interaction is appropriate, it is usually most helpful to respond initially in a therapeutic manner. If you later decide that such a stance is inappropriate, it is easy to adopt another mode of interaction, such as interviewing. If, on the other hand, you respond first to facts, as in an interview, you may communicate an unwillingness to consider feelings and thus block the opportunity to respond therapeutically.

Second, you must acknowledge the feelings expressed and/or problems discussed as real and as the property of the other person. With the best intentions and skill in the world, you cannot elicit different feelings or solve a personal problem effectively for someone else. Change must come from within that person. In recognition of the individual's integrity, worth, and ability to solve his or her own problems, the nurse acts as a facilitator, not the solver of a problem.

The next step is to concentrate on the process of interaction itself. Creating a relationship conducive to a therapeutic interaction is one of the initial responsibilities of the nurse. This may be done partly by meeting the patient's physical needs and thus creating a basis for trust. More important is being open and accepting of the person as he or she is, a matter not of offering judgments but of offering yourself. You may simply offer to spend time with the individual, or pause in your tasks to convey nonverbally that you have time to listen. Acknowledging the person's feelings as real and indicating your awareness of these feelings sets the stage for effective interaction.

Facilitating responses

Responses that facilitate communication on the part of another person have been called "therapeutic techniques" (Hays, 1964) and "active listening" (Gordon, 1970). We will here use the term *facilitating responses*, because it is the total interaction that is therapeutic, not a single statement made during that interaction. Facilitative techniques are tools for the skilled nurse and should not become ends in themselves: the nurse who concentrates on saying "the right words" but whose nonverbal behavior does not convey true concern and interest may fail to assist the patient. The purpose of facilitating responses is to encourage and support the individual's own communicating and problem-solving processes.

One of the first goals of therapeutic interaction is to encourage the other person to recognize and then express his or her own feelings and ideas. Bringing them to the patient's attention allows them to be dealt with. Sometimes this step alone decreases anxiety. *Nondirective comments*, those that simply encourage the person to continue talking, often accomplish this goal. Comments such as "yes. . .," "go on," and "mm-hmm" are known as general leads. *Reflecting*, or simply restating as a question what the person has just said, is also nondirective. For example, the patient says, "I just can't stand staying in bed any longer!" and the nurse replies, "You can't stand staying in bed any longer?" This response allows the other person to hear what he or she is saying and think about it. Overuse can, however, make the patient uncomfortable and self-conscious. An alternative nondirective response is *restating*, or repeating what the person has said in different words or terms. This technique helps the person recognize the meaning he or she is conveying. If the patient says, "I need a stronger sleeping pill," the nurse may reply, "Your present sleeping pill is not effective?"

When your goal is to help the person explore a situation more fully, nondirective comments may be supplemented by *exploratory responses*. You might help the person place events in a *time sequence* by asking "Was that before or after. . ?" or "What happened next?" or you might *focus* on a statement that appears to be important, saying something like, "You said your brother is helpful. Could you explain more about that?" *Encouraging comparisons* may help the person weigh and evaluate the significance of something: "Is this like . . . ?" Or you may *seek clarification*—a clearer understanding of something said—with comments such as, "I don't quite understand what you mean. Could you explain more fully?" If you think you understand but want to *validate* your statement, you can ask, "Do you mean. . . ?"

Responses That Facilitate Communication

RESPONSE	EXAMPLE
Nondirective comments	
General leads	"Yes," "Go on," "um-hmmm"
Reflecting	Person: "I'm really scared." Nurse: "You're really scared?"
Restating	Person: "I just can't seem to sit still." Nurse: You're feeling nervous?"
Exploratory responses	
Placing in time sequence	"When did that happen?" "Was this before or after . . . ?"
Encouraging comparisons	"Was this similar to . . . ?" "Are there differences this time?"
Focusing	"You said . . . Could you explain that more fully?" "This seems to be an important point."
Seeking clarification	"What would you say is the main concern?"
Validating	"What I understand from what you said is . . . Is that correct?"
Aids to decision making	
Serving as a resource	"Children under 14 can visit if special arrangements are made."
Pointing out information	"Have you considered . . . ?"
Reviewing	"Now you said the main concerns are . . ."
Considering consequences	"If you do . . . what might happen?"
Encouraging formulation of a plan	"What do you think you might do?"

There are several ways to help another person establish goals and explore solutions or possible courses of action, avoiding the temptation to provide a solution or give advice on the appropriate course of action. You may serve as a *resource person* by providing information that makes possible an informed decision. This must be done without expressing personal judgments. For example, "If you wish to leave before your doctor discharges you, you must sign a legal release relieving the hospital of responsibility for the consequences of your action." *Pointing out information* the person has failed to consider—"Have you thought about . . . ?"—can help in decision making, as can *reviewing* what has been said—"Now these were the main points you seemed to be considering. . ." You might *encourage formulation of a plan* by asking such questions as, "What do you think should be your next action?" or "You have said that . . . is the problem. What do you think might help to solve it?" When a solution is proposed, you may help the person to *think through the consequences* of the action by saying, "If you do . . . how will your wife feel?" If you exercise care, you might be able to *point out the consequences* yourself in a nonjudgmental way: "If you don't do the exercises, the result will be . . ." This is another way of serving as a resource person.

Of course, these techniques make it possible that the individual will decide on a course of action other than the one you or the health care team prefers. In the past, health care personnel have been reluctant to allow this freedom to patients. As you become more open and more aware of individuals rights, you will become more content with functioning in a supportive rather than a directive role. You can have the satisfaction of helping individuals to direct their own lives.

Blocking responses

When considering therapeutic interaction, it is helpful to recognize comments that tend to block communication or damage the problem-solving process. Such remarks will be referred to as *blocking responses*. Some of these responses are commonly used in social conversation and when confronting others' problems. They are not wrong or inappropriate in themselves, except when they prevent the interaction from achieving its purpose.

Giving reassurance is usually considered comforting, but comments such as "Everything will be all right" give the impression that you do not recognize the seriousness or importance of the situation.

Responses That Tend to Block Communication

RESPONSE	EXAMPLE
Giving reassurance	"You'll be just fine."
Approving	"I'm glad to see you're cheerful today."
Disapproving	"Now don't be so glum."
Agreeing	"That's right. You do need to look at the bright side."
Disagreeing	"I don't think you understand." "No, you're wrong about that."
Rejecting	"Don't think about that, it's too depressing."
Denying	Person: "I'm not worth bothering with." Nurse: "Of course you are."
Belittling	Person: "I don't want to live like this." Nurse: "You'll feel differently in the morning."
Interpreting	"Underneath, you really feel . . ."
Making a stereotyped comment	"Chin up." "It's for your own good."
Introducing an unrelated topic	Person: "Am I going to die?" Nurse: "Oh, your wife will be here shortly. We have to get you straightened up."
Challenging	"It isn't possible for that to happen."
Demanding an explanation	"Why do you feel that way?"
Defending	"Now you have a very good doctor. He certainly wouldn't do anything that wasn't in your best interest."

True reassurance is conveyed not by such statements but by pointing out specific indications of improvement or progress.

Giving approval or disapproval can also have a blocking effect. By approving of one emotion or feeling, you are indicating disapproval of the opposite emotion or feeling. Thus, if it is "good" to be cheerful, it is "bad" to be depressed, and your goal is to communicate acceptance of all feelings. Agreeing and disagreeing with feelings and opinions can convey the same undesirable message.

If you reject the person's comments—"I don't want to discuss that!"—or deny the truth of what is said—"Of course, your family cares. You're just upset"—you also communicate that such feelings are not acceptable to you and ought not to be expressed. Your comments do not change the person's feelings, however; you have only prevented the person from dealing with them in an open way.

Nurses sometimes unwittingly *belittle* feelings with comments such as "Everyone feels like that sometimes" or "I was depressed once but I got over it." Such responses may convey the message that the other person's feelings are not serious or important to you.

When helping someone explore a topic, you need to avoid *probing* by asking for specific personal history. Allow the person to decide what he or she wants to share by using general leads or nondirective responses. The person may also feel a sense of violation if you offer *psychological interpretations*, such as "Unconsciously you are saying . . ." or "What you really mean is . . ." You may or may not know what the person really means. Let the person decide what he or she means.

When anxiety is high, the nurse may inadvertently stifle communication by introducing an unrelated topic, such as commenting on the flowers when the patient mentions dying, or by making a stereotyped comment such as "Keep your chin up." This usually occurs because the nurse wants to say something and cannot think of anything else to say. In such a situation, it is better to remain silent than to make inane remarks.

When the other person expresses opinions, they should be accepted, not challenged: a response like "You know that's impossible!" prevents further communication but does not change the person's opinion. When the health care team or the facility is criticized, you may have to stifle a desire to defend those criticized. Both such responses put you in the position of adversary, rather than that of a member of a team trying to deal with a problem.

If you are trying to help an individual explore feelings or problems, be careful not to *demand an explanation*. The individual may not

know the source of a feeling or attitude. In fact, the goal of the interaction may be precisely to discover its source.

It is important to recognize that the use of facilitating responses and the avoidance of blocking responses does not guarantee
a successful interaction. Much depends on the previously established trust, the person's own readiness to proceed, and the nonverbal messages you communicate. Techniques are tools, and the goal is
therapeutic effectiveness.

Health teaching

Teaching is a specialized purpose of communication. Because
of its increasing importance to the health care consumer, health
teaching is assuming a larger place in the activities of the registered
nurse. The teaching process is considered in detail in Chapter 8.

Written communication

Written communications are used constantly in the health care
setting. The nurse is expected to know what ought to be recorded
and to do so in a manner clearly understandable by others on the
health care team. Thus written communication is a central concern
for the practicing nurse.

One of the most obvious characteristics of written communications in the health care field is the use of abbreviations and initials.
As you move from facility to facility, you will discover that, although
some are used in one place and not another, the great majority of
medical abbreviations are standard and used everywhere. You will
want to begin your study of abbreviations with those most commonly used in the facility where you work. Frequently, a list of approved abbreviations is made available by the facility. A list of some
of the most common abbreviations is provided in Appendix A.

You will also notice that many health care records do not contain complete sentences. Information is often given in as brief a form
as is consistent with understanding. Articles (a, an, the) are commonly omitted and simple forms of verbs are used. When you begin
recording, always check what you have written to make sure that it
says what you intended, and that the desire to be brief has not caused
you to sacrifice clarity.

Although nurses use many forms and methods of written
communication, this discussion will focus on the two most fre-

quently used: the written nursing care plan (frequently referred to as "the Kardex") and the patient record or chart.

Nursing care plans

The primary purpose of written nursing care plans is to communicate to the entire nursing care team what is to be done for the patient. Secondarily, written nursing care plans serve as evidence that the nursing process is proceeding and that the patient is receiving appropriate nursing care. Written evidence has become increasingly important because of the increased participation of the federal government (through Medicare and Medicaid) and insurance carriers in evaluating health care. Nurses are also increasingly using written records—both the care plan and the chart—as aids in improving patient care. This process may be undertaken by nursing review committees within an employing institution.

Since the nursing care plan is the nurse's responsibility, it is important that both content and form be critically appraised by the nurse to ascertain whether it is fulfilling its purposes adequately. In evaluating any written nursing care plan, the following questions may be used as guidelines:

1 Are the goals or objective of care, both immediate and long-term, identified?

2 Can the patient's current problems be quickly discerned?

3 Are the prescribed nursing actions paired with the problems they are intended to alleviate, so their effectiveness can be evaluated?

4 Are the prescribed nursing actions stated clearly enough that anyone responsible for care can follow them accurately?

The written nursing care plan may be in a card index (Kardex), on a separate sheet on the chart, or in a variety of other locations. The only requirement is that it be kept where it is available to those who care for the patient. In some settings, nursing care plans are erased and changed, and eventually discarded when the patient is discharged. This procedure makes it easier to change the care plan as the patient's needs change, but greatly hampers ongoing review of the situation and subsequent evaluation.

Patient records

The patient's record—or chart, as it is commonly called—is a tool for communication within the health care team about the patient's illness, therapies, tests, and response to care. As such, it is the legal record of care. The nurse has a responsibility to record on it: (1) assessment data, including subjective and objective information obtained; (2) problems identified; (3) nursing actions carried out; and (4) evaluation of the effectiveness of actions undertaken.

Traditional patient records provide separate forms for each discipline caring for the patient, such as the doctor's progress notes, physical therapy record, and the like. There are also separate forms for specific data, such as the laboratory report sheet and graphic sheets for vital signs. On the traditional form, nurses record on the sheet labeled "Nurse's Notes." These records are usually organized chronologically, or in order of time of occurrence. Traditional nurse's notes provide for an effective record of the entire nursing process.

Many health care settings are reorganizing their record keeping, and encouraging all health team members to use a problem-solving approach to patient care, by instituting the "Problem-Oriented Medical Record" (POMR) defined by Weed (1970). The basic components of the POMR are (1) the data base, (2) the problem list, (3) the initial plan, (4) progress notes, and (5) flow sheets.

The data base is the core of information about the patient, including a record of physical examination, the patient's medical history, the nursing history, the laboratory reports, and reports of tests and diagnostic procedures. The data base is meant to be comprehensive in scope so that changes will be recognizable. Weed has recommended a standardized format for each item in the data base, so that any health care provider may quickly find the information needed and the patient may move with ease through different components of the health care system.

The problem list serves as a combined table of contents and index of the record. Each problem is titled and numbered. Problems are stated in terms of what is currently known. As more data is gathered, items on the problem list may be revised, eliminated, or resolved. The numbering system is constant, so that a number is not reused even if the problem it refers to is resolved. As problems are defined, some may be subdivided. Each institution determines independently which health care personnel may add to or alter the problem list. Usually the physician makes the initial list, after which, other health care providers participate in the areas of their expertise.

Initial plans are made in response to each problem identified. Emphasis is on current management of the problem, but the plan also outlines further studies or information to be gathered, patient education, and follow-up. The latter two items are included at the outset to encourage long-range planning and the inclusion of the patient in both processes.

Progress notes contain four components: (1) identification of the problem being discussed, by number and title; (2) current data, both subjective and objective, about that problem; (3) impressions or judgments on the meaning of the data; and (4) the plan for action. Some progress notes may not contain all four components; this is up to the person making the note.

Flow sheets are limited records for the purpose of monitoring rapidly changing parameters or recording data in a more convenient form. They may be graphs or charts, or take any form that meets the current needs of the patient and the health care team. Flow sheets might also be used to record the progress of an on-going activity, such as patient teaching.

If you use a problem-solving approach to the nursing process, you should find that you are able to adapt to any charting system and record those components of the process that are significant to the patient's care.

Conclusion

Because communication includes all the means that people use to convey meaning to one another, you will be a more effective nurse if you understand the processes involved and are skillful at using various techniques of communication. Continuing effort and practice will be necessary to develop real skill in these processes.

CARE STUDY / A therapeutic interaction

Mrs. Shadle is a seventy-five-year-old patient in an extended care facility for care following the repair of a fractured hip. Mrs. Langley is the registered nurse in charge of the unit. As she enters Mrs. Shadle's room on her nursing rounds, Mrs. Langley notes that Mrs. Shadle is sitting in a wheelchair with her hands in her lap, hair uncombed, shoulders down, and head bowed. Mrs. Shadle emits a long sigh and does not look up as the nurse approaches.

Nurse: "Mrs. Shadle, you look like you're feeling down this morning."

Patient: "Who wouldn't? I'll never leave this awful place."

Nurse: "Never leave this awful place?"

Patient: "That's right—I can't ever go home because I can't walk, can't do a thing." (With this, tears start to flow down her cheeks.)

Nurse: (She sits down beside Mrs. Shadle and takes her hands.) "Mrs. Shadle, do you mean that you believe you won't be able to walk again?"

Patient: "That's right—and I can't be home in this thing." (She points at the wheelchair.)

Nurse: "You are going to Physical Therapy. Can you tell me what you did there yesterday?"

Patient: "I stood up between those bars and tried to walk—but I could only go halfway and I got so tired."

Nurse: "Yesterday you went halfway. Do you remember what you were doing in Physical Therapy last week?"

Patient: "That was when I first started going. It took two of them to hold me up."

Nurse: "So last week it took two people to hold you up and this week you walked halfway down the bars."

Patient: "I guess that is better, isn't it? But it goes so slowly."

Nurse: "It's a slow process but it has been steady. What do you suppose you might be doing next week at this time?"

Patient: "Maybe I'll be able to walk the whole way." (Her face brightens.)

Nurse: "You may even be using a walker so you can walk around the room." (Mrs. Langley has communicated with the Physical Therapy Department and knows that this is the plan.)

Patient: "Really? I might be able to go home if I could use a walker."

Nurse: "Mm-hmm"

Patient: "I guess this isn't such a bad place for a while."

Nurse: (She gives Mrs. Shadle's hand a squeeze and stands up.) "I'll have Miss Johnson, the aide, help you comb your hair and clean up to go to Physical Therapy. I'll be back to check on how you are getting along. If you get to feeling down again, call me. O.K.?"

Patient: "Thank you, Mrs. Langley,"

Study terms

blocking responses
  agreeing-disagreeing
  approving-disapproving
  belittling
  challenging
  defending
  demanding explanations
  denying
  interpreting
  introducing an unrelated topic
  making stereotyped comments
  rejecting
communication
  nonverbal
  verbal
facilitating responses
  clarifying

general leads
nondirective comments
problem solving
reflecting
restating
interviewing
  structured
  unstructured
Kardex
nursing care plan
Problem Oriented Medical
  Record (POMR)
silence
socializing
touch
validating

References

NONVERBAL AND VERBAL COMMUNICATION

Burnside, I. M. 1973. Caring for the Aged: Part 5, Touching Is Talking. *American Journal of Nursing* 73:2060-2063.

Chappelle, M. L. 1972. The Language of Food. *American Journal of Nursing* 72:1294-1295.

Egolf, D. B., and Chester, S. L. 1976. Speechless Messages. *Nursing Digest* 4:2:26-29.

Epstein, C. 1974. Breaking the Barriers to Communication in the Health Care Team. *Nursing '74* 12:63-68.

Fast, Julius. 1970. *Body Language*. New York: Simon and Schuster.

Field, W. E., Jr. 1972. Watch Your Message. *American Journal of Nursing* 72:1278-1280.

Goldsborough, Judith. 1970. On Being Non-Judgmental. *American Journal of Nursing* 70:11:2340.

Gordon, T. 1970. *Parent Effectiveness Training*. New York: Wyden.

Hays, J., et al. 1964. *Interacting with Patients*. New York: Macmillan.

Orlando, I. 1961. *The Dynamic Nurse-Patient Relationship*. New York: G. P. Putnam's Sons.

Radulovic, P. O. 1973. Under the Cover of His Charm. *American Journal of Nursing* 73:1731-1737.

Robinson, L. 1972. The Crying Patient. *Nursing '72* 12:2:16-20.

Travelbee, J. 1966. *Interpersonal Aspects of Nursing*. Philadelphia: F. A. Davis.

Veninga, R. 1973. Communications: A Patient's Eye View. *American Journal of Nursing* 73:320-322.

WRITTEN COMMUNICATION

Ansley, B. 1975. Patient-Oriented Recording. *Nursing '75* 5:9:52-53.

Atwood, J., *et al*. 1974. Symposium on the Problem-Oriented Record. *Nursing Clinics of North America* 9:2 (June 1974).

Henderson, V. 1973. On Nursing Care Plans and Their History. *Nursing Outlook* 21:378-379.

Howard, F., *et. al*. 1973. Problem-Oriented Charting: A Nursing Viewpoint. *Canadian Nurse* 68:34-37 (Aug. 1973).

Kerr, A. H. 1972. Nurses' Notes: Making Them More Meaningful. *Nursing '72* 9:6-11 (Sept. 1972).

Schell, P. L. 1972. POMR—Not Just Another Way to Chart. *Nursing Outlook* 20:510-514.

Skinner, R. 1975. Quick Directory of Medical Abbreviations. *Nursing Update* 6:1-3 (Aug. 1975).

Weed, L. L. 1970. *Medical Records, Medical Education, and Patient Care*. Cleveland: Western Reserve University Press.

Woody, M., *et al*. 1973. The Problem Oriented System for Patient Centered Care. *American Journal of Nursing* 73:1168-1175.

8 Health Teaching

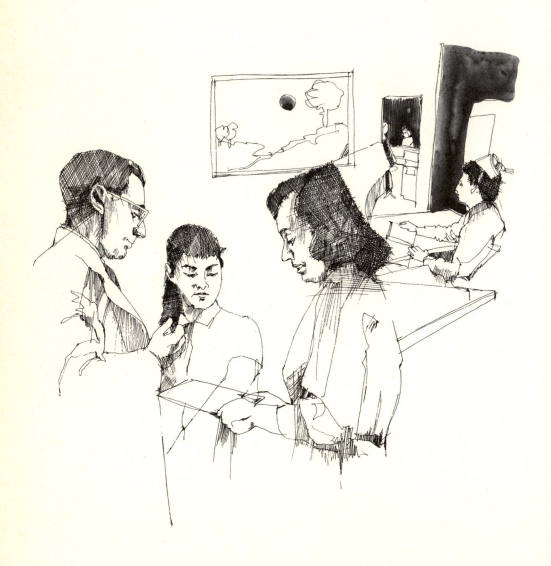

Objectives

After completing this chapter, you should be able to:

1 Identify patient situations in which a need for health teaching exists.

2 Assess the patient's readiness to learn.

3 Plan health teaching to meet the identified learning needs of the patient, taking into consideration appropriate techniques and procedures.

4 Carry out a health teaching plan.

5 Evaluate the effectiveness of the teaching in light of preestablished objectives or goals.

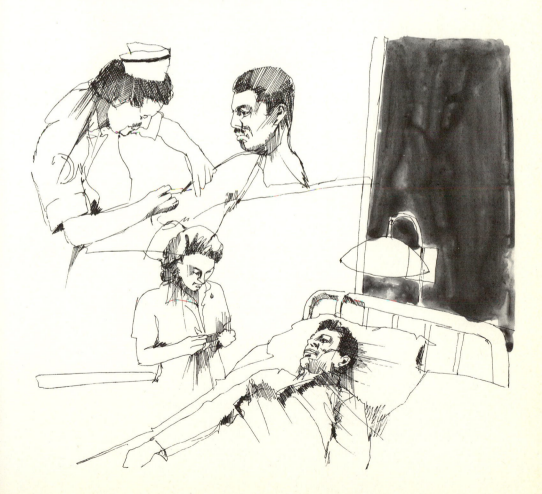

H EALTH TEACHING is an important function of the registered nurse. As more and more people must learn to live with complex regimes and chronic illnesses, while others need knowledge about maintaining their own and their families' optimum health, the responsibilities of the nurse continue to grow. Entire courses are devoted to the teaching/learning process in teacher education programs, and we do not expect this short presentation to provide all the information you need to be an excellent teacher. Instead, it is a base for your future growth.

Because you will usually work with a single individual, rather than a group, teaching will be a simpler task for you than for the public school teacher. Although the processes are identical, it is less confusing to a beginning teacher to work with one learner at a time. Your knowledge of health and illness and the opportunity to establish a close relationship with the patient provide you a unique opportunity to (1) assess the patient and the situation to determine learning needs, (2) assess the patient's readiness to learn, (3) set goals or objectives and devise a teaching plan to meet them, (4) implement the plan, and (5) evaluate the effectiveness of your teaching.

Assessing learning needs

Learning can be defined as any change in behavior that is not due to growth or fatigue. *Behavior*, in this context, means both observable activities (taking medications, eating special foods) and unobservable activities (thinking, planning, and the like). A *learning need* is a need for a change in behavior. In assessing a patient's learning needs, you must consider a wide variety of health-related factors. The following questions will help you do so.

Is the patient required to perform a new task or use a new skill? For example, a person on crutches must walk in an unfamiliar way. Stairs, ramps, and doorways all require new movements and means of balance. Instruction in these skills is needed. Similarly, the mother of a first baby will be expected to bathe, change, and feed the infant when she goes home. Does she know how? Has she ever done it before? Situations such as these abound in a hospital.

Will the patient's pattern of daily living have to change? A woman with a serious heart problem may need to rest during the day and to avoid strenuous activities. What is she allowed to do? What specific exertions should be avoided? The diabetic needs to adopt a stable pattern of meals and activity. Does this mean that each day must be exactly the same? How are necessary variations provided for? Of course, teaching the patient to establish a new life style is not your only responsibility. You must also help the person to deal with the feelings aroused by such a change, as outlined in Chapter 7.

Does the patient need information on which to base judgments? The diabetic may be instructed to carry candy or sugar for use in an emergency. What constitutes an emergency? How much candy is enough? When must a physician be called? Many similar, if less dramatic, judgments need to be prepared for. A mother must decide when a child is ill enough to require a visit to the physician. She must decide when to increase an infant's food intake. The health-related decisions we make throughout our lives need to be based on sound information.

Will the current problem be of continuing concern? Short-term problems call for very different teaching than do long-term problems. Joint disability due to a sprain requires different adaptations and planning than does joint disability due to rheumatoid arthritis, which is a lifetime health problem.

Is the immediate situation unfamiliar to the patient? A person who is to undergo a diagnostic test needs to know what is to be done, how it will feel, what he or she is expected to do, the time involved, and perhaps other things about the test. The person scheduled for surgery needs to know about preparation for surgery, what will happen afterwards, and expectations for his or her behavior. It has been documented that individuals who have had thorough pre-operative teaching have fewer postoperative complications.

Common learning needs involve medications to be taken after discharge, special diets or activities that must be continued at home, symptoms that need to be reported to the physician, and the continued management of a chronic illness.

After you have determined that a learning need exists, it is necessary to find out whether the patient also sees it as a need. In doing so, you will find the techniques of therapeutic interaction helpful. This is a situation in which the patient must do the problem solving. If the patient does not perceive a learning need, your best efforts at teaching may be unsuccessful.

Setting goals and objectives

When a learning need has been agreed on, specific goals and objectives must be established in cooperation with the patient. Nurses commonly err by trying to impart to the patient all the information they possess. The patient may be able to tell or indicate nonverbally to you what information he or she will use and is able to absorb at the current time. The patient who is very worried about giving himself an injection may be uninterested in considering any other aspect of his care until he has mastered that skill. Immediate needs must be addressed first.

It may be necessary initially to outline with the patient a series of objectives, recognizing that you are only beginning the teaching process. The patient who is a full partner in the teaching/learning process may then continue learning at a later time, either independently or with another teacher. For example, the patient who has a complicated medication regime to understand may spend an hour discussing her learning needs and formulating objectives with you. The next day she might initiate further discussion with the nurse who administers her morning medication. The nurse working in the evening might help her plan a means of keeping track of when medications are due. Thus the entire team would be involved.

Such team involvement may be planned in advance, and facilitated by a health teaching flow sheet on the patient's record. The objectives are listed on the flow sheet, and each nurse involved in teaching records what has been accomplished. The more specifically the goals and objectives are stated, the easier it will be for the patient to plan and participate in learning and to measure and evaluate progress. A goal as general as "to learn about the prescribed medications," while accurate, does not provide much direction to someone who does not know what is important to know about medications. More specific objectives might be (1) to know the name and dosage schedule for each medication, (2) to know the purpose of each medication, and (3) to know what untoward signs and symptoms should be reported to the physician. This kind of objective enables the patient to ask appropriate questions and to evaluate his or her learning: the patient can review the medications and determine whether or not more learning is needed. The patient who is discharged from the hospital before completing the objectives will be able to continue learning with a nurse in the physician's office, a public health nurse, or someone else involved in his or her health care.

Planning patient teaching

Planning for teaching requires an understanding of some basic information about learning. Although there are several theories of learning, most educators consider the following factors important in the learning process.

Internal influences on patient learning

Internal characteristics of the learner are the first considerations in planning patient teaching. These internal factors are the learner's (1) previous education and life experience, (2) physiologic status, (3) vocabulary level, (4) anxiety level, and (5) motivation.

Previous education and *life experience* make a great deal of difference in the patient's approach to learning. An individual who has enjoyed school and other types of learning may enjoy this new challenge. But a person for whom learning has been difficult and surrounded by failure will be hesitant to embark on new learning. A patient whose college work included extensive study of the biological sciences will respond very differently to learning how illness is affecting the body's functioning than will a person who has avoided anything scientific and knows little about normal functioning of the human body. A person with three small children has a very different background for learning to care for a handicapped baby than does a person who has never cared for an infant. Sometimes the desired learning will occur only if you provide the necessary background, such as teaching normal nutrition in order to teach about a special diet.

A person's *physiologic status*—fatigue, hunger, lack of oxygen, altered blood components, or drugs—can strongly affect learning. This is a factor of special concern to nurses, since patients frequently have physiologic problems, and many adaptations must be made in teaching to accommodate them. In order not to tire the patient, learning may need to be undertaken in small segments. You may need to explain to the patient that slow learning is a result of illness and fatigue, and not an indication of lack of ability or effort. A slow pace may arouse frustration in both the patient and the nurse, and teaching may have to be postponed until the patient's condition improves. A patient whose mind is absorbed with the effort of breathing is not likely to be interested in learning about a new diet. By planning for rest, providing medication for pain relief, and promoting comfort, you may be able to minimize the effects of physiologic factors. Immediate needs must be met before secondary needs.

The extent and level of the learner's *vocabulary* may affect his or her ability to understand written material or oral explanations. The individual may interpret some words differently than you do. As a beginning nursing student encountering a new vocabulary, you may have a heightened sensitivity to the patient's unfamiliarity with medical language. But all too quickly your own vocabulary will be filled with such terms as *void*, *feces*, *emesis*. Sometimes the desired learning will occur only if you first explain terms to be used.

A mild level of *anxiety* may facilitate learning by causing the learner to focus more completely on the task. Higher levels of anxiety interfere with learning by diffusing attention or focusing it on only part of the situation. An individual who is very anxious may leap from one thought to another, unable to concentrate on a single idea. Also, high anxiety tends to orient the individual to the present rather than the future. However, the sharpened acuity of mild anxiety focuses attention and speeds learning. A therapeutic interaction may help to lower the patient's anxiety. Sometimes anxiety-relieving medications are given to make learning more effective. If, on the other hand, the patient demonstrates total lack of anxiety and concern, pointing out potential problems that could be solved by the proposed learning may arouse enough anxiety to facilitate learning.

Motivation may be thought of as an internal tendency or desire to learn. Motivation is greatest when the individual feels a need and recognizes that the learning would meet it. The individual in a strange country needs to learn its language in order to relate to others. Because the need to learn is great, effort and attention will be correspondingly great. But needs for new knowledge are often much less readily obvious. A male patient who is to eat a special diet at home and who expects his wife to plan and cook all meals may not perceive a need to know about the diet. In such a case, the effort and attention given to learning would be minimal. Trying to motivate an individual to learn is a challenging task. Pointing out a person's needs does not mean that they will be perceived as needs. The most effective strategy is usually to help the person think through the situation and arrive at an independent decision that a need exists.

The teacher, as facilitator of the learning process, is responsible for assessing the variables described above and determining the patient's degree of "readiness to learn." "Readiness to learn" is the state brought about by the combined effect of the internal factors, which makes an individual able or unable to learn. It may be necessary to postpone teaching if readiness is at a very low level. In other instances, the teacher can alter or affect these internal factors sufficiently to enable the person to learn.

External influences on patient learning

In addition, the teacher can facilitate learning by changing or adapting factors *external* to the learner, such as (1) physical environment, (2) other persons in the environment, (3) time of teaching, (4) the teacher's vocabulary, and (5) strategies involved in teaching.

The *physical environment* may need to be manipulated to insure that temperature, light, noise, heat, and the like are at levels that promote optimum functioning. It may be necessary to find another setting for teaching or to consult with those responsible for the physical plant. Simply opening windows or doors to provide ventilation may help. If the learner will need to read or to examine a fine scale, such as on a syringe, the lighting should be evaluated.

The nature of the task or material to be taught should be considered in light of the patient's probable feelings about another person overhearing the information or seeing the task practiced. It may be necessary to wait until the patient's roommate is absent or visitors have left in order to provide privacy. In other cases, however, it may be helpful if a family member is present during the teaching. Sometimes closing the curtains or shutting the door insures adequate privacy. A task such as a colostomy irrigation may be taught in a bathroom whose door can be locked to protect privacy.

Too frequently, the *timing* of teaching is determined by the convenience of the nurse, rather than by its appropriateness for learning. The arthritic who is very stiff and sore when first arising may need to learn manual skills later in the day. The elderly diabetic who always arises very early, while other patients are still asleep, may learn best then, when he or she is freshest and most alert. Such matters as the schedule for diagnostic tests should be taken into account. Of course, if your teaching concerns the test itself, it should be scheduled prior to the test. If it concerns another matter, the patient's preoccupations with the test may make the period before the test inappropriate for teaching other material. Teaching scheduled too far in advance of the person's need for the information imparted may be seen as unimportant or may produce anxiety. If the teaching is scheduled immediately before the knowledge is needed, there may not be sufficient time for learning.

The teacher should alter the *vocabulary level* used in explanations to suit the understanding of the learner. Many otherwise well-educated people do not understand such medical terms as "void," meaning *urinate*. Rather than asking whether the patient understands the words you are using, you might ask him or her to restate what you have said. This approach reveals whether you are conveying your message satisfactorily and provides you with a sample of the patient's vocabulary. You might also consider the patient's education and socioeconomic background, as well as cultural factors, when determining what vocabulary to use. It is the teacher's responsibility to use words that can be understood by the learner.

An example of the problems vocabulary can cause is the following situation, in which a student nurse once found herself. A very elderly man hospitalized for diagnostic tests was very friendly and anxious to please, but his English was broken and difficult to understand. A stool specimen was ordered by the physician. For an entire week, the nurses carefully explained this to the patient, who smiled, nodded, and later walked to the bathroom where he had a bowel movement and flushed it down the toilet. Everyone was becoming upset. The student reviewed her information on the patient, and found that he had worked at manual labor all his life and had had very little education. Deciding that he probably did not understand what was wanted, she tried a variety of terms—to no avail. Finally, in desperation, she said, "Shit in the pan," and pointed at the bedpan. The patient's face lit up. He said, "Sure!" and the problem was solved. This was not the student's customary vocabulary—but it *was* the patient's.

The following teaching strategies have been shown to affect learning. You can consider them as you plan your teaching and use them to guide you in selecting methods and materials.

Reinforcement, a reward given to the learner for making the desired response, is considered by many theorists to be the primary basis for learning. Anything the learner perceives as rewarding can be a reinforcement. Praise is the most common reinforcement, since most

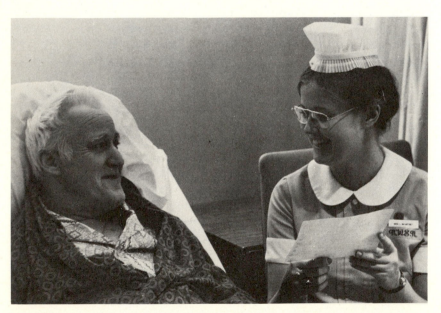

Lynn McLaren, courtesy of Newton-Wellesley Hospital

people have learned to value it. For some individuals, more tangible rewards—such as reading a story to a child or allowing a teenager extra time to talk on the telephone—may be more appropriate. The most effective reinforcement follows immediately after the desired response, without delay. Punishment for inappropriate responses has less effect on behavior than does reward for appropriate responses. In fact, many theorists believe that ignoring inappropriate responses is a more effective way of eliminating them than is punishment.

Frequent opportunities to *practice* new skills will increase the rate of learning. Practice spaced out over time is more effective than a single long session, in which fatigue can undermine performance. Practice immediately after instruction is more helpful than delayed practice because less is forgotten. *Feedback*—comparison of the individual's performance during practice to the desired objective—will make learning easier and more rapid.

Active participation appears to facilitate learning by allowing the learner to exercise several modes of input: touch, motor action, hearing, sight, and so on. This can be accomplished by having the learner practice each segment of the skill as it is explained. Writing down important points is another means of active participation on the part of a learner who will benefit from doing so.

Audiovisual aids are an alternative mode of communication that can enhance direct verbal interaction. They are most helpful if they relate to the learner's previous knowledge or experience. Many audiovisual aids for health teaching, including slide/tape presentations, films, and posters, are produced commercially and by voluntary associations. Anatomical models may help the person to understand better the parts of the body being discussed. Some hospitals provide many such aids and also stock a number of pamphlets and books appropriate for health teaching. It is a nursing responsibility to determine what audiovisual aids are needed and to communicate these needs to the administration of the health care facility. This may be done individually or by serving on special patient care committees.

The *sequence* in which material is presented can have a direct effect on the rate and extent of learning. Proceeding from familiar to unfamiliar material helps the learner put new information in perspective. In order to make this possible, you must first find out what the learner already knows. Never make assumptions about a person's level of knowledge. Whether the patient is a doctor or a laborer, an individualized assessment is needed. A dermatologist may be totally unfamiliar with the routine preparations for kidney x-rays in a particular hospital, while a laborer may formerly have worked as an orderly in the same hospital and helped prepare others for the same x-ray. Validate your impressions of the patient's knowledge before proceeding. In general, progressing from simple to complex ideas, from normal to abnormal, and from well to ill helps the learner absorb new information in an orderly way.

Writing the plan

When learning needs are long-term, a written plan for teaching is needed. The more specific the plan, the more easily it will be carried out by various members of the team. The plan should specify the material to be taught, the objectives or goals to be reached, the methods to be used, and the time span in which it is to be accomplished. The more detailed your treatment of external factors that are subject to manipulation, the greater will be the continuity of the teaching/learning process.

When the learning need is short-term and may easily be provided for by a single individual, a written plan may not be necessary. This does not mean that *no* plan is necessary; it means that, because the plan is less complex, you can carry it in your mind.

Evaluating the results

It may be necessary to devise tests or trials in order to evaluate learning adequately. Such tests may be return demonstrations, recitations, or the successful assumption of certain responsibilities. To be most helpful, progress in learning should be evaluated during the teaching process. Remember that, in doing so, you are evaluating the actual learning that has occurred, not the success or failure of the teaching plan.

An opportunity for feedback should be provided at each step. Otherwise, the person may learn misinformation or practice incorrectly. Success should be praised freely, since praise tends to motivate the learner to achieve further. Praise should also focus on specific accomplishments and learning. Thus, you might say to a child learning to give an injection, "You did a good job of measuring the medicine. You showed real skill!" *Not* "Good girl!" Enlarge your vocabulary to include a variety of terms for praise.

Be cautious with regard to failure. After pointing out errors, encourage renewed efforts in a nonthreatening way; failure can lead to depression and withdrawal. Criticism may be interpreted as personal rejection if it is not phrased with care.

The learner should be encouraged to evaluate his or her own learning, which necessitates knowing what the objectives are. The learner may need your assistance in comparing his or her performance with the desired objectives.

If learning fails to occur or if the rate of learning is too slow, you need to reassess the internal and external factors affecting the teaching/learning situation and to replan your teaching.

Conclusion

As you progress in nursing, you will have increasing opportunities for involvement in health teaching. It is a mistake to undertake very large projects independently until you have had a chance to teach on a limited scale or with someone else. As individuals in your care become increasingly self-directed as a result of skills and information you have taught them, you will begin to understand why some writers consider health teaching the most important function of the nursing practitioner.

CARE STUDY / Teaching about an upper g.i. x-ray

Mr. Stokes has been admitted to the medical unit for diagnostic tests. His admitting problem is "recurrent epigastric pain"; his orders included "upper G.I. series in a.m.—routine preparation."

Mr. Kyle, a registered nurse, is assigned to care for Mr. Stokes. As part of the admitting process, Mr. Kyle takes a nursing history. He notes that this is Mr. Stokes' first hospitalization, that he is quite upset, and that Mr. Stokes has had a high school education and is currently employed as a salesman. The nurse sits down to discuss with Mr. Stokes his concerns about the next day's tests and his understanding of what is to happen. Mr. Kyle then formulates a plan and discusses it with the patient.

Nurse: "Mr. Stokes, it seems that you would like to know a little more about what is going to be happening."

Mr. S.: "Sure would!"

Nurse: "Right now I must pass four o'clock medications, I'll come back at five and we'll discuss the preparation you will have this evening, what will be done here before you go to x-ray, and exactly what will happen in x-ray. While I'm gone, you can think of any specific questions you'd like to ask. I'll leave a pencil and paper so you can jot things down if you'd like."

When Mr. Kyle returns, he gives Mr. Stokes a printed form outlining the preparation for an upper G.I. x-ray and goes over it point by point with him.

Later that evening, Mr. Kyle again approaches Mr. Stokes to ask him to review what they discussed earlier. At this time, Mr. Kyle clarifies a few points that were not clear to Mr. Stokes.

Mr. Kyle then records his assessment of the learning need, the teaching undertaken, and the patient's learning.

Study terms

active participation
audiovisual aids
environment
external factors
feedback
internal factors
learning
learning needs
motivation
objectives

practice
readiness to learn
reinforcement
sequence
   known to unknown
   normal to abnormal
   simple to complex
teaching/learning process
vocabulary level

References

Aiken, L. H. 1970. Patients' Problems are Problems in Learning. *American Journal of Nursing* 70:1916.

Ballantyne, D. J. 1974. Closed Circuit T.V. for Patients. *American Journal of Nursing* 74:263-264.

Brylski, E., and Gillin, J. 1972. Audio-visuals Made to Order. *Nursing Outlook* 20:6:385-387.

Collins, R. D. 1968. Problem-Solving: A Tool for Patients, Too. *American Journal of Nursing* 68:7:1483-1485.

Conant, R. K., Jr., *et al.* 1973. Health Education: A Bridge to the Community. *Nursing Digest* 1:7:4-11.

Haferkorn, V. 1971. Assessing Individual Learning Needs as a Basis for Patient Teaching. *Nursing Clinics of North America* 6:1:199-209.

Murray, R., and Zentner, J. 1976. Guidelines for More Effective Health Teaching. *Nursing '76* 6:2:44-53.

Palm, M. L. 1971. Recognizing Opportunities for Informal Patient Teaching. *Nursing Clinics of North America* 6:4:669-678.

Piepgras, R. 1969. All Nurses are Teachers. *Nursing Outlook* 17:49-51 (Oct. 1969).

Redman, B. K. 1971. Patient Education as a Function of Nursing Practice. *Nursing Clinics of North America* 6:4:573-580.

———. 1968. *The Process of Patient Teaching in Practice*. St. Louis: C. V. Mosby.

Sharp, A. E. 1974. Four Steps to Better Patient Teaching. *RN* 37:5:62-63.

Smith, D. 1971. Writing Objectives as a Nursing Practice Skill. *American Journal of Nursing* 71:2:319-320.

Wood, M. M. 1974. 300 Valuable Booklets to Give to Patients and Their Families: A Source Guide. *Nursing '74* 4:4:43-50.

9 Spiritual Needs of the Patient

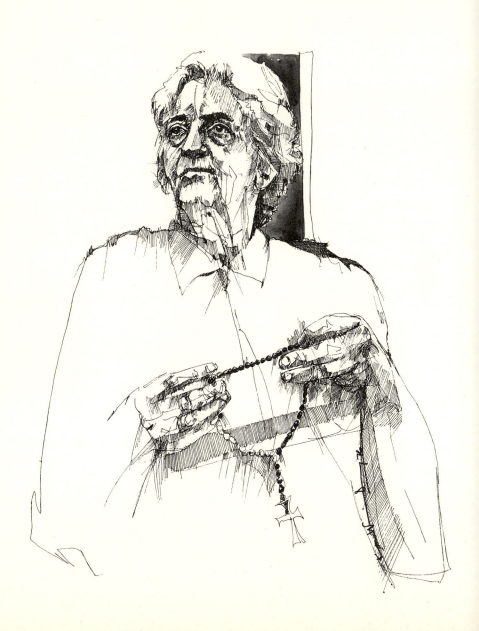

Objectives

After completing this chapter, you should be able to:

    1 Outline the major characteristics of the following religious groups as they directly affect health care: Roman Catholicism, Protestantism, Eastern Orthodoxy, Judaism, Islam, and Buddhism.

    2 Discuss the role of the clergy on the health care team.

    3 Assess the individual patient's spiritual needs.

    4 Initiate action, including appropriate referrals, to meet the spiritual needs of a patient.

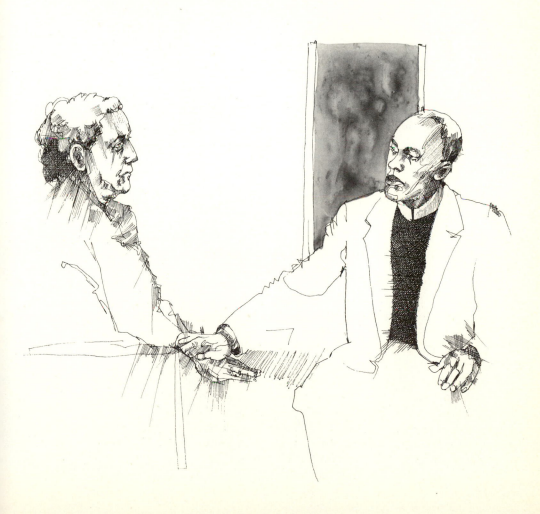

THOSE IN SCIENTIFIC DISCIPLINES often overlook the spiritual or religious sphere of life. In the broadest sense, the spiritual aspect of life is our wish to know its ultimate meaning and purpose. Organized religion may provide such direction and meaning, as may a variety of philosophical and ethical systems. Most of the following discussion will center on the major religious groups in the United States, with which most Americans maintain at least nominal affiliation, but we will briefly discuss other belief systems.

Religions and beliefs that affect health care

Although individual members of the same faith differ in adherence to its tenets, it is helpful for the nurse to have a general familiarity with specific religious beliefs as they relate to health care. An understanding of theology is not expected of the nurse.

Roman catholicism

The Roman Catholic Church is a single uniform religious body characterized by fairly formalized ways of dealing with health care problems. The specificity and uniformity of its guidelines facilitates action on the part of health care workers.

Three of the sacraments are of special significance to the ill Catholic. The first is Baptism. Baptism is considered essential and is usually performed on the young infant. If an unbaptized person wishes to be baptized, a priest will be willing to come and perform the rite. If the patient is in danger of dying, the priest will come immediately, for it is the Church's wish that no one die without Baptism. If Baptism is truly desired and it appears that the person will die before a priest arrives, *any* person may perform this rite. Baptism has three essential components: (1) the sincere intent to baptize on the part of the person performing the rite; (2) sprinkling or pouring of water over the head (any clear water can be used); and (3) recital of the words "I baptize you in the name of the Father, the Son, and the Holy Spirit" while the water is being sprinkled. The Baptism is then recorded on the chart, and a priest is notified immediately. If a Roman Catholic staff member is present, it is appropriate but not necessary for that person to perform the rite. Crises requiring such action probably occur most commonly in obstetrics, when a newborn child dies or a fetus is aborted. If the family is Catholic, the product of conception is baptized when there is any possibility that life is present. If it is known that the family is Catholic, Baptism might be performed even if the parent cannot be consulted first (if, for example, the mother is under anesthesia and the father is not present). The fetus is buried by the family, and special arrangements must thus be made.

The second sacrament important to the Roman Catholic patient is Holy Communion, which must be administered by a priest. When Communion is planned, the patient should be made presentable, the unit straightened, and a clean cleared table provided for the patient's use. The table may be covered with a linen hand towel if one is available. The patient may eat before Communion. Privacy is necessary during the priest's visit because the patient may wish to make a confession in conjunction with Communion. Communion may not be administered to the patient who is not allowed food, because the communicant eats a bread wafer. An exception to the prohibition on food may be made by the physician for the eating of a Communion wafer.

The third important sacrament is the Anointing of the Sick, which is performed by a priest to bring comfort and a sense of God's presence to the patient. It is always administered to a Catholic who is gravely ill. If a dying patient is known to be Catholic, a priest is always called even if the patient is unable to authorize such a call. The Anointing of the Sick may be administered to an individual more than once, but is usually administered only once in a particular epi-

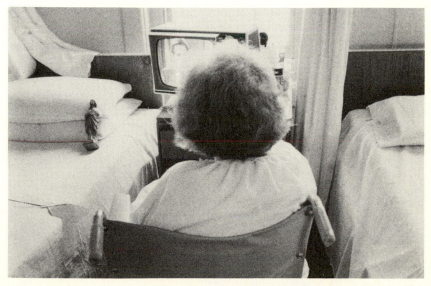

John Goodman

sode of illness. In the past this sacrament was called "Extreme Unction" or "Last Rites" and was commonly given only to those about to
die. For this reason, many patients still become very frightened
when this sacrament is suggested, viewing it as evidence of impending death. The nurse should be prepared for such a response, especially from the older patient. A note should be made in the patient's
record after this rite has been administered.

The Roman Catholic patient may use a rosary, which is a specially constructed chain of beads used as a guide to prayer, and may
have various religious medals. These items may be very important to
the patient, and special care is needed to guard against their loss in
the hospital.

Protestantism

Protestant religious groups account for the largest number of individuals in the United States. It is difficult to make specific statements about Protestant religious beliefs because there are many
denominations, each with its own beliefs and practices. Even
within a single denomination, individual beliefs and practices differ; therefore, it is especially important to consult the individual
about his or her wishes.

Most Protestant groups have no dietary restrictions. One exception is the Seventh-Day Adventists, who strongly advocate an
ovolacto-vegetarian diet (see Chapter 14). The Latter-day Saints
Church, commonly called Mormon, does not approve of drinking
coffee, tea, chocolate, or cola beverages, because they all contain
stimulants. Many Protestant groups disapprove of drinking alcoholic
beverages.

Baptism is a sacrament in most Christian churches. Some
Protestant groups believe in infant baptism, and might wish to have
a gravely ill infant or child baptized. Others, notably the Baptist
churches, believe baptism should be deferred until the child reaches
an age of responsible decision making, usually about twelve or thir-
teen years old. Thus infant baptism is not undertaken without explicit directions from the family. Communion, a sacrament in the
majority of Protestant denominations, is conducted at a church with
the congregation present. Although rarely performed for an individual patient in the hospital, communion may usually be provided if
the person desires it. Most Protestant groups do not routinely anoint
the sick, but some may do so in special instances. Many Protestants
take great comfort in reading the Bible. Visiting of the sick by members of the church is a common practice.

Religious beliefs concerning health care may affect nursing

care. Christian Scientists believe that physicians and medicine are not necessary to healthful living or to the cure of illness; they believe that prayer, faith, and proper living will solve health problems. A Christian Scientist who does seek medical care may feel guilt for inadequate faith or for failure to adhere to his or her beliefs. This guilt may, in turn, seriously affect the individual's response to care. Jehovah's Witnesses do not believe in blood tranfusions. This belief is based on interpretation of the Bible and is not to be reasoned away. A Jehovah's Witness may prefer death to a transfusion. Beliefs of this type are very difficult for health care providers to accept and invariably create a great deal of tension. Allowing others to control their own lives according to their own belief systems is not always easy.

Eastern orthodoxy

There are several Eastern Orthodox churches, each with a specific national background, such Russian Orthodox and Greek Orthodox. Because these churches are governed and function independently, the Eastern Orthodox patient will prefer a priest from his or her own church if a spiritual counselor is needed. If a community has no religious body of the individual's national background, the patient can be asked whether another Orthodox church should be called. These churches do constitute a single faith, and in an emergency any Orthodox priest will serve the needs of an Orthodox patient.

The priest may perform confession and communion (or Holy Eucharist, as it is frequently called in the Orthodox Church) at the patient's bedside. There is also an ordinance for anointing of the sick, which is called Holy Unction. Preparation for these observances is the same as for the Roman Catholic sacraments.

Judaism

There are several Jewish groups, which differ in the strictness of their adherence to the laws of Judaism. The Orthodox Jew is the most strict, and will usually wish to observe the *kosher* laws concerning food (see Chapter 14). Reformed and Conservative Jews are less strict. The only Jewish ritual that might be performed in the hospital is circumcision of the male infant. Because a number of Jewish men, in addition to the rabbi, are present during the circumcision, special arrangements must be made. In areas where ritual circumcision is commonplace, a routine has usually been established. If not, planning in consultation with the rabbi is appropriate. Such a plan must also be approved by the physician in charge of the infant's care.

The death of an Orthodox Jew presents a unique concern: bur-

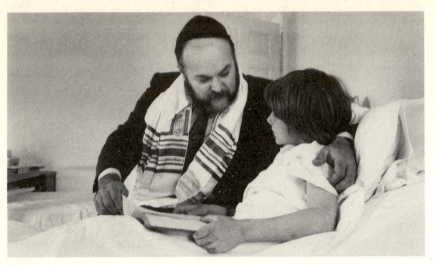

Chris Maynard

ial should take place before the Sabbath, which begins at sundown
on Friday. If the death occurs early in the week, this is not difficult,
but a death on Friday requires prompt action. Orthodox Jews usually
do not permit autopsies to be performed.

Islam

Islam—or the Muslim faith, as it is sometimes called—is rare in Europe and North America, but is the major religion in the Near East
and North Africa. Islam emphasizes very precise individual rituals
and prayers, and the Islamic patient will wish to carry out these individual devotions in private. The only Islamic dietary restrictions
are disapproval of alcoholic beverages and of pork. There is a fas-
ting period in the Muslim calendar, but the ill are exempt from this
requirement.

The nation of islam

The Black Muslim movement in the United States combines strong
social attitudes and race consciousness with religious beliefs that are
similar in some ways to those of Islam. It is, however, a separate religion. Self-determination and maximizing one's own potential are
important components of the Black Muslim belief system and are
highly compatible with health care workers' efforts to assist patients
toward rehabilitation and independence. The emphasis on racial

separation and black independence encourages the Black Muslim to look for health care that is provided and controlled by the black community. White health care workers need to be aware that these beliefs may limit their personal usefulness to the Black Muslim patient.

Buddhism

There are growing numbers of Buddhists in the United States. Many are of Asian background; others are young people who have converted to Buddhism in recent years. Like Christianity, Buddhism has many variations. Many Buddhists are vegetarian. Most believe that one's current actions will affect later life and rebirth, and thus generally attempt to be peaceful and cooperative in their daily living. This system of belief encourages calm acceptance of whatever life has to offer, and as a consequence the patient may not express needs or ask for care. The nurse must be especially alert to nonverbal indications of needs and problems.

Philosophical systems

Some philosophical systems view life as completely predetermined: "That's fate" and "What will be will be" are expressions that reflect this viewpoint. Adherents of such systems may not be willing to change their diets or life styles to improve health, in the belief that the future cannot be altered. Although concentrating on the present may enable you to assist such a person, you may not be able to change this attitude. A right to respect for one's philosophical beliefs is one of the rights of the patient.

An agnostic is a person who believes that human beings cannot know whether or not God exists. An atheist does not believe in the existence of God. A person who holds either of these beliefs bases ethical decisions on his or her philosophy of life. Such an individual will usually not wish to consult a member of the clergy, but may wish to discuss concerns with an interested, caring friend.

Assessing the patient's spiritual needs

Nurses are often reluctant to ask about patients' religious needs or concerns, believing their questions may be interpreted as prying or may lead patients to erroneous assumptions about the seriousness of their illness. If you believe that support of the whole person is a nursing function, concern for spiritual needs will be a part of your nursing plan.

When a nursing history is taken on admission to the hospital, you might ask if the patient wishes a religious adviser, pastor, or church notified of his or her illness. The response will provide some information about the patient's spiritual concerns.

Observation of the patient's behavior provides additional information. Does the patient read the Bible or a prayer book? Does the patient wear religious medals or insignia or use religious objects, such as a rosary?

In conversation, does the patient discuss God or God's will? Does the patient ask questions about the meaning and purpose of his or her existence? These are religious questions in the broadest sense. Expressions of guilt or a troubled conscience are often dealt with best by recognizing them as religious problems.

The hospital admission form frequently provides a space in which to indicate religion. If the religious affiliation noted there would in some way affect health care, it should be taken into consideration when planning care. The family can usually give you specific information about the patient's religious practices when he or she is unable to communicate.

Meeting the patient's spiritual needs

The role of the clergy

Many large hospitals have a chaplain, who serves as a member of the health care team to identify and, if possible, meet the spiritual and religious needs of the patient. The modern chaplain has usually had a special education in dealing with the spiritual needs of those who are ill. Familiar with a wide variety of religious beliefs, the chaplain is prepared to contact clergy in the community when patients have specific needs. Furthermore, the chaplain's understanding of health care makes him or her a valuable partner on the health care team. Some very large hospitals may even have more than one chaplain, representing various religions.

Chaplains' methods of operation may vary, depending on the philosophy of the hospital. Often, the chaplain visits each newly admitted patient. Although an ordained member of the clergy in a particular faith, the chaplain does not restrict his or her attention to members of the same faith. During the initial visit, the chaplain greets the patient and explains the role of the chaplain. A patient who has religious needs will often indicate them to the chaplain at this time. The chaplain is also available for referrals from the nurse or consultations with the staff about patient problems related to religious needs. The chaplain may spend time with the patient simply visiting, reading scripture, or ministering in a variety of ways. A skilled chaplain assesses the patient's needs and relates in the way that is most helpful to the patient. In some settings the chaplain also helps the staff cope with the stresses of caring for patients who are critically ill.

When there is no hospital chaplain, the clergy in the community usually undertake to meet this need. Since they are not usually in the hospital and are often unfamiliar with its routine, they may need special assistance from the nurse in planning what they will do. If the patient wishes to see a member of the clergy, the patient, the family, or the nurse (with the patient's permission) may call one. If the patient is affiliated with a specific church, synagogue, or group, it is best for its clergy to be called. If the patient is far from his or her own congregation or does not belong to one, you may ask a few questions to ascertain the patient's general beliefs and then suggest several churches with similar beliefs whose clergy have expressed willingness to serve the needs of the sick.

Not all those with strong religious affiliations wish a member of the clergy to visit. For example, the Jewish clergy or rabbis, are basically teachers to the congregation and have few special religious powers exceeding those of other Jews. Thus, a Jewish patient may wish to see his or her own rabbi but be uninterested in seeing any other rabbi.

Some religious groups do not have ordained clergy, the Latter-day Saints and Christian Scientists among them. Within such religious groups there are usually persons whose role it is to minister to the sick, and their religious function should be recognized by the health care worker. In Christian Science, this role is undertaken by the "reader."

Occasionally, a clergy member from the community may lack skill in dealing with the sick. A visit may upset rather than support the patient. In such a case, the nurse must explain this tactfully to the clergy member and suggest that he limit or abandon his or her visits.

Well-intentioned but misguided members of some religious groups sometimes wish to visit many patients without regard for the individual patient's wishes. The patient who would deny strangers entry into the home often feels unable to control access to his or her hospital bedside. Thus it is the nurse's responsibility to protect the patient's privacy.

Quiet rooms

The majority of hospitals have a chapel or quiet meditation room for use by patients, families, and staff. This room is usually nondenominational so that a wide variety of people will feel comfortable using it. Of course, this may not be the case if the hospital is sponsored by or affiliated with a specific religious group. Such a room can be of value to those who need a few moments of quiet thought, as well as to those who wish to worship in more conventional modes. It may be the only place where privacy and refuge from the hectic pace of the hospital are available to the family that has just lost a loved one. Wise use of this peaceful environment will be supportive to many people. Staff members, too, may need a few moments' refuge to gather strength to meet a difficult situation.

Worship services

Some large hospitals and nursing homes allow for worship services to be held in the facility. These services may be nondenominational, or separate services may be held for different religious groups. If such services are held, the nurse should offer information about them to the patient and the family. It is also the nurse's responsibility to plan the patient's care so that attendance is possible. A desire to attend religious services should be treated as a special need when determining priorities for care.

Potential difficulties

Sometimes a patient requests that a nurse read scripture to him or her. Most people would not consider this participating in a religious observance, but the individual nurse must decide how to respond in light of the specific situation. Often a volunteer will read scripture, or the patient's congregation will locate a member willing to do so.

If the patient has religious symbols or medals, their loss can, as we have said, seriously upset the patient. Every effort should be made to note these items and to insure that they are not inadvertently lost. On occasion, a patient will request permission to take a religious object to the operating room. Although not common practice, arrangements to do so can usually be made with the surgeon, operating room staff, and recovery room staff. This alone may make a significant difference in the patient's ability to tolerate severe stress.

Patients may ask you as a nurse to pray for or with them. If your religious beliefs coincide, you might join the patient in prayer.

If your religious or philosophical beliefs differ greatly, you might simply offer to stay while the patient prays. If you find this difficult, you can seek another staff member who would be more comfortable in this role. If the patient asks you to pray on his or her behalf and you do not feel that it is appropriate for you to do so, you might say that you will continue to keep the patient in your thoughts and offer to contact a clergy member or other person who could meet this need.

If a person feels guilt, with regard either to illness or to some other aspect of life, a clergy member is often best able to assist in its resolution. Some religions have prescribed means of absolving guilt; in others the process is less formalized. Nevertheless, all major religions address issues of guilt and conscience and attempt to assist the individual in confronting them. The serious anxiety that guilt can arouse may be a barrier to healing. Thus resolution of guilt, which is a religious problem, contributes to recovery from physical illness.

Occasionally patients behave in ways related to their religious beliefs that create problems for the nurse. If a patient attempts to convert the nurse to his or her own religious beliefs, the nurse faces the difficult task of simultaneously maintaining a helpful nurse-patient relationship and personal religious or philosophical integrity. Acknowledging the importance of the patient's beliefs and redirecting the conversation to focus on the patient's needs is an effective way to deal with this problem.

When a member of the clergy or other person in a religious vocation, such as a nun, becomes a patient, health care workers may have unrealistic expectations of their behavior. Such an individual is sometimes expected to continue to act in a supportive way toward others, and to be exemplary in behavior and free from anxiety. This expectation is far from realistic. Clergy are people, with varying degrees of ability to tolerate and deal with the stresses of illness. Natural feelings of anxiety will be present, and the support and aid of others will be needed. Reducing staff expectations of exceptional behavior and carefully assessing the individual will insure realistic care.

Conclusion

The spiritual dimensions of patient care may easily be overlooked. Patients often feel that their spiritual lives and beliefs must be kept separate from their health care. This feeling most often originates with health care workers who feel that spiritual matters are not their concern. Recognizing and meeting spiritual needs, or making referrals to those who can meet them, is an aspect of caring for the whole patient, and may significantly enhance the patient's ability to deal successfully with the major stress of illness.

Study terms

agnostic

Anointing of the Sick

atheist

Baptism

Buddhism

chaplain

clergy

Eastern Orthodoxy

Holy Communion

Islam

Judaism

kosher

Muslim

Protestantism

quiet room

rabbi

reader

religious medals

Roman Catholic

rosary

sacrament

scripture

References

Berkowitz, P., and Berkowitz, N. 1967. The Jewish Patient in the Hospital. *American Journal of Nursing* 67:2335.

Damsteegt, D. 1975. Pastoral Roles in Pre-Surgical Visits. *American Journal of Nursing* 75:1336-1337.

Delespesse, M. *Church and the Community*. Notre Dame, Indiana: Ave Maria Press.

Dickinson, Sr. C. 1975. The Search for Spiritual Meaning. *American Journal of Nursing* 75:1789-1793.

Dillenberger, J., and Welch, C. 1955. *Protestant Christianity*. New York: Charles Scribner and Sons.

Inman, K., *et al*. 1957. If You Ask Me: What Specific Assistance Has a Clergyman Given You in Helping a Patient Meet His Problems. *American Journal of Nursing* 57:737.

McKnight, E.T. 1961. A Chaplain Interprets His Work. *Canadian Nurse* 57:1139-1141.

Morris, K.L., *et al*. 1972. Team Work: Nurse and Chaplain. *American Journal of Nursing* 72:2197-2199.

Naiman, H.L. 1970. Nursing in Jewish Law. *American Journal of Nursing* 70:10:2378-2379.

Patients' Religious Beliefs—Nurses' Responsibility. 1974. *Regan Reports on Nursing Law* 14:2 (April 1974).

Pederson, W.D. 1968. The Broadening Role of the Hospital Chaplain. *Hospitals* 42:9:58.

Piepgras, B. 1968. The Other Dimension: Spiritual Help. *American Journal of Nursing* 68:2610-2613.

Raciappa, J.D. 1973. A Total Ministry. *American Journal of Nursing* 73:645.

Recognizing Your Patient's Spiritual Needs. 1975. *Nursing Update* 6:7:1-2.

Taking Patient's Spiritual History is Called Important by the Surgeon. 1973. *O.R. Reporter* 8:12:11.

Ware, T. 1972. *The Orthodox Church*. Baltimore: Penguin Books.

Westberg, G.E. 1955. *Nurse, Pastor and Patient*. Rock Island, Ill.: Augustana Press.

10 Dependent Nursing Functions

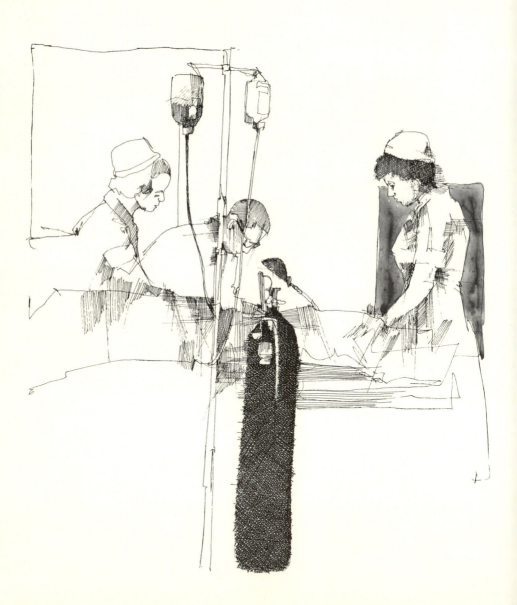

Objectives

After completing this chapter, you should be able to:

1 Discuss the various dependent functions of the nurse.

2 Identify the nurse's responsibility with regard to drug therapy.

3 Identify the nurse's responsibility with regard to treatments and procedures.

4 List the steps in performing any procedure or treatment.

5 Teach the patient about the diagnostic or treatment therapies to be performed.

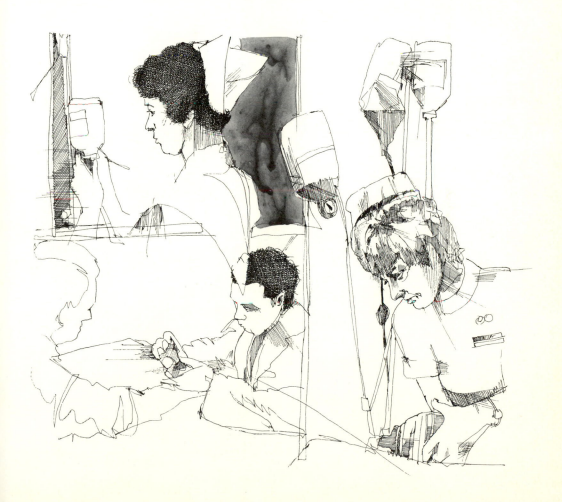

T HE NURSE HAS MANY dependent responsibilities related to the medical plan of care, which include implementing drug therapy, performing special treatments and therapeutic measures ordered by the physician, helping the physician perform diagnostic and therapeutic measures, preparing the patient for diagnostic and therapeutic measures to be carried out by other members of the team, and caring for the patient afterwards.

Administering drug therapy

Implementing drug therapy ordered by the physician involves far more than administering medications.

Knowledge of drugs

The nurse's first responsibility is to understand the drug itself—its purpose, the way it acts, contraindications to its use, and possible side effects. Acquiring a basic knowledge of drugs takes a great deal of time and effort, and even then the task is not over. Because new drugs are constantly being produced, familiarizing yourself with the drugs you administer is an ongoing responsibility. Such knowledge is important because it enables you to consider a given drug's potential and actual effect on an individual patient. Although the physician is responsible for ordering medication, the system is strengthened by the double-check provided by a knowledgeable nurse.

Knowledge of the patient's condition

The patient's physical condition, diagnosis, and history should be available to the nurse whenever medications are to be administered. Unless you have this information, you will not be able to make correct judgments about medications or to discern changes caused by drugs.

The nurse's responsibilities

Information about the patient should be considered in conjunction with information about the drug, paying particular attention to contraindications to the drug's use. Attention to possible allergies to medications can prevent unfortunate and sometimes tragic mistakes.

Thus, if the medication ordered is contraindicated for patients with glaucoma (an eye disease) and checking reveals that the patient has glaucoma, it is the nurse's responsibility to bring this circumstance to the attention of the physician. If the physician is aware of the conflict, the nurse should request an explanation of the rationale for giving the medication. If, after hearing the rationale, the nurse is still reluctant to give the medication, the nursing supervisor may be contacted for advice and direction. It is the privilege and responsibility of the nurse not to administer a medication that the nurse firmly believes will be harmful to the patient.

Another responsibility of the nurse is to evaluate the effectiveness of medications given. In order to do this, you must know the expected reaction and criteria must be established for ascertaining its effectiveness. For example, you need to know that codeine is given to reduce pain in order to plan a method of evaluating its effectiveness for the patient. Knowing the length of time it takes a medication to be effective also helps you to establish specific criteria, such as "pain relief obtained within thirty minutes."

Side effects and allergies to drugs are a common complication of drug therapy. Familiarity with the problems that can result from a given medication will enable the nurse to note their presence in a patient. The earlier a problem is recognized, the sooner appropriate action may be taken to combat it. It may be necessary to lower the dosage, discontinue the medication altogether, or even order other medications to counteract a given reaction.

It is another responsibility of the nurse to know the correct dosage of a medication. Errors can occur because of incorrect transcription of orders from one place to another, poor penmanship, and simple human fallibility. The nurse who knows the correct dosage and checks the order is often able to catch such errors and contact the physician to correct them. This is a particularly important task for nurses working with children. Children's dosages are so much smaller than adult dosages that even slight errors can cause serious problems.

Routes of administration

The way in which a medication is applied to or enters the body significantly affects the speed with which it works and the area of the body affected.

Oral medications are those that are swallowed. Some medications taken orally are absorbed in the stomach. Because they must be dissolved before absorption, liquids are usually absorbed more quickly than solids. However, some solids (such as aspirin) dissolve so rapidly that this advantage is not significant. Some oral medications are destroyed by stomach secretions, and must therefore be coated to allow them to pass into the small intestine where absorption will occur. This coating is called *enteric* coating.

Some medications are held against the mucous membranes of the mouth, where they dissolve slowly and are absorbed by the mucous membrane. Those held next to the cheek are called *buccal* medications; those held under the tongue are called *sublingual*.

Topical preparations, those applied to external surfaces of the body, include powders, lotions, and ointments. Also included in this category are eye (ophthalmic) and ear (otic) preparations. Because a few medications are absorbed from the skin, topical application may have systemic effects.

Some medications can be administered *rectally*. Many of these are prescribed for local effect on the bowel, but some medications can be absorbed by the large intestine and thus have a systemic effect.

Parenteral medications, those that are injected into body tissue, are categorized according to the tissue into which the medication is injected. *Intradermal* medications are injected into the skin, and *subcutaneous* medications into those tissue layers under the skin that lie over the muscle. *Intramuscular* injections go directly into the muscle tissue. *Intravenous* medications are directed into the bloodstream by way of a vein. *Intra-arterial* injections go into an artery. *Intracardiac* medications are injected directly into the heart (done only with emergency drugs in life-threatening situations). *Intrathecal* injections go directly into the subarachnoid space, to combine with the cerebrospinal fluid, by way of a lumbar puncture.

The faster a medication enters the circulatory system, the sooner a systemic result will occur. Thus, topical medication is the slowest to have a systemic effect since it is absorbed very slowly, if at all. Rectal absorption is faster, and oral medications faster still. Buccal and sublingual absorption is faster than oral because of the rapidity of absorption from the mouth. As for the parenteral medications, the deeper the tissue, the more vascular and thus quicker to absorb it is. Thus, intravenous is fastest, followed in descending order by intramuscular, subcutaneous, and intradermal. Many intradermal medications are not systemically absorbed at all. Intrathecal medications are administered for local effect in the cerebrospinal fluid, and there is little systemic absorption.

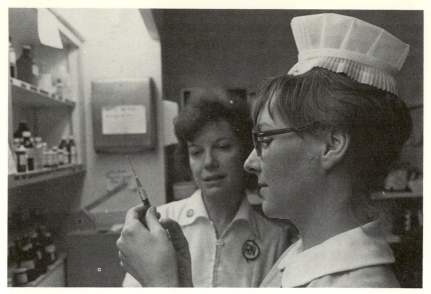

Lynn McLaren, courtesy of Newton-Wellesley Hospital

The five rights

In addition to general responsibilities with regard to medications, the nurse must give medications according to very rigid guidelines established to assure that the *right patient* receives the *right medication* at the *right time* in the *right dosage* by the *right route* of administration. These guidelines are sometimes referred to as "the five rights."

The cycle begins when an order for a medication is written by a physician, osteopathic physician, or dentist. A written order is usually required, to lessen the possibility of error. In emergency situations, however, verbal orders are given; errors are minimized if the emergency order is repeated exactly as heard before it is carried out. In some settings orders are given to the nurse over the telephone; such an order should be written down as it is given and read back to check for error. Both emergency verbal orders and telephone orders are recorded in the patient record, with a notation of the origin of the order ("Telephone order, A. J. Smith, M.D."), and signed by the person receiving and writing the order ("by J. Jones, R.N."). This written record is checked and countersigned at the earliest opportunity by the physician who gave the order.

After receiving the order, the nurse has many further responsibilities with regard to it. The order must be transcribed from the patient record to the Kardex, chart, and/or medication cards consulted when giving medication. In some places this step is eliminated by writing the order directly on the record from which the medication is given. In other settings the task of transcribing is assigned to the ward secretary or clerk. Nevertheless, the ultimate responsibility for checking the correctness of the transcription belongs to the nurse.

If the order has previously been transcribed, a routine for checking the accuracy of the duplicate record may have been established. This is especially likely when small cards are used to record each medication for administration. Such cards are easily misplaced, and failure to check them against an original record could result in medication errors.

Once you have ascertained that you have the correct information, you may begin the procedure of administering the medication. Whatever its structure, the system of drug administration is designed to provide the right patient with the right medication in the right dosage, by the right route, at the right time. You will need to learn the exact system or procedure of any facility in which you are employed. Some systems, such as the Brewer system, have been commercially designed, while others originate in the hospitals that use them. Still others, such as medicine cards, have been in use for so many years that no one may know how they originated. Whatever the system, it is the nurse's responsibility to perform it correctly so that the chances of error are minimized.

After administration of the medication, a recording is made of the medication, dosage, time, and route (oral, I.M., I.V., or whatever). This legal record must be signed by the person administering the medication. The importance of accurate recording cannot be overemphasized. Failure to record might result in a patient's receiving an ordered medication twice, with potentially serious effects. Omission of a medication must also be recorded, along with the reason for omission.

Medication errors

Because of the complexity of modern medication regimes, errors do occur. Whenever any *one* of the five rights is not observed, an error has been made. There are errors of commission, such as an incorrect medication or dosage, and errors of omission, such as failure to administer the correct medication or inadequate dosage.

However a medication error occurs, your immediate concern

must be the well-being of the patient. The patient is assessed in light of the nature of the error. If there was an overdosage, are there signs of adverse reactions? If a medication was omitted, are there possible adverse consequences for the patient? When the immediate status of the patient has been assessed, the nurse must plan the course of action. Notes may be made on the nursing care plan or Kardex to alert other nurses to look for particular problems. Sometimes immediate measures should be taken. When, for example, a medication to relieve muscle spasm was to have been given at 8:00 a.m., and the nurse discovered at 10:00 a.m. that it had been omitted, the nurse elected to give the medication immediately because the patient needed relief. Other errors may require other types of action.

The plan of action must always include notification of the physician. When notification is made, the nurse should be prepared to give the physician a complete assessment of the patient's condition and a summary of any action taken, and to consult with the physician on further action. If the problem is not serious, notification may be postponed until the physician's next visit. Otherwise, notification should be made immediately. If the physician is not available, the nursing supervisor and another physician may be called.

Another part of the nurse's plan will be to fill out a special incident form for the hospital or facility. The primary purpose of such forms is to gather data on errors so that steps can be taken to eliminate them. They also serve as a legal record for the facility.

Performing treatments

Many specific treatments are ordered by the physician in the course of the medical plan of care, and these treatments are very frequently implemented by the nursing staff. It is the nurse's responsibility to check orders and to understand the treatment's purpose, correct technique, expected outcome, and possible untoward reactions in much the same way as is the case for a medication. In general, treatments can be performed by following the ten steps listed in the Procedural Checklist and described in the following pages.

1. Check the order

As for a medication, it is necessary to have an order for a treatment. The order must be checked, verified, and transcribed accurately.

Procedural Checklist

  1 Check the order.
  2 Review the procedure.
  3 Gather the equipment.
  4 Prepare the patient psychologically.
  5 Prepare the patient physically.
  6 Perform the procedure.
  7 Evaluate the results.
  8 Make the patient comfortable.
  9 Care for the equipment and the specimen.
10 Record the data.

2. Review the procedure

Treatments you perform often will be familiar to you, and can be re-called simply and quickly. Any procedure with which you are unfa-miliar can be checked out in a procedure book or reference text. Sometimes it is necessary to consult a more experienced nurse to learn the details of a procedure. When a procedure has not been es-tablished, you can often design an appropriate one on the basis of the treatment's purpose and your background knowledge of the sci-ences and nursing theory. As you move to a new area of the country or even to another hospital in the same city, you may find that proce-dures are carried out differently. Review the new procedure with an eye to its conformity with basic principles of care. If these principles are observed, minor variations in procedure are not significant. For example, some facilities use prepackaged disposable sets for chang-ing dressings, which contain some instruments and sterile gloves; others do not have prepackaged materials, and the nurse has to de-termine what items are needed and plan to provide them. Although the procedures differ, it is possible to perform a dressing change with excellent sterile technique by both methods.

3. Gather the equipment

Many procedures in the modern hospital are performed with pre-packaged disposable equipment, which saves a great deal of time that was formerly spent gathering supplies. It is important to recog-nize that sets of equipment differ, and to study their labels to determine exactly what is contained and what is not. For example, some sets for urinary catheterization contain all of the equipment necessary for the procedure, including the catheter and the drainage bag. Other sets contain everything except these items. In addition to the prepackaged set, you may need a blanket for draping the patient, a light, and a pencil and paper on which to make notations.

When no prepackaged set is available, the task is more complex. While reviewing the procedure, you might make note of the equipment needed for each step so that you remember to provide it.

The major reason for organizing equipment ahead of time is to lessen the patient's anxiety. Making numerous trips for forgotten equipment is distressing to the patient and erodes confidence in your ability to perform the procedure correctly. Organizing your work also saves you many steps, lessens fatigue, and makes it possible to accomplish more in the same amount of time.

4. Prepare the patient psychologically

People are more able to handle a stressful situation if they have some knowledge and understanding of it. Therefore you will want to explain to the patient exactly what is to be done. Details are provided only if needed by the patient and unlikely to arouse un-

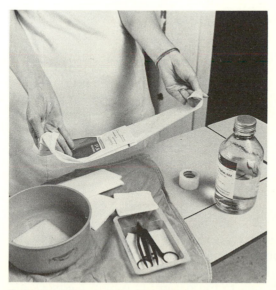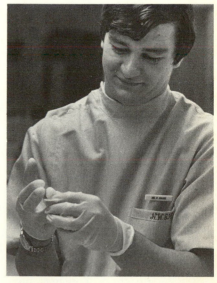

Setting up for a sterile treatment
Left: *Dan Bernstein*; Right: *Lynn McLaren, courtesy of Newton-Wellesley Hospital*

due alarm. Thus patients having bladder irrigations should be told
that they may experience some pressure during the procedure.
They need not be told all about the sterile technique you will use
or the possible adverse consequences of improper technique. If
pain is likely to occur, the patient is usually less frightened if told
that discomfort is expected at a certain point in the procedure.
Otherwise the patient might fear that something is seriously
wrong. On the other hand, a description of the extent and severity
of the discomfort might only increase anxiety. Of course, the patient's specific questions should always be answered.

In addition to conveying direct information, you should be
alert to questions and feelings the patient would like to express or
work through before the procedure begins. The techniques of therapeutic interaction are used in such instances (see Chapter 7).

5. Prepare the patient physically

When the patient understands what is to be done, you proceed to
make physical preparations. These preparations may include providing privacy, positioning the patient, changing the position of the
bed, moving tables and stands, draping the patient, and providing
proper lighting. Sometimes you might consider giving medication
for pain or a tranquilizer to prepare the patient for the procedure.
Judgments on when PRN (whenever necessary) medications are to
be given is an important nursing responsibility.

6. Perform the procedure

Once everything is prepared, you can proceed with the procedure as
planned, paying careful attention to detail. It is important that you
observe the patient's responses closely. There may be times when
the procedure must be changed, delayed, or even halted because of
the patient's response. A very common failing of inexperienced
nurses is to become so engrossed in technical details that the patient
is neglected.

7. Evaluate the results

Some evaluation is performed during the procedure, but a more
complete evaluation of both its effectiveness in accomplishing its
goal and the patient's response to it is undertaken when you have
finished. You may have to talk to the patient to obtain feedback on
his or her response. Consider the purpose of the treatment when
evaluating it. If a hot pack is used to reduce pain and inflammation of

a swollen arm, but the patient experiences no relief from discomfort, the procedure is not considered completely successful even if performed correctly. Sometimes evaluation cannot be completed immediately after the procedure, but criteria and a plan for evaluation can be established at that time.

8. Make the patient comfortable

Before moving on to other tasks, you should make the patient as comfortable as possible. Doing so may entail rearranging bedding, changing the patient's position, returning tables and stands to positions convenient for the patient, and consulting the patient about his or her immediate needs. Again, the possibility of a need for pain medication and the patient's psychological well-being should be considered. The patient may wish to talk about the experience, or may prefer quiet and privacy to regain composure if the procedure has been particularly long and/or difficult.

9. Care for the equipment and the specimen

Equipment and supplies must be taken care of in the manner prescribed by the facility. Disposable equipment may need to be disposed of in a particular place to avoid endangering housekeeping persons with needles and sharp instruments. Nondisposable equipment may need to be cleaned according to a particular routine or sent to a department where such cleaning is performed. Nurses are expected to demonstrate care with the many costly pieces of equipment used in the modern health care setting.

    If a specimen was obtained in the course of the procedure, it must be labeled carefully so that no errors occur. It is then processed in whatever way is appropriate for such a specimen to prevent deterioration, which would render it useless. In certain instances, for example, a stool specimen must be kept warm so that organisms present can be identified in the laboratory; urine must sometimes be refrigerated to slow chemical decomposition. Some specimens must be placed in special preservatives or treated containers. Information on the care of a specimen for a specific purpose should be available from the laboratory.

10. Record the data

Data on the treatment itself, the patient's response, the effectiveness of the treatment, and the disposition of the specimen (if any) are usually recorded on the patient's medical record. A flow sheet is sometimes used to record repeated treatments in much the same way that medications are charted. In other instances, treatments are recorded on nurses' notes in a narrative fashion. Whatever the format, a clear record is needed.

You will find that you can easily adapt these ten steps to both simple and complex procedures. For a simple procedure, such as taking a temperature, you will perform the steps very rapidly: you might gather your equipment, enter the patient's room, explain your purpose, rearrange the pillow, and take the temperature in less than five minutes. You have simply telescoped the steps, performing some almost simultaneously. For a longer and more complex procedure, you might isolate each step and enter the patient's room twice in the course of the procedure, once to prepare the patient and again to bring the equipment to the bedside. Thus, the procedural checklist is a tool for your use, not an implacable formula.

Assisting with diagnostic tests and procedures

A variety of special tests and procedures are performed by the physician and other members of the health care team, and the nurse is frequently called on to assist with them. The same procedure checklist will be of value in this situation. In reviewing the various steps, you can decide which will be performed by others and which will be your responsibility. For a diagnostic study or procedure to be undertaken in another department, the process may be as follows: (1) Check the order. (2) Review the procedure in order to decide what you need to do and explain it to the patient. (3) Equipment may be taken care of by the other department. (4) Prepare the patient by teaching about and discussing the procedure. (5) Physical preparation may be performed in the other department or by you. (6) The procedure is carried out in the other department. (7) Evaluate the patient on his or her return. (8) The other department will take care of the equipment used. (9) The other department will record its own procedures or treatments, but you will record those portions you have performed. (10) Make the patient comfortable on his or her return. (See the Care Study on page 172.)

In some situations, such as a diagnostic procedure performed by the physician, you may find that you perform all the steps except the procedure itself. While the physician is performing the procedure, you will assist by making equipment available, positioning the patient, and helping the patient tolerate the procedure.

Tables 10.1 through 10.6 describe some of the common procedures and tests performed by other members of the health care team, and will enable you as a beginning student to participate in the patient's care with greater understanding. Specific aspects of these procedures will vary from place to place, and the procedure manual for your institution should be consulted for details. A medical-surgical nursing text should be consulted for information on understanding the results of the test and on providing more skilled care if it is required.

Conclusion

Nursing is characterized by many modes of functioning and of relating to others. As a nurse, you will exercise your decision-making ability constantly as you function independently. Working effectively with other health care team members and carrying out delegated tasks requires the same kind of capable functioning. The nurse cannot simply do as directed. Both the law and those who depend on nurses expect informed, thoughtful action in every situation.

TABLE 10.1 SPECIAL VISUAL EXAMINATIONS (ENDOSCOPY) Hollow organs that open to the body's exterior surface are examined by means of a hollow tube and a light. These "scopes" are of two basic types: the rigid and the fiberoptic. The rigid scope is a metal or plastic tube, and the passageway into the organ must be straightened to allow entry of the tube. The light allows the inside of the organ to be visually inspected. It is also possible to insert a special instrument to take a specimen of tissue. This procedure is called a *biopsy*. The

	ORGAN STUDIED	PREPARATION
BRONCHOSCOPY	Bronchi and (with fiberoptic scope) lung segments	NPO and sedatives. If general anesthesia, routine preop. If local, special explanation of procedure.
COLONOSCOPY	Entire large bowel (with fiberoptic scope)	Measures to cleanse bowel completely begun evening before and completed morning of test.
CYSTOSCOPY	Bladder	Same as for bronchoscopy.
ESOPHAGOSCOPY	Esophagus	Same as for bronchoscopy.
GASTROSCOPY	Stomach (with fiberoptic scope)	Same as for bronchoscopy.
LARYNGOSCOPY	Larynx	If general anesthesia, routine preop. If local, special explanation of procedure.
PROCTOSCOPY	Rectum	Measures to cleanse bowel completely begun evening before and completed morning of test.
SIGMOIDOSCOPY	Sigmoid colon and rectum	Same as proctoscopy

TABLE 10.1 SPECIAL VISUAL EXAMINATIONS (ENDOSCOPY)   161

fiberoptic scope is a flexible tube containing a bundle of fibers that reflect light. These fibers are so perfectly aligned that the image at the bottom of the tube is seen clearly at the top. Fiberoptic scopes can conform to the shape of the passage or organ and can thus be inserted into areas of the body not accessible to metal scopes. They cause less discomfort than do rigid scopes, and also have attached instruments to take tissue samples.

SPECIAL NURSING CONCERNS

If performed with local anesthesia, do not give fluids or food until gag reflex returns. Complications to watch for include bleeding due to tissue trauma, laryngospasm, and respiratory distress.

Bleeding due to trauma

Urinary tract irritation from scope. Possible infection. Encourage fluids.

If performed with local anesthesia, do not give fluids or food until gag reflex returns.

Same as for esophagoscopy

If performed with local anesthesia, do not give fluids or food until gag reflex returns. Complications to watch for include bleeding due to tissue trauma and laryngospasm.

Bleeding due to trauma

Same as above

TABLE 10.2 X-RAY EXAMINATIONS X-rays produce a negative-type film that shows images of the outlines of various structures whose different densities allow varying amounts of radiation to penetrate through to the film.

Most x-rays are simple images of body parts; examples are x-rays of the chest and of the extremities to check for fractures. The view or patient position is usually designated by the physician.

Some organs do not appear on routine x-rays because they are not suffi-

	ORGAN STUDIED	PREPARATION
ANGIOGRAM	Blood vessels. Usually used to examine a system of veins and arteries within an organ.	Usually NPO. Sometimes surgical prep of site.
ARTERIOGRAM	Arteries (but often used as a synonym for angiogram)	Same as for angiogram
BARIUM ENEMA (LOWER BOWEL)	Large intestine	Measures to cleanse bowel completely begun evening before and completed morning of test.
BRONCHOGRAM	Bronchi	NPO. Routine preop. General anesthesia usual.
CYSTOGRAM	Bladder	None usual
CHOLECYSTOGRAM (GALL BLADDER SERIES)	Gall bladder	NPO. Fat-free meal evening before. Oral contrast pills evening before as directed.
CHOLANGIOGRAM	Bile ducts	NPO. Preparation for surgery. Usually done during gall bladder surgery.
INTRAVENOUS PYELOGRAM (IVP)	Kidney, ureters, and bladder	NPO. Measures to cleanse bowel completely evening before test.
MYELOGRAM	Spinal canal	NPO. Sedative given. Usually not general anesthesia.

TABLE 10.2 X-RAY EXAMINATIONS   163

ciently dense to block any radiation. In these cases *contrast studies* are performed: a contrast material (radio-opaque substance) is introduced into the organ so that a clear outline of it can be seen on the x-ray. The functioning of an organ can sometimes be studied by taking a series of x-rays as the contrast material moves through the organ. Intravenous dyes (contrast materials) are potent and can cause severe allergic reactions.

METHOD	SPECIAL NURSING CONCERNS
Catheter is threaded into artery (often the femoral), and dye is injected under pressure into the organ's vascular system.	Allergic reaction to dye. Bleeding from puncture site. Thrombus formation.
Same as for angiogram	Same as for angiogram
Barium is given as enema. Large plug is inserted in rectum to prevent loss of barium.	Barium causes severe constipation or even obstruction, if not removed by means of enemas or laxatives.
Dye is inserted through bronchoscope, then suctioned out.	Same as for bronchoscopy. Also irritation from dye causes increased secretions. Retained dye may cause pneumonia.
Patient is catheterized and dye inserted through catheter.	Encourage fluids to prevent infection.
Material excreted in bile is given in pill form. X-rays are taken to determine whether gall bladder contains the material. Then a fatty liquid is given, and further x-rays are taken to observe function of gall bladder.	Pills often cause nausea and vomiting. Vomiting of pills makes test invalid. Burning on urination as dye is excreted.
Dye is injected into bile ducts themselves. May give dye IV just before test.	None usual
Dye is injected intravenously and excreted by kidneys. A series of x-rays made of entire urinary tract.	Dye can cause urinary irritation. Encourage fluids.
Lumbar puncture is done, some spinal fluid removed, and dye injected into canal. Patient is positioned on tilt table, which is tilted to allow dye to flow to desired level.	Same as for lumbar puncture. (See Table 10.6.) Allergic reactions to dye.

Table 10.2 cont.

	ORGAN STUDIED	PREPARATION
PNEUMO-ENCEPHALOGRAM	Ventricles of brain	NPO. Sedative given. Full: 100 cc. of air, general anesthesia. Limited: 10-15 cc. air, local anesthesia.
RETROGRADE PYELOGRAM	Kidney	NPO. Laxatives to clear bowel.
UPPER G.I.	Esophagus, stomach, duodenum	NPO after midnight
VENTRICULOGRAM	Ventricles of brain	Complete surgical preparation as for neurosurgery.

TABLE 10.3 MEASUREMENT AND RECORDING OF ELECTRICAL IM-PULSES Some organs of the body undergo changes in electrical potential in

	ORGAN STUDIED	PREPARATION
ELECTROCARDIOGRAM (EKG or ECG)	Heart	None usual
ELECTROENCEPHALOGRAM	Brain	None usual
ELECTROMYOGRAM	Muscles	None usual

TABLE 10.3 MEASUREMENT OF ELECTRICAL IMPULSES 165

METHOD	SPECIAL NURSING CONCERNS
Lumbar puncture is done, some spinal fluid removed, and air inserted. Air rises to ventricles when patient is placed in upright position.	Headache until air is absorbed. Pain medications are given.
Cystoscopy is performed. Ureteral catheters are inserted, films taken of catheters, and dye is then injected into renal pelvis for films.	Same as for cytoscopy
Barium is swallowed. Films are taken as material fills upper gastrointestinal system.	Same as for barium enema
Burr holes are drilled in skull and cannula is inserted to inject contrast medium into ventricles.	Complete postop. care for a neuro patient. (See a medical-surgical textbook.)

the process of functioning. These changes in electrical potential can be of significance in evaluating the functioning of the organ.

METHOD	SPECIAL NURSING CONCERNS
Electrodes are secured to the chest wall with electrode paste and tape or suction cups. Other electrodes are attached to the extremities. The machine then records the electrical activity of the heart.	None
Electrodes are attached to the scalp with small needles or paste. The patient is at rest in a darkened room, and may be asked to deep-breathe (hyperventilation) or watch a flashing light (photic stimulation) at certain times.	None
Electrodes are attached to the muscles tested with small needles or paste and the electrical impulses are recorded.	None

TABLE 10.4 MISCELLANEOUS TESTS OF SPECIFIC BODY FUNCTIONS   A great many tests have been devised to examine the functioning of body processes. Those listed here are only a few of the more common tests.

	PURPOSE
BASAL METABOLISM RATE (BMR)	To test the rate at which the body uses oxygen at complete rest (not sleep) in order to measure metabolic rate
GASTRIC ANALYSIS	To measure the stomach's production of gastric juices
GLUCOSE TOLERANCE TEST (GTT)	To measure the ability of the body to metabolize a glucose "load"
INDIRECT GASTRIC ANALYSIS (TUBELESS GASTRIC ANALYSIS "DIAGNEX BLUE," "AZUREA")	To measure the production of gastric acid by determining the rate at which the dye material is absorbed and excreted

TABLE 10.4 MISCELLANEOUS TESTS OF SPECIFIC BODY FUNCTIONS 167

PREPARATION	METHOD
NPO. Test performed first thing in the morning. No activity allowed preceding test.	The nose is clamped; the patient breathes through a mouthpiece so that oxygen consumption can be measured.
NPO	A nasogastric tube is inserted into the stomach. All gastric contents are aspirated and saved over a period of time. Samples are taken at specified time intervals according to laboratory procedure.
NPO	A fasting urine sample is obtained, and a blood sample is drawn for a fasting blood sugar test. Then a solution containing a known amount of glucose is drunk by the patient. At intervals specified by the laboratory, urine samples are taken and blood samples are drawn (usually by the laboratory technician).
NPO	Dye material is given as directed by the manufacturer. Urine is saved for 24 hours and sent to the laboratory for analysis. Urine will continue to be blue for several days after the test.

TABLE 10.5 TESTS USING RADIOACTIVE MATERIALS In these tests, small amounts of radioactive substances are injected or ingested into the body and a scanning device that registers the presence of radioactive particles is used to determine their distribution. Some substances are simply circulated in the blood stream to allow circulatory pathways, and changes or interruptions in

	ORGAN STUDIED	PREPARATION
BRAIN SCAN	Brain	None
I^{131} UPTAKE	Thyroid gland	NPO before test. Meals are resumed after taking iodine preparation.
LIVER SCAN	Liver	None
LUNG SCAN	Lung	None

TABLE 10.5 TESTS USING RADIOACTIVE MATERIALS   169

those pathways, to be seen. In other tests, differential rates at which the radioactive substance is absorbed by different tissues allow rates of activity, types of tissue, and ability to function to be determined. The amounts of radiation are so small that they pose no hazard to personnel or patient.

METHOD

Material is injected IV and the scanner is used to trace the circulatory pattern of the brain. Because some tissues will absorb more of the material, abnormal tissue can be located.

An oral solution containing this radioactive isotope of iodine is given. The thyroid is scanned to determine its rate of metabolism of the iodine 24 hours after the I^{131} is ingested.

Material is injected IV and the scanner is used over the liver. Areas of obstruction result in increased uptake of the material.

Material is injected IV and scan films are taken of the lungs. Circulatory patterns are apparent and diseased areas often show up as blocks in circulation on the scan.

TABLE 10.6 TESTS INVOLVING INTRODUCTION OF A LARGE NEEDLE INTO AN ORGAN OR BODY CAVITY These tests are all performed by a physician with the careful sterile technique appropriate to minor surgical procedures.

	PURPOSE
ABDOMINAL PARACENTESIS	To remove fluid that has accumulated in the peritoneal cavity
BONE MARROW BIOPSY	To obtain a sample of bone marrow tissue to examine its production of blood components
LUMBAR PUNCTURE	To puncture the spinal subarachnoid space to remove a sample of fluid for study or to inject dye for a contrast x-ray
THORACENTESIS	To puncture the pleural space to remove fluid or allow for the insertion of chest tubes

TABLE 10.6 TESTS INVOLVING A LARGE NEEDLE   171

Because of the size of the needle, a local anesthetic is administered. If the patient is especially anxious, some sedation may be given before the procedure is begun.

METHOD	SPECIAL NURSING CONCERNS
With the patient in a sitting position, the needle is inserted through the abdominal wall. A 3-way stopcock, syringe, and tubing may be attached to the needle to allow aspiration of the fluid.	The patient should void first. Shock may occur during the procedure. (See a medical-surgical text.) The wound must be dressed afterwards.
The patient is lying down. The sternum or the iliac crest is commonly punctured.	The procedure may be very upsetting to the patient. Some pain is felt when the bone is entered, and the aspiration of tissue may be painful. The sound of bone penetration may be upsetting. Afterwards, pressure is applied for 5 minutes to prevent bleeding.
The patient lies on a side in a flexed (bowed) position to allow access to the lower spine. During the procedure, a measurement of spinal fluid pressure is made.	Afterwards the patient is kept flat for a time. The prone position is preferred to allow "welling" of the puncture site, preventing further loss of fluid. Fluids are encouraged to facilitate replacement of spinal fluid. Headache occurs infrequently as a complication.
With the patient usually sitting up and leaning over a table; the puncture is made in the lower posterior chest to remove fluid and in the upper anterior chest to remove air.	Possible respiratory distress and pain during aspiration

CARE STUDY / Assisting with a physical therapy treatment

Mrs. Jones, an elderly woman with severe arthritis in both hands, is a newly admitted patient. Mrs. Schultz, the registered nurse, checks the physician's orders (step 1) and notes that physical therapy treatment involving the application of hot wax to both hands are to take place daily. Mrs. Schultz calls the Physical Therapy Department to arrange appointments for Mrs. Jones, and at the same time inquires about the exact manner in which the procedure will be carried out (step 2). This is Mrs. Schultz's first experience with such a treatment since her employment at General Hospital.

After obtaining the information, Mrs. Schultz goes into Mrs. Jones' room to explain the treatment (step 4). Mrs. Schultz also plans for morning care to be given to Mrs. Jones after treatment so that the pain relief afforded by the treatment can become effective before Mrs. Jones tries to perform self-care.

The next morning Mrs. Schultz prepares Mrs. Jones to go to the Physical Therapy Department. Assessing Mrs. Jones' abilities, the nurse determines that a wheelchair is the most appropriate means of transportation (step 5).

The treatment is carried out by the physical therapist (steps 3 and 6), who records complete information on Mrs. Jones' chart (steps 7 and 9).

When the patient returns to the unit, Mrs. Schultz makes her comfortable (step 8) and notes her fatigue level. She inquires about the pain relief experienced and watches for any untoward results, such as skin irritation (step 7). Mrs. Schultz then records her observations on Mrs. Jones' record (step 10) in the following manner: "Upon return from P.T., appeared pale and exhausted. Stated the hot wax had decreased pain in hands. Skin appears pink and smooth. No irritation of skin noted." H. Schultz, R.N.

Study terms

allergy
contraindication
diagnostic test
dosage
drug therapy
"five rights"
medical plan of care
procedure
routes of administration
  buccal
  intra-arterial

intradermal
intrathecal
oral
parenteral
rectal
subcutaneous
sublingual
topical
side effect
treatment

References

Bermock, L. S., *et al.* 1973. Do We Practice What We Teach? *Nursing '73* 3:9:26-32.

Brunner, L. S. 1971. Standards on Policies and Procedures and How to Write Them. *Association of Operating Room Nurses Journal* 13:5:39-55.

Budd, R. 1971. We Changed to Unit Dosage System. *Nursing Outlook* 19:116-117.

Burkhalter, P. 1972. Medication Errors: Let's Eliminate Them! *Supervisor Nurse* 3:11:58-59.

DelBueno, D. J. 1972. Verifying the Nurse's Knowledge of Pharmacology. *Nursing Outlook* 20:462-463.

Harmon, M. L., *et al.* 1971. Fiber Optics Photography in the Stomach. *RN* 34:7:46-51.

Levine, R. 1970. Breaking Through the Medication Mystique. *American Journal of Nursing* 70:799.

Siegler, A. M. 1971. Trends in Laparoscopy. *RN* 34:11:OR-1-4.

Standing Orders and Nursing Judgment. 1970. *Regan Reports on Nursing Law* 11:1 (Nov. 1970).

11 Infection

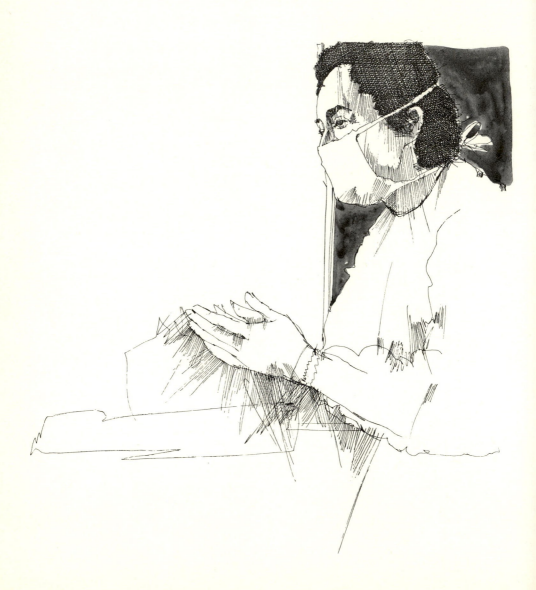

Objectives

After completing this chapter, you should be able to:

1 Define the key terms relating to infection and infective agents.

2 List the factors that predispose individuals to infection.

3 Diagram and explain the movement of pathogens through the infection chain.

4 Outline the nursing actions necessary in caring for the patient with an infection.

5 Name the types of isolation and the general requirements of each.

6 Provide for effective isolation and carry out the nurse's responsibilities.

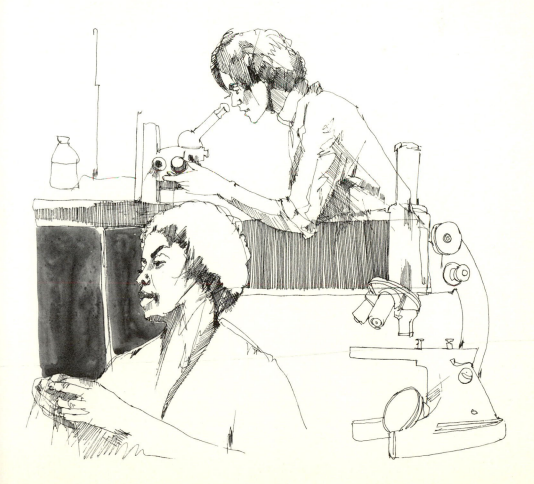

NFECTION POSES A serious problem to the hospitalized patient. Many patients are admitted to the hospital because of the presence of an infection. And, more often than we would like, patients who are in the hospital for the treatment of a medical condition or for surgery develop secondary infections. Thus a major aspect of nursing care is the prevention, management, and treatment of infection. You need a basic knowledge of infection control, and as a nurse you must make a continuing effort to prevent transmission of infection.

A brief history of the treatment of infection

As long as human beings have existed, their wounds have been accompanied by infection. Thus, though attempts were made to contain it, infection was long thought to be a natural aspect of healing. The ancient Romans dressed wounds with mixtures of molds and yeasts spread on cloth, called poultices. These mixtures appeared to slow the infection process. Not until the twentieth century did Sir Alexander Fleming, an English bacteriologist working on the mold theory, discover penicillin, now the most commonly used antibiotic in the world.

In the interim, then, effective measures to combat infection, as well as specific knowledge of how infection was transmitted from person to person, were both lacking. In the nineteenth century Louis Pasteur, a French chemist, proved beyond a doubt the germ theory of disease. About the same time Ignaz Semmelweis, an obstetrician, found that germs could be transmitted from the hands of one person to another person. Physicians routinely examined pregnant women immediately after examining cadavers, without washing their hands, and Semmelweis observed that these women became infected and often died of what was known as "childbed fever." Knowledge of infection and its control has thus expanded gradually, giving rise to modern scientific concepts with important implications for the entire health care team.

Definition of terms

To discuss infection, we need to define a few key terms. Extremely small animals and plants called *micro-organisms* exist throughout the human body. Many of these tiny organisms are beneficial, but some are not. Those that are beneficial prevent the growth of disease-producing micro-organisms within a certain area of the body, such as the nose, throat, intestinal tract, and vagina. Disease-producing micro-organisms are called *pathogens*. When pathogens multiply to a point at which they cause signs and symptoms in a person, that individual is said to have an *infection*. In other words, all of us carry pathogens, but we remain infection-free unless they multiply sufficiently to cause disease.

Pathogens are divided into roughly five categories. It is important to know these categories, since the type of pathogen causing an infection suggests the type of infection control that is appropriate. Many pathogens are *bacteria*, single-cell organisms that cause a variety of infections in man. Some bacteria form *spores*, a dormant type that is extremely difficult to kill. *Viruses* are the smallest pathogens, some only recently observed microscopically. Viruses are often non-responsive to drugs, and many of the infections they cause must "run their course." *Fungus*, a moldlike pathogen, can also cause difficult-to-subdue infections in patients. *Protozoa* are simple single-cell organisms responsible for infections such as malaria. Infections caused by *parasitic worms* are termed *helminthic* infections.

The origin of infection

An infection contracted while in the hospital is called *nosocomial*. It is these types of infection that are most worrisome to hospital personnel. Hospitals are not, despite their appearance, clean places. Many persons, from many different home environments, are confined to a fairly constricted facility in which contact with one another can hardly be avoided. And patients have other health problems that weaken their resistance to infection. Many patients have open wounds, which offer entry for pathogens. Most hospitals have formed "infection committees" to study the origin of nosocomial infections. Nurses often serve on these committees; because they are directly involved in care, nurses can provide valuable input.

Some persons are more susceptible to infection than others, for one or a number of reasons. Age is a major factor, since the very young lack the immune mechanisms developed later in life and may develop infections more easily. The general condition of any patient is important in that it may heighten susceptibility. The elderly, who are weakened by the infirmities of old age, have a high incidence of infection. Specific disabilities sometimes contribute to the occurrence of infection. For example, the patient whose bladder does not empty completely may be subject to repeated bladder infections. Patients whose state of nutrition is adequate are less prone to infection than are the malnourished. The presence of another disease can allow an infection to develop, as in the case of the patient with chronic obstructive lung disease who contracts pneumonia. Certain medications encourage infection, most notably the drugs used in blood diseases like leukemia. Such drugs, in conjunction with the patient's already decreased ability to fight infection, make infection an ever-present danger. Investigators now know that persons under stress have an increased incidence of infection. This may be due to the interaction between physical and psychological coping.

Knowing the various contributory factors to infection in any individual suggests to the nurse which of a group of patients should be guarded most closely against infection. If a person has more than one predisposing factor, the chance of infection multiplies accordingly. All patients should be protected from infection in the hospital, and some should be given special care.

The spread of infection

Now let us examine the manner in which pathogens move from one person to another. Understanding this process will help you to perform effective infection control.

The *infectious agent* is the pathogen. As we have said, it must multiply sufficiently to cause an active infection. The person in whom the organism is present is called the *host*. In some persons the pathogen never reaches a level high enough to cause an active infection, but is harbored and can be passed along to someone else. Such a person is called a *carrier*. A famous carrier was a food handler, later labeled "Typhoid Mary," who caused numerous cases of typhoid fever in persons to whom she served food but never developed the disease herself. The *reservoir* is the place in or on the body where growth or multiplication of the pathogens takes place. This reservoir could be the throat, skin, bowel, a wound, or even a specific organ. The point at which the pathogen leaves the host is called the *portal of exit*. The respiratory, urinary, and intestinal tracts are common portals of exit; the blood and wound drainage are less common. The pathogen must also have a *means of transmission* or movement from the host to another person. Nurses should take special interest in this factor in infection, for all isolation techniques are based on interrupting the means of transmission. If you can identify the portal of exit

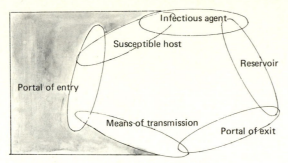

FIGURE 11.1   THE INFECTION CHAIN
Adapted, with permission, from V. W. Greene, "Microbial Contamination: Control in Hospitals," Hospitals, Journal of the American Hospital Association 43, no. 78 (October 16, 1969).

and the means of transmission, it is not difficult to determine the appropriate isolation technique. Some pathogens are borne purely on the air; others are carried through the air in droplet form and can be either inhaled or contracted by contact. Excreta and secretions are passed only through contact. The pathogen enters a new susceptible host through a *portal of entry*, perhaps the same portal through which it left its last host. For example, the respiratory organism may enter the next victim's respiratory tract. Or the portals of exit and entry may differ, as when an organism that leaves a bowel enters an open wound.

Unfortunately, the infection chain (see Figure 11.1) is continuous and ever-present when human beings live in community with one another. Constant vigilance is required to prevent and control communicable disease.

Asepsis: the prevention of infection

Asepsis means the state of being free from pathogens. Because the term is general in nature, nurses and other health care team members differentiate between two kinds of asepsis. *Medical asepsis* is designed to reduce the number of pathogens and decrease the likelihood of their transfer. It is often referred to as *clean technique*. Micro-organisms may continue to be present, but a threshold of safety has been established. The daily practice of hygiene falls into this category, as does the administration of oral medications, tube feedings, enemas, and many other treatments. The aim of *surgical asepsis*, on the other hand, is not simply to reduce the number of pathogens but to make the object or person free of all pathogens. This practice of *sterile technique* is reserved primarily for such procedures as changing sterile dressings, performing catheterizations, and surgical procedures in the operating room.

Methods of maintaining asepsis

The nurse plays a vital role in asepsis, and must accept it as one of the responsibilities inherent in nursing. A nurse's hands may touch numerous patients and a variety of equipment, perform various procedures, and attend to personal needs during a given day. Each contact or task represents a potential transfer of microorganisms. Because nurses must move quickly from patient to patient, it is easy to forget to wash hands properly between patients. It is hard but necessary for beginning student nurses to remember.

HANDWASHING   Handwashing, the primary barrier to infection, must always be the last task performed before going to the patient and the last upon leaving. The hands must be washed with flowing warm

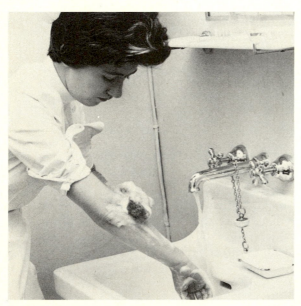

Lester V. Bergman & Assoc., Inc.

water over a basin. A good soap or detergent is accompanied by brisk friction. If the hands are dirty, they are rinsed from the wrist downward, with the elbows held high to allow micro-organisms to be rinsed off the fingers into the bowl. This procedure is called *medical asepsis handwashing*. If, on the other hand, the hands are uncontaminated and are being washed prior to sterile gloving or working within a sterile field *surgical asepsis handwashing* is performed. The hands are thoroughly washed, sometimes with a brush, and rinsed with the elbows low over the sink so that the fingers are rinsed first and the water flows off the elbows into the basin. This procedure makes the fingers the cleanest part of the hands.

CARE OF LINENS   Linens fresh from the laundry are relatively free of pathogens due to the strong detergents and bleaches used in the laundering process and the hot automatic ironers. In order to prevent contamination of linen, a clean place should be provided for them prior to use. Linen intended for one patient should not be put down at the bedside of another, if the transfer of micro-organisms from one patient to another is to be avoided. Shaking clean or dirty linen spreads micro-organisms by creating air currents, and should be avoided. Linen dropped on the floor must be discarded, regardless of how wasteful this may appear, because the floor is usually heavily contaminated with dirt and with the many organisms that settle out of the air. To prevent contamination of the nurse's uniform, used linen should be firmly bundled and carried away from the clothing. Hands are to be washed immediately after depositing soiled linens in the appropriate bag or hamper.

CARE OF EQUIPMENT   Shared equipment must be appropriately cleaned before being moved from one patient to another. Thermometers, blood pressure cuffs, and deep breathing machines fall into this category. Again, proper cleanliness prevents cross-contamination.

ARRANGEMENT OF THE PATIENT'S UNIT   The physical arrangement of patients' units varies considerably; some arrangements promote cleanliness better than others. The self-contained unit is the most effective in minimizing the likelihood of cross-contamination. Patients in these units have their own thermometers, bathing basins, emesis basins, bedpans, and urinals at their bedsides. These items are not shared with other patients. Even in self-contained units, however, nonhygienic practices that encourage the spread of pathogens do occur. Bedpans and urinals should never be placed on a bedside table or stand. Instead, they are kept in the compartments of the stand nearest the floor, where the most micro-organisms reside. The top-most drawers and compartments are reserved for the cleaner items used by the patient, such as toothbrushes, cosmetics, eyeglasses, and books. This arrangement allows micro-organisms to move or set-tle downward from the cleanest to the dirtiest areas.

CARING FOR MORE THAN ONE PATIENT   When two or more patients express a need for a service simultaneously, it is best to determine which re-quest is the most urgent and to respond to that patient first. After washing your hands, you may meet the second patient's need. This approach is necessary because it is very difficult to avoid spreading some degree of contamination from one patient to the other when carrying objects to and from more than one patient.

CLEANING METHODS   Dishes and other objects may be washed with hot water and soap, as well as friction, to eliminate pathogens and attain medical asepsis. Although no longer practical and less effective than other methods, direct exposure to sunlight reduces pathogens and was used in early hospitals for antisepsis. Objects may also be soaked in solutions that retard or kill pathogens. *Antiseptics* inhibit the growth of pathogens, and many are mild enough to be used on the tissues of the body. *Disinfectants* also inhibit the growth of patho-gens, are usually chemical in nature, and can be harmful if directly applied to tissue. Neither disinfectants nor antiseptics may be effec-tive against spore-forming bacteria. *Bactericidal* agents kill all micro-organisms, pathogens and nonpathogens alike.

In the operating room, other methods are frequently used to sterilize gowns, drapes, dressings, and surgical instruments. Cen-tral supply departments, which supply procedure trays that must be sterile, use similar methods. Usually such objects are subject to *autoclaving*, a process of steaming under high pressure for a specif-ic period of time. A special tape, with which you should be famil-iar, is used on the wrappings. When the object being autoclaved has been exposed to the prescribed time, temperature, and pres-sure required to render it sterile, the tape will show a particular marking, often but not always a black diagonal stripe. If a sterile packet is not designated sterile in some such way, it should be im-mediately returned for exchange. If autoclaved packets are not dry from the steam in the autoclave, they must be considered contami-nated since dampness allows for the transfer of pathogens. Some hospitals use gas sterilization, which exposes the object to a toxic gas, for objects that cannot be autoclaved.

Aseptic conscience

Of all things you learn in nursing, the most valuable will be the development of an *aseptic conscience*, or the state of being the strictest and most rigid judge of whether or not you have deviated from technique. Aseptic conscience can apply to medical or surgical technique. If, for example, you have begun to prepare the patient's tray for feeding and suddenly remember that you have not washed your hands since leaving the patient in the next bed, you have an aseptic conscience if you leave the tray and go directly to the nearest basin to wash, offering your patient at least partial protection from pathogens. If, while performing a catheterization, you inadvertently touch the surrounding unsterile drape with the tip of the catheter, your aseptic conscience directs you to secure another catheter and discard the first.

To remedy deviations from technique—and each nurse does at times fail to conform to technique—often takes additional time and is at best inconvenient. Much of the time, the patient will not develop an infection as a result, but the outcome cannot be predicted; the patient may be subjected to pain and further suffering due to infection resulting from just such a lapse. A nurse who knows that medical or surgical technique has been broken and does not rectify it is unfit to practice nursing. If you observe technique broken by someone else, you are equally obligated to see that the lapse is rectified to protect the patient. Simply commenting that contamination has taken place and offering to secure new equipment is usually sufficient. Sometimes the other person does not know that a lapse has occurred and will appreciate your intervention. Even if the nurse only *suspects* that technique has been deviated from, steps must be taken to correct the possible lapse. In asepsis, nothing is assumed.

The control of infection with drugs

Decreasing the number of pathogens within a host decreases the likelihood of a spread of infection. Although modern drugs are very effective in infection control, it is mistaken and often dangerous for nurses to believe that the need for precaution is less if a patient is on one of these medications.

There are at present several hundred such *antimicrobial* drugs, many simply variations of each other. Antimicrobials are, in turn, subdivided into three large categories. The *sulfonamides,* low-cost synthetics usually given orally, have an antibacterial effect. The second group are the *antibiotics*, both natural and synthetic. Natural antibiotics are derived from yeasts and molds that have a destructive effect on the more virulent pathogens. The third group, the *antifungals*, are agents used specifically against resistant fungal infections.

When you administer these preparations, it is your responsibility to know not only their actions but also their contraindications and side effects (see Chapter 10). Because these drugs have varied and potentially dangerous side effects, close observation is always in order. Besides watching for the allergic reactions that may occur in response to antimicrobials, you will observe the effect of a particular drug on the patient and his or her progress. You might note, for example, a diminishing fever, loss of the general malaise that frequently accompanies an infection, the improved appearance of an infected wound, or the patient's verbalization of a feeling of increased well-being.

Nursing care for infection

Whether the patient has a generalized or a localized infection, there are measures the nurse can take to help fight the infection process. As we have said, the ill person needs adequate rest, and the ill person with an infection needs additional sleep and rest. It sometimes requires ingenious planning of nursing care to provide for such rest. Infection makes increased demands on the body, and for this reason the diet must not be deficient. The intake of protein and carbohydrates is especially important; the protein helps in healing damaged tissue, and carbohydrates serve to meet the increased metabolic requirements caused by infection. High fluid intake prevents dehydration resulting from fever and aids in the excretion of toxins from the body.

Meticulous hygiene should be observed with the patient suffering from an infection. Such patients are often diaphoretic (perspiring) due to fever, which necessitates frequent bathing. General malaise may prevent the patient from performing adequate self-hygiene. Infection can also cause foul odors, unpleasant to the patient and staff alike, which can be alleviated through the practice of good hygiene. For example, the patient with a suppurating (pus-discharging) wound needs frequent dressing changes and cleansing of the wound area. (This is done, however, only on the physician's order.) The patient suffering a severe throat infection needs extra oral care. Finally, but importantly, the patient with an infection needs emotional support from the nurse. Infection is an assault on the body, psychologically as well as physically. It is often interpreted by the patient as meaning that things are not going well or as planned. Infection is frequently called a "complication," which understandably makes the patient anxious. The nurse can offer needed explanations of the vigorous efforts being undertaken to treat and control the infection.

Isolation

When a patient is known to have an infection, or to be especially susceptible to infection, special precautions are used to separate him or her from other patients. These precautions are called *isolation*.

Types of isolation

Isolation has two main purposes: to protect the environment from the pathogens infecting the patient or to prevent pathogens from infecting the patient. There are four types of isolation designed to protect others from the pathogens infecting the patient: *strict isolation, respiratory isolation, wound and skin precautions,* and *enteric isolation*. Protecting the patient is called *protective isolation* or *reverse isolation*. The requirements of the various types of isolation are listed in Table 11.1.

In most settings the physician determines the type of isolation to be put into effect and the length of time it is to last. The presence of an infection is determined by examining the laboratory findings, which specify the type of organism or pathogen present, its virulence, and its route of transmission. In such cases the goal is to protect others from infection. If the patient has a condition, such as severe burns or leukemia, that lessens resistance to infection, the physician will choose protective isolation until the patient's own resistance becomes adequate.

ISOLATION TO CONTROL INFECTION   *Strict isolation* is observed to restrict pathogens that may be transmitted through the air or by contact. A private room free of all unnecessary equipment and furniture is arranged. The door is kept closed. Gowns and masks must be worn by all individuals, including visitors, entering the room. Hands are washed at a basin within the room on entering and leaving. Depending on the virulence of the organism, gloves may be required of all persons entering the room and discarded inside the room before leaving, or they may be worn only for dressing changes and direct

TABLE 11.1 REQUIREMENTS OF ISOLATION

	STRICT ISOLATION	RESPIRATORY ISOLATION
ROUTE OF TRANSMISSION	Air and contact	Air
ROOM ASSIGNMENT	Private with door closed	Private with door closed
GOWNS	Worn by all persons	Unnecessary
MASKS	Worn by all persons	Worn by all persons
HANDS	Washed by all persons on entering and leaving room	Washed by all persons on entering and leaving room
GLOVES	Worn by all persons	Unnecessary
ARTICLES	All must be wrapped or discarded with care	Precautions for those with secretions

contact. All linens and other articles: whether thrown away or returned to another department in the hospital, must be *double-bagged* and clearly marked as contaminated. Double-bagging is discussed on pages 187-188.

Respiratory isolation is designed for the control of pathogens that are exclusively air-borne. Again, a private room whose door is closed at all times is necessary. Gowns and gloves are not needed, but masks are a necessity and should be discarded on leaving the room. Hands are washed on entering and leaving. Any article contaminated with excretions must be carefully disinfected or double-bagged for disposition. Individuals with known respiratory ailments or predispositions should be discouraged from visiting.

Enteric isolation is observed when the pathogen is transmitted by direct contact and the mode of transmission is the gastrointestinal system. The physician writes such an order. A private room is desirable for adults and a necessity for children because of the difficulty of controlling children's natural social tendencies. Gowns and gloves are worn by those who have direct contact with the patient, but masks are not necessary. Hands are carefully washed when entering and leaving the room. Linen should be double-bagged, and

WOUND AND SKIN PRECAUTIONS	ENTERIC ISOLATION	PROTECTIVE ISOLATION
Contact	Contact	Air and contact
Private is desirable	Private if a child	Private with door closed
Worn by all persons having direct contact	Worn by all persons having direct contact	Worn by all persons
Unnecessary except when changing dressings	Unnecessary	Worn by all persons
Washed by all persons on entering and leaving room	Washed by all persons on entering and leaving room	Washed by all persons on entering and leaving room
Worn by all persons having direct contact with dressings	Unnecessary	Worn by all persons having direct contact
Special handling of linens, dressings, and instruments	Special handling of articles contaminated with urine or feces	All articles entering room must be as clean as possible, often sterile items required

any items contaminated with urine, feces, or vomitus must be carefully discarded or disinfected. The substances themselves should be disposed of in an adjoining private toilet facility. (Urine is considered contaminated because of its proximity to the intestinal tract and the rectum.)

Wound and skin precautions, taken if there are micro-organisms in a wound that may be spread by contact, do not require the patient to be isolated; however, a private room is desirable. This procedure is sometimes called *dressing isolation*. Gowns must be worn when in direct contact with the patient, and gloves are mandatory when in direct contact with the infected area. Hands are always washed on entering and leaving the room. Special precautions must be taken with instruments, linen, and dressings. These items are double-bagged to be sent to central supply or the laundry or discarded.

Double-bagging is performed by two persons, a nurse who has been ultimately caring for the patient and a "clean" partner, who stands outside the isolated unit with a bag whose size depends on the object to be double-bagged. Cuffing this outer bag and placing the hands safely under the cuffing, the partner prepares to receive the contaminated bag. The nurse closes the contaminated bag and drops it directly into the receiving bag, making sure that it does not open. The partner then folds over the top of the outer bag, closes it securely, and disposes of the parcel. The outer linen bags are usually clearly marked with a wide red stripe of fabric sewn to the bag. If not so marked, you can mark them yourself by pinning on a note or labeled tape. Trays or dishes, if not disposable, can also be double-bagged. In fact, this method is a safe way of transporting many items. Specimens can be placed in small plastic bags for transport to the laboratory. It is health care workers' responsibility to protect each other, as well as patients, from infection. Only an unsafe practitioner knowingly allows contaminated materials to be passed unmarked to other workers. Even trash is double-bagged for this reason.

ISOLATION TO PROTECT THE PATIENT   Protective isolation requires the practices outlined above, and some others as well. The nurse garbs to protect the patient from any pathogens that could be carried to the patient on the body or clothing. Cloth boots over the shoes may be required. Any object introduced into the room is considered a potential hazard to the patient. For example, a newspaper taken from inside the stack offered for sale is likely to be freer of

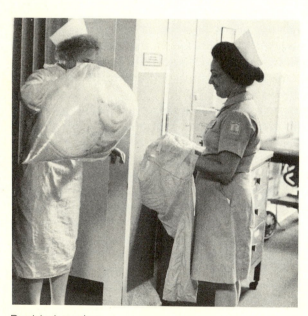

Double-bagging
Elizabeth Wilcox

pathogens than those on the outside. In some facilities, food trays are handled and prepared by a single worker to prevent cross-contamination of food. Bottled or canned beverages are poured directly into paper containers held by the nurse just inside the door of the room, or the containers themselves are sponged with hot water and soap or alcohol. Paperback books and magazines must be chosen with care from newsstands to assure that they are clean (hardback books are discouraged because they are difficult to clean). The nurse's wristwatch is not considered clean, and should be removed, pinned under the gown, or carried in a clean plastic bag. Studies have shown that pathogen growth is minimal on metal watchbands, due to the properties of the metal, but extensive on plastic or cloth bands. Money and mail envelopes can also carry harmful pathogens. Money should be kept at the nursing station for the nurse to spend on the patient's behalf when requested, and only the contents of envelopes should be given to the patient for perusal.

Because the room used for protective isolation is considered clean, all items and equipment can be safely removed and disposed of or cleaned in the usual manner. Double-bagging is not needed.

Some of the practices described above will seem extreme, and all will not be employed in every case. Individual need will determine how stringent isolation must be. However it is helpful for you to keep in mind the purpose of these measures: the patient for whom an infection could prove fatal needs every protection.

PSYCHOLOGICAL ISOLATION   Because communication is difficult through masks, and because of the inconvenience of garbing for isolation, the isolated patient rarely receives the attention and interchange afforded nonisolated patients. Holding the hand of a severely ill or depressed patient through a glove is not a wholly satisfying experience for either nurse or patient. As a result, such patients can become irritable, restless, and depressed. Psychological support for the patient throughout this difficult experience is an essential part of total care.

The role of the nurse in isolation technique

The nurse has an important and definitive role in isolation technique. You must also have the same understanding as the physician of cases of infection, so that you will know the rationale for specific practices and be able to explain it to visitors and other personnel. All isolation techniques are designed to create barriers to interrupt the transmission of disease. *Isolation technique is only as effective as the least careful person*. Therefore, a total effort must be made by everyone having any contact whatsoever with the patient, including not only the health care team but also the family, visitors, the chaplain, the newspaper deliverer, the housekeeper, the librarian, and others. You must be certain that everyone has the same information, observes the same technique, and is fully instructed on the necessary routine.

It is essential that isolation rooms be unmistakably marked for all to see. In most hospitals, cards are affixed to the door of the room to identify the type of isolation being observed. Plain white cards, cards color-coded for various types of isolation, cards with complete instructions or simply the word "Isolation" are used. It may even be necessary for you to make your own sign; if so, it is wise to print in large letters the type of isolation being observed and, below, the five or six requirements for carrying it out. Sometimes an additional sign, asking all visitors to report to the nurses' station for instructions, is posted. This is a particularly good idea, since it gives the nurse an opportunity to instruct in technique and perform health teaching with regard to infection, as well as to make contact with the family and friends of the patient.

Regardless of the type of infection or isolation, a small stand containing items needed to carry out effective isolation technique is usually placed outside the room. It may contain gowns, masks, protective caps, gloves, or even cloth boots. Equipment such as thermometers, blood pressure cuffs, materials for hygiene, and other items needed by the patient can be kept in the room itself. A laundry hamper is kept in the room.

The nurse should remove watches and other jewelry, since pathogens can be carried in the crevices and even under tight-fitting wedding bands. For the same reasons, fingernails should be closely trimmed.

Staff and visitor acceptance of isolation

Patients do not enjoy being isolated, and the staff and visitors derive no pleasure from participating in such practices, which are inconvenient, bothersome, and at times purely uncomfortable. The visitor may, in frustration, pull the mask below the nose or remove a cap covering the hair, which he or she construes as looking silly. It is up to you, then, not just to remind the visitor of the agreed-on precautions but also to back up such admonitions with kindly explanations.

Conclusion

The patient with an infection has a multitude of problems: problems of hygiene, threatened health status, and the burden of becoming a potential threat to others in the environment. The patient being protected from infection feels equally burdened. The nurse who knows both the theory and the skills of infection treatment and control can be most helpful to the patient in this situation. It is also rewarding to the nurse to grasp the relationship between the patient and the environment and to perform those nursing actions that will provide safety. Isolation is a unique situation in which health teaching, care planning, and skills evolve directly from an understanding of the invisible world of micro-organisms.

Study terms

antibiotic
antifungal
antimicrobial
antiseptic
asepsis
   medical asepsis
   surgical asepsis
aseptic conscience
autoclaving
bacteria
bactericidal
barrier
carrier
complication
disinfectant
double-bagging
fungus
handwashing
helminthic
host
infection
infectious agent

isolation
   enteric
   protective
   respiratory
   strict
   wound and skin precautions
means of transmission
micro-organisms
nosocomial
parasitic worms
pathogen
portal of entry
portal of exit
precaution
protozoa
reservoir
spore
sulfonamide
suppurating
susceptible host
virus

References

Birum, L. H., *et al*. 1971. Catheter Plugs as a Source of Infection. *American Journal of Nursing* 71:11:2150-2152.

Castle, M. 1975. Isolation: Precise Procedures for Better Protection. *Nursing '75* 5:5:50-57.

De Groot, J., and Kunin, C. M. 1975. Indwelling Catheters. *American Journal of Nursing* 75:3:448-449.

Greene, V. W. 1969. Microbial Contamination: Control in Hospitals. *Hospitals* 43:11:78.

Hardy, C. S. 1973. Infection Control: What Can One Nurse Do? *Nursing '73* 3:8:18-24.

Langford, T. L. 1972. Nursing Problem: Bacteriuria and the Indwelling Catheter. *American Journal of Nursing* 72:1:13-15.

Lee, R. V. 1973. Antimicrobial Therapy. *American Journal of Nursing* 73:12:2044-2048.

Roueche, B. 1947. *Eleven Blue Men and Other Narratives of Medical Detection*. Boston, Mass.: Little, Brown.

Rowson, L. 1970. The Lateral Position in Catheterization. *Nursing Clinics of North America* 5:1:189-190.

Selwyn, S. 1972. Changing Patterns in Hospital Infection. *Nursing Times* 5:643-646.

Streeter, S., *et al*. 1967. Hospital Infection—A Necessary Risk? *American Journal of Nursing* 67:5:526-533.

Wheeler, M. O. 1970. Surveillance, the Key to Infection Control. *RN* 33:12:38-40.

12 Hygiene

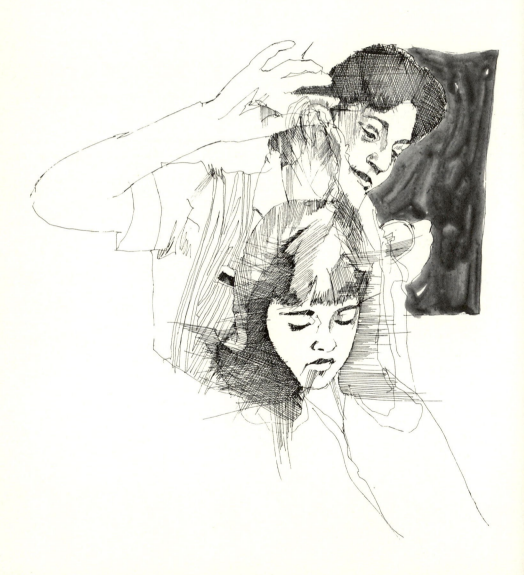

Objectives

After completing this chapter, you should be able to:

1 Name those practices that usually constitute hygienic care for the patient.

2 Indicate when in the hospital day hygiene should be administered to the patient.

3 Discuss the safety factors specific to each type of bathing procedure.

4 List the characteristics of a comfortable and safe bed.

5 Assess and plan hygiene for an individual patient, making adaptions for specific needs.

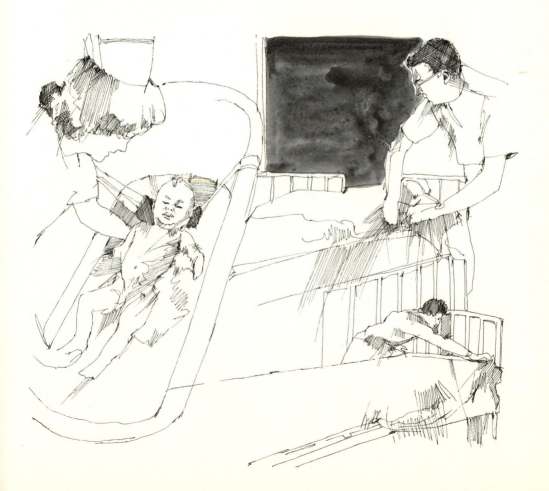

HYGIENE MAY BE DEFINED as all those practices that bring about personal cleanliness, comfort, and a feeling of well-being. Such practices vary greatly in our society and wherever you practice, it is important to be cognizant of the prevailing hygiene habits and general life style. In the hospital setting, being clean, tasteful, and neat conveys to the patient that you know the importance of good personal hygiene. In urban and rural outpatient settings, where standards of hygiene and general appearance are very different from those of hospitals, nurses' wearing apparel and hair styles may conform to those of the facility's clients. If you administer skillful and knowledgeable hygiene, the patient's confidence in your ability to perform other tasks will be enhanced. Helping patients maintain hygiene tells them that you care about their comfort.

Culture and hygiene

One has only to walk through European palaces and castles to realize that cold and dampness kept their early occupants from bathing frequently. Burning herbs and fragrances was a common practice, both to ward off disease and to disguise unpleasant odors caused by poor hygiene. As late as the first part of this century, bathing was infrequent; in fact, many people believed that frequent bathing was injurious to health.

People have become much more hygiene-conscious in the last few years. The development and sale of hygiene products has become an enormous national business. Central heating and ample supplies of hot water have made daily bathing more feasible than in the past, and the traditional "Saturday night bath" is no longer a way of life. Showers have become popular and supplement or replace bathtubs in many homes. Deodorants, shampoos, oils, powders, lotions, and a wide variety of soaps, some antibacterial in nature, enhance individual hygienic practices.

Among the many patients who do not regard a daily bath as healthful or necessary may be the economically disadvantaged persons whose dwelling does not provide proper bathing facilities or privacy and the older person who chills easily and perspires very little. Dry skin is a chronic problem for many persons, young and old, perhaps partly because of the warmth and dryness typical of American homes. Unless oils are used, daily bathing can aggravate dry skin. Finally, some people were not taught as children to bathe daily, and have thus never made it a practice as adults.

The nurse's personal hygiene

Many of the functions nurses perform are physical in nature, and thus cause more perspiration than do sedentary tasks. And synthetic uniforms, which do not "breathe" as do cotton fabrics, allow perspiration to remain on the skin and deteriorate, which can sometimes cause unpleasant odors. Personal cleanliness is essential for nurses, regardless of the work setting. Many nurses are careful to bathe immediately after arriving home from work, to remove any pathogens that might have been transmitted to them. This is a prudent practice.

It is advisable to wear a uniform only once before laundering, and to remove it immediately on arriving home. This practice prevents pathogens from being spread to the home environment. Concern for the welfare of others also suggests that a uniform worn in the hospital should not be worn in other settings, such as stores or offices. Your uniform should also be clean when you enter the clinical area, to prevent bringing micro-organisms to the susceptible patient. Some hospitals provide locker facilities where nurses may change clothes. Pediatric units have pioneered in the use of large apron-like smocks, which are worn over the uniform and can be changed during the day as needed. They are usually provided and laundered by the hospital.

The nurse should also practice good oral care. Brushing the teeth regularly leaves the mouth clean and odor-free. Caries (cavities) can be prevented; if they do occur, however, they ought to be repaired promptly by a reputable dentist. Carious teeth create a persistent mouth odor that is not relieved by brushing or mouthwash. Smokers must be certain that their breath is not unpleasant, and perhaps ought to brush even more frequently than nonsmokers. The use of chewing gum to mask mouth odor is discouraged, for it is distracting to patients and other workers; breath mints and mouthwashes are preferable.

Hair should be worn short or secured at the back of the head to prevent it from falling forward and obscuring your vision. As well as being convenient and neat-looking, these styles make it unnecessary to use your hands often to arrange your hair, which is unhygienic since it transmits micro-organisms from hands to hair and vice-versa and can scatter organisms about the immediate surroundings. Also, long loose hair will hang over patients' food as trays are served and over open wounds as dressings are changed, posing a general hazard of transmitting micro-organisms. Men's beards should be short and well-groomed for the same reasons. Regular shampooing gives all hair a shiny, healthy look.

Fingernails that are well-trimmed and filed are hygienic in that they are much easier to keep clean. Long fingernails are also likely to scratch the patient. Nail polish can chip and fall into a patient's bed or, worse, a sterile area. If polish is worn, it must be in good repair and ought to be of an undistracting pale hue.

Hospital routines for hygiene

In most hospitals it has long been the policy for each patient to be completely bathed every day. In nursing homes, where staff-patient ratios are lower, patients are necessarily bathed less frequently. Some hospitals are beginning to modify the rigid policy of bathing patients daily.

Complete morning care usually consists of a bath or shower; special perineal care; a backrub; and care of the mouth, hair, and nails. All bed linens are changed. The unit is tidied and unused items are discarded or put aside, with the patient's permission.

Partial care involves washing of particularly soiled areas of the body, usually the face, neck, hands, axilla, and perineum. Oral care and hair care are also provided, and a backrub may be included. The unit is made neat, and soiled linens are changed. It is a thoughtful practice to change the pillowcase so as to give the patient a sense of freshness.

Both complete care and partial care are sometimes referred to as "a.m. care." Unfortunately, the practice of bathing patients in the morning disregards the wishes of the individual who prefers to bathe in the evening or just before bedtime. A few facilities are beginning to offer baths at times other than the morning. This practice helps to relieve the strain on staff time during the busy morning hours and accommodates the patient who sleeps well after an evening bath.

"Early a.m. care," often provided by the night staff before the nurses' report in the morning, is preparation for the morning meal. Toilet facilities are offered and the face and hands are carefully washed. The stand is straightened and cleared to make room for the diet tray. Oral hygiene may accompany the cleaning of teeth or dentures. It is also appropriate to clean eyeglasses before giving them to the patient.

"H.s. care" (evening or bedtime care) is given in the evening just before sleep. If you think of the things you like done before sleep, you will recognize their importance to the patient. A clean gown or pajama is often appropriate. The face, hands, and back are washed and a relaxing backrub is given. Glasses and dentures are carefully put away for the night and soiled dressings or linens are replaced. Oral care is given.

There are times other than those specified when hygiene is appropriate. After using a bedpan, urinal, or toilet, the patient should be given the opportunity of washing the hands in order to remove micro-organisms. If the nurse has assisted, the nurse's hands should also be washed. Handwashing before eating should also be encouraged.

Assessing the patient's hygienic needs

The administration of hygiene has three main goals. First is the maintenance of healthy skin. Massaging and cleansing increases cellular nutrition and circulation, and thus keeps the skin intact as a line of defense against infection. Second, hygiene provides for the removal of transient micro-organisms from the body, decreasing the chances of infection. The third and in no way least important factor is the comfort of the patient. A subjective feeling of well-being occurs when the patient is refreshed and clean. An added advantage, if not a primary goal, of good hygiene is that it promotes self-esteem. Lipstick for an elderly lady in a nursing home and a shave for a businessman incapacitated by a heart attack can both enhance self-valuation.

Patients are individuals, with specific wishes and needs pertaining to hygiene. And hygiene also involves expectations of privacy. Some privacy must be sacrificed when a person becomes a patient, but the more the nurse can offer the patient the better.

You should realistically and carefully assess the hygienic needs of each of the patients assigned to you on any given day. If, for example, you are to administer a.m. care, you should determine which patients need a complete bath and which might appropriately be given a partial bath (assuming, of course, that your facility allows you to make such decisions and does not require daily morning baths for all patients). In fact, if you are to administer morning care to as many as five or six patients, it would be difficult to give each a complete bed bath. Often patients can undertake part of their own care. Allowing patients to participate in their own care helps maintain a feeling of independence, and can thus be very beneficial psychologically. Some patients who are free of drainage and excess perspiration do not need a complete bath daily. Others may need bathing more than once a day. Although the patient's needs should determine what is done, the nurse's time must also be considered. Often, the two factors must be weighed together in order to use your time as effectively as possible for the patients under your care.

The tasks of hygiene provide the nurse an opportunity to assess the patient. Physical assessment can focus on the patient's general appearance or on such factors as relative strength and the presence or absence of stiff joints. Muscles may be observed for turgor, and skin for color, dryness, and the presence of lesions. The condition of the hair, nails, teeth, and gums may also become apparent during care. Psychological assessment is no less important. The time spent with the patient can be an occasion for interaction, allowing you tactfully to explore the patient's feelings and concerns. States of confusion, depression, contentment, or elation can all become obvious to the nurse who is sensitive to others' feelings.

General hygienic measures

The bath also affords generalized physiological benefits to the patient. The activity and movement it elicits stimulate the respiratory system and improve circulation. The movement of muscles and joints maintains and promotes mobility. Since the muscles are relaxed by exposure to warm water, it is appropriate for the patient to perform range-of-motion exercises in the bathtub. Cellular nutrition and circulation are enhanced by the application of friction to the skin, and some micro-organisms and dead epithelial cells are thereby removed from the skin.

Baths

KINDS OF BATHS   The methods of bathing a patient are the bed bath, tub bath, conventional shower, and chair shower. The bed bath is performed by the nurse, who bathes the patient in bed using basins of warm water. Special draping prevents the patient from being chilled or unduly exposed. Washing is accomplished in long, smooth strokes, moving from the cleaner parts of the body to the more soiled parts. A variation of the bed bath is the towel bath, which is performed with very large towels or flannel bath blankets. The folded towels are placed in a large plastic bag containing hot water and a small amount of a special antiseptic solution that need not be rinsed from the skin. Wringing out the towels and placing them on the patient, the nurse lightly massages the patient from the feet upward, advancing the clean top sheet as the bath progresses. The back is then washed in the same fashion. Because the massage is beneficial to patients incapable of much exercise, this type of bath might be alternated with a complete bed bath. Its advantages are that the patient is not likely to be chilled if the bath is properly performed and that the skin is rendered quite moist and soft.

The tub bath is the same as the bath one takes at home. Special handles on some tubs help the patient get into and out of the tub. The tub must be disinfected well after each use.

The conventional shower is also identical to that taken in the home, the patient standing beneath an overhead shower head.

A chair shower is administered in a cabinet that allows the patient to remain seated in a shower chair. A waist-high partition may enclose the shower area, permitting the nurse to assist while remaining dry. It is questionable, however, whether the nurse can give an effective shower from such a position. A newly available device consists of a horizontal shower cabinet that allows the bedridden patient to be showered on a special stretcher.

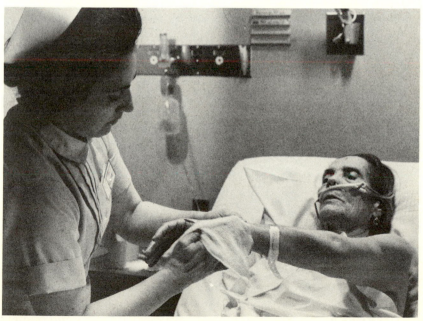

Elizabeth Wilcox

The method of bathing chosen will be determined not only by the patient's preference but sometimes also by his or her condition or the physician's orders. For example, a patient with a full leg cast cannot shower or take a tub bath, and a patient on strict bed rest or in isolation also has a restricted choice.

ADMINISTERING THE BATH Whatever method of bathing is chosen, certain general principles must be adhered to in the interests of efficiency, comfort, and safety. Following the Procedural Checklist on page 154 will make the bath, like any other procedure, easier to perform. It is essential to elicit the patient's cooperation and participation in the procedure; only the unconscious patient cannot be an active participant.

Water temperature always poses a hazard and must be carefully checked. Tubs are filled and showers run *before* the patient enters, and water for the bed bath is checked before being applied to the patient. A bath thermometer is sometimes difficult to find but, if you are unsure of the temperature, an ordinary thermometer can be used. With practice, most nurses become quite adept at recognizing safe temperatures by testing water on the wrist; but until you become skilled at doing so, always test the water with a thermometer. It is advisable to ask patients whether or not they use soap on their faces: soap can be irritating, and dangerous to the eyes, if not used with care. Many soaps are drying, and oil might be added to the bath water for patients with obviously dry skin. The patient who showers could apply a small amount of oil after the shower.

Safety is a major factor in a patient's bath or shower. Most facilities have installed handrails in the tub or shower area, and the patient should be encouraged to use them. A towel placed in the bottom of a tub or on the floor of a shower provides for more secure footing. The extremities should be washed from the *distal*, or farthest, point from the body to the *proximal*, or nearest, point, thus increasing the venous return of blood. For specific directions on administering the various types of baths, the procedure manual of the facility or a skill module may be consulted.

USING DEODORANTS, BATH POWDERS, AND SOAPS Individuals respond differently to products such as deodorants and bath powders. If a person has used a product for a certain period of time, there is probably no danger of toxicity. But, if such a product is new to the patient, it is prudent to use it sparingly until its safety has been established.

The active ingredient in many antibacterial soaps and hygiene products is hexachlorophene. In the early 1970s a study revealed that the use of this chemical in high concentration caused brain lesions in newborn monkeys. Though such serious effects have not been demonstrated in humans, the U.S. Food and Drug Administration issued a warning that hexachlorophene in concentrations of more than 3 percent should not be used on newborn infants. This policy has expanded to most hygiene products on the over-the-counter market today, making them safe to use.

Increasingly meticulous hygiene has been accompanied by growing popularity of what advertisements call "feminine hygiene sprays." These products are, in fact, perineal deodorant sprays whose value is questionable. They are quite irritating to many women, and have been proven to cause severe reactions in some.

Shaving the patient

Daily shaving is necessary for many men to appear and feel well-groomed. Even some men with beards shave the edges of the beard to give it the shape they desire. Furthermore, some patients develop skin irritations if they do not shave; the hairs hold perspiration on the skin, causing a fine rash. Male patients quite often bring their own razors to the hospital, but some hospital units have electric razors available for patients' use. The blades of such communal razors must be soaked in disinfectant solution between patients. Alternatively, disposable safety razors designed for one-time use are very efficient to use. If you stretch the skin slightly taut, shaving a patient is not a difficult task. Using warm towels to moisten the skin before shaving makes it easier. The shaving soap the patient customarily uses will be the best choice. Bed patients should always be shaved before the bottom linen is changed, since small hairs that fall into the bed can cause discomfort.

Perineal care

The perineal area requires meticulous care, due to its heavy concentration of bacterial growth. This phenomenon is due to the excretion of feces and urine and to the deep creases of the groin, which provide bacteria moisture and warmth in which to grow. A thick, cheesy substance called *smegma*, a secretion largely composed of dead epithelial cells in the area of the perineum, can act as a reservoir for bacteria. Cleansing ought always to be done from front to back, or from the urinary orifice to the intestinal orifice, to prevent contamination of the urinary tract with intestinal organisms. Good perineal care is thus a matter of careful cleansing. It is important to emphasize the necessity of frequent perineal care for the patient who has an indwelling catheter in place. The region around the catheter should be cleaned well before cleansing the remainder of the area.

If able, patients should be given the opportunity to perform their own perineal care. While providing the bed patient with clean water, soap, a cloth, and a towel, you might ask, "Would you like to finish your own bath now?" " . . .wash between your legs," " . . . wash your genitals," or " . . . wash the crotch area." Use words the patient is likely to understand, and then allow sufficient time and privacy. If the patient is unable to perform this task, undertaking it in a professional, efficient manner will help relieve anxiety or embarrassment on either side. This aspect of care may discomfit the inexperienced student, but practice makes it a more routine matter; the patient will become more relaxed as you do.

A *douche* is an irrigation of the vagina. The fluid used may be any of a variety of commercial products, a mild vinegar solution, or tap water. Because douches can destroy the normal flora of the vagina, leading to infection, douching is regarded as unnecessary for the normal healthy woman.

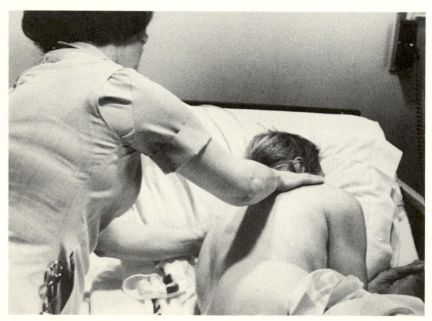

Elizabeth Wilcox

The backrub

The backrub is a nursing art much cherished. It is thus disconcerting when a nurse pours a bit of lotion on the hand, briskly rubs up and down the patient's back, and considers the patient to have had a backrub. A backrub or massage is given for two purposes: stimulation and relaxation. A rub after a morning bath may be given to stimulate the skin and muscles; before sleep, a soothing, relaxing backrub encourages rest. If the patient falls asleep during a backrub of the latter type, the nurse should feel a sense of success. Both the extent of the backrub and the type of stroke used, including the amount of pressure, will determine the effect on the patient.

It is always good practice to keep the hands in constant contact with the patient's skin, using long smooth strokes. There are various correct methods of massage, in all of which the main focus is on the coccyx and buttocks and the full length of the spinal column. The nurse's hands radiate upward and over the shoulders, giving extra treatment to the muscles of the neck, which become quite taut when the patient spends a lengthy time in bed. Lotions are the most popular lubricants to use for massage: they replace the moisture lost in the skin, have a pleasant odor, and allow the hands to move smoothly. Powder also makes for a smooth rub, but it is both drying to the skin and potentially dangerous if inhaled. If powder is used, care must be taken to prevent inhalation by patient or nurse. If the patient has a fever, alcohol is occasionally used; it evaporates quickly and cools the patient. On cooling, however, it becomes sticky in consistency and makes strokes jerky unless more alcohol is added. Alcohol also has a drying effect on the skin.

The backrub is a part of the administration of the bath, and should be considered as such. Often, when a backrub is offered, the patient declines on the basis that "it's too much trouble" for the nurse. The nurse should explain that it is no trouble because the patient's skin, which is in contact with the bed, needs such care. In addition, most patients very much enjoy backrubs and many ask for such attention. Because it brings such pleasure to the patient, the nurse may also enjoy it. It is often an opportune occasion to talk quietly with the patient, and conveys a caring attitude.

Oral care

Oral care consists of assessment, treatment, and care of the teeth, mouth, and gums. It is important for every patient, but particularly so for the unconscious or immobilized patient. Illness and contingent problems involving diet and fluids cause the patient's mouth

to need almost constant attention. The patient becomes uncomfortable if the mouth is dry and unpleasant-tasting, due largely to the
accumulation of sordes. *Sordes* are composed of mucus, epithelial
cells, and bacteria that adhere to the teeth and inside the mouth.
The lips or tongue may develop painful cracks or fissures, and a
foul odor may be present.

Patients who are in relatively good health can perform oral
care as they would at home. For those who must be given oral care,
the nurse must assess what is needed. In general, the teeth are
brushed and the inside of the mouth and the lips cleaned and moist-
ened. Dentures can be brushed with a special denture brush or an
ordinary toothbrush. Commercial powders and creams are sold for
this purpose but, if the patient does not have these items, toothpaste
or even plain water can be used. Dentures may be stored overnight
in a safe container, immersed in a solution or dry, depending on
their composition. Mouthwashes, though pleasant and refreshing,
do not kill micro-organisms. Dental hygienists tell us that the use of
dental floss is as effective or more so than brushing, and removes
sordes that cannot be removed with a brush. Another recent aid to
oral hygiene is the high-pressure water appliance known as a Water
Pik. Though improper use can cause gum damage, its effectiveness
has now been proven.

For patients unable to undertake their own oral care, a number of techniques are needed. If the patient is able to hold water
in the mouth and spit it back out without choking, the nurse may
perform regular oral care with a toothbrush and dental floss. If the
patient is unconscious, oral care becomes both more difficult and
more necessary, since sordes accumulate rapidly when a person
mouth-breathes and cannot swallow saliva. If conventional flush-
ing techniques are used, however, the patient may aspirate fluid.
Thus the teeth are cleaned with cotton swabs dipped in a solution.
You may wish to make up an oral hygiene tray containing various
solutions, all clearly labeled, as well as cotton swabs. Whether you
use commercially made swabs or make your own, care must be
taken that the gauze or cotton is secure and cannot be inhaled or
ingested. Nurses have different preferences on solutions to use for
oral care. Buttermilk was popular until it was proven to promote
the formation of caries. A mixture of glycerine and lemon is still
widely used, but lemon can damage tooth enamel if used for a
long time. Glycerine, rather than moistening the mouth, can absorb moisture from mouth tissues, contributing to damage of the
mucous membranes. A diluted solution of hydrogen peroxide,
with a small amount of mouthwash added for esthetic purposes,
has good cleaning properties.

If the lips are dry, a light coating of water-soluble oil may be applied. (Oils used around the nose and/or mouth should always be water-soluble so as not to be harmful if inhaled into the lungs.) The patient receiving oxygen needs oral care more often than usual. Oxygen is very drying and patients with oxygen hunger tend to mouth-breathe, which dries the tissues of the mouth and increases the accumulation of sordes.

Nail and hair care

Complete general hygiene also involves attention to the nails and hair. Orange sticks are usually kept on hospital units for cleaning under patients' nails, since ill patients can collect secretions, loose skin, and pathogens there. It is the policy of many institutions for only the head nurse or podiatrist to trim the nails of diabetic patients, in view of the fact that diabetics are very prone to difficult-to-heal infections. The very slightest nick may have such a consequence. Filing the nails of diabetic patients is thus often safer than cutting. Filing is also preferable in the case of the older patient with extremely hard and thick toenails, which can be almost impossible to cut with scissors or clippers. Soaking the nails before cutting is usually beneficial. It is

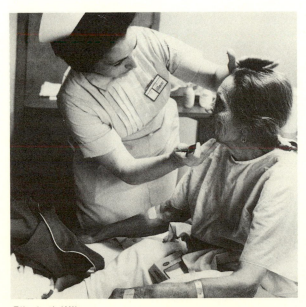

Elizabeth Wilcox

important to examine the patient closely for rough nails, which can cause abrasions of the skin.

Hair can become a significant problem in the hospital, for both the patient and the staff. Long hair quickly becomes matted from rubbing against bedding. A small amount of alcohol or vinegar applied to the hair, and subsequent brushing, will often remove such tangles, but alcohol dries the hair and should only be used occasionally. It is advisable to arrange the hair in an attractive and convenient manner of the patient's choosing soon after admission to avoid problems. (Braids or pigtails are popular ways of arranging long hair.) You can usually assess the frequency of the patient's need for shampooing. Most hair does not need to be washed every day. Dry shampoos may be used with bed patients, but can cause itching of the scalp and discomfort; some such patients can be placed on a stretcher and taken to a basin where, with padding under the head, the scalp and hair are washed. Using a device that combines a funnel with a plastic or rubber sheet, you can wash the hair of the patient unable to be removed from bed. The need to have the hair shampooed can become a major concern for patients, especially women with long hair.

Care of the patient's bed

The patient's bed is, in many cases, his or her environment. Precisely because of the long periods patients must spend in bed, nurses must exert their efforts to make the bed a place of comfort and safety.

Proper placing of linens such as draw sheets, incontinent pads, and turn sheets allows the bed's cleanliness to be easily maintained and saves the nurse and the patient the inconvenience of having to change the entire bed. For the patient who cannot turn without help, a turn sheet can be made from a bath blanket folded in quarters or a draw sheet folded in half and placed under the heavier portion of the patient's body. It is much easier for nurses to turn a patient by grasping the sides of this device than by grasping the patient's extremities. This method is also more comfortable and safer for the patient.

When making a bed, whether the patient is in the bed at the time or not, four goals should be kept in mind. First, the surface under the patient should be smooth and free of wrinkles. The patient with sensitive skin can develop pressure sores, or decubitus ulcers, because of the slightest wrinkle. Even wrinkles in the underbedding—such as the mattress pad, bottom sheet, or plastic sheet—must be smoothed to prevent such occurrences. Second, all surfaces that touch the patient must be meticulously clean. To protect the patient from micro-organisms, the linens that are nearest to the body must be changed as needed. Third, enough bedding should be used to keep the patient warm. The physical work you do may make you feel quite warm, but you should not assume that the patient resting quietly in bed is equally so. A good index is to ask patients how many blankets they want. A single blanket is usually enough, since hospitals are kept quite warm. Finally, the well-made bed must give the patient room for adequate movement. An overly neat bed that constricts movement is not a service to the patient. Loosening the bedding over the feet is especially important so that, when the patient is lying on the back, the feet are not in constant extension but remain in anatomical position, the toes pointing upward.

Comfort and safety are more important considerations, but a neat appearance should be strived for in making a bed. It is possible to make a neat bed without ignoring the more important factors.

Conclusion

In giving hygiene, you are usually performing tasks the patient would undertake if able. To the patient, conscious or unconscious, this is a valuable service. In learning the skills that comprise good hygiene, you, as a beginning student, will gain needed confidence in your own abilities. The performance of these skills combines theory and practice in many areas of nursing, such as asepsis, control of infection, maintenance of mobility, and physical and psychological assessment. Hygiene represents total patient care, and is never an isolated task. To leave a formerly soiled, disheveled, and uncomfortable patient in a state of cleanliness, comfort, and repose is a reward in itself.

Study terms

backrub

bed bath

caries

cavities

chair shower

coccyx

crotch

dental floss

dentures

deodorant

deterioration

douche

epithelial cells

fissure

flora

genitals

hygiene

hydrogen peroxide

massage

mouthwash

oral hygiene

orange stick

orifice

perineum

podiatrist

range-of-motion exercises

shower

smegma

sordes

swabs

taut

towel bath

tub bath

turn sheet

water-soluble

Water Pik

References

Davis, B. D. 1947. A Patient's View of Back Rubs. *American Journal of Nursing* 47:2:112.

Davis, E. D. 1970. Giving a Bath? *American Journal of Nursing* 70:11:2366-2367.

Gibbs, C. 1969. Perineal Care of the Incapacited Patient. *American Journal of Nursing* 69:1:124-125.

Greenleaf, J.; Staley, R.; and Payne, P. A. 1974. Portable Shower for Bed Patients. *American Journal of Nursing* 74:11:2021.

Johnson, B. 1965. The Meaning of Touch in Nursing. *Nursing Outlook* 13:2:59.

MacKenzie, A. 1970. Effectiveness of Antibacterial Soaps in a Healthy Population. *Journal of the American Medical Association* 211:2:973-976.

Newton, M. 1967. Feminine Hygiene. *Nursing Fundamentals*. Dubuque, Iowa: Wm. C. Brown, pp. 141-147.

Rietz, M., *et al*. 1973. Mouth Care. *American Journal of Nursing* 73:10:1728-1730.

Should Genital Deodorants Be Used? 1972. *Consumer Reports* 37:39-41 (Jan. 1972).

Tassmann, G. C.; Zayon, G. M.; and Zafran, J. N. 1963. When Patients Cannot Brush Their Teeth. *American Journal of Nursing* 63:2:76.

Temple, K. D. 1967. The Back Rub. *American Journal of Nursing* 67:10:2102-2103.

Warning Issued Against Some Uses of Hexachlorophene. 1972. *American Journal of Nursing* 72:2:342.

Wiley, S. B. 1969. Why Glycerine and Lemon Juice? *American Journal of Nursing* 69:2:342-343.

Part Three
Physiological Needs of the Patient

13 Basic Vital Functions

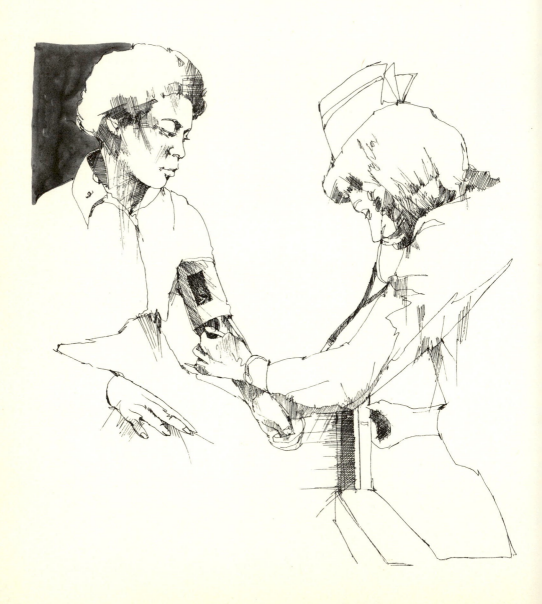

Objectives

After completing this chapter, you should be able to:

1 Discuss the bodily processes called *basic vital functions*.

2 Define the terms used to report on basic vital functions.

3 Recognize when observations and measurements of vital functions are necessary.

4 Learn the skills involved in measuring basic vital functions.

5 Integrate measurements of vital functions with general observations to make a complete assessment of vital functions.

6 List the four levels of awareness and the assessments appropriate to each.

7 List the observations that should be made in checking neurological signs.

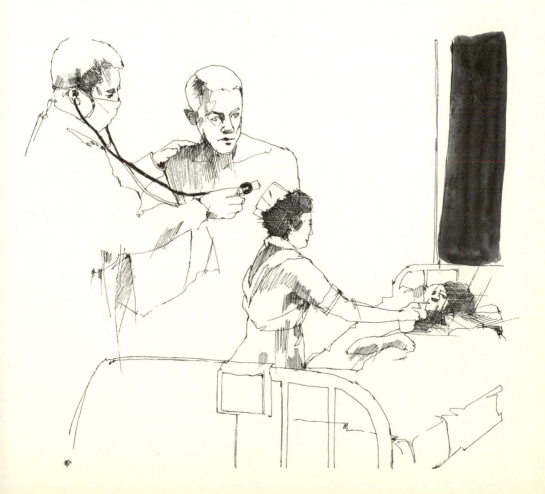

I N A SENSE, every life function is vital but there is a group of functions without whose activity the body is unable to survive more
than a short time. These are the *circulatory, respiratory*, and *neurological* functions. *Temperature regulation* will also be discussed
here, because of its close affinity to the other vital functions and because its disturbance is similarly life-threatening, though not so
quickly.

Measurements that indicate the functioning of circulation,
respiration, and temperature regulation are commonly called *vital
signs*. In some places they are referred to as "the cardinal signs." Observations of neurological functioning are called simply *neuro signs*
(neurological signs).

Circulation

The function of the heart is to pump blood through the vessels, in order to transport oxygen and nutrients to, and to remove
waste products from the cells. Failure of the heart to function will result in death within a few minutes. Furthermore, if circulatory function is not restored within three to five minutes, irreversible brain
damage can occur. Because the heart responds to the condition of
other parts of the body, observation of its functioning can also provide information about such other phenomena as infection, shock,
and anxiety.

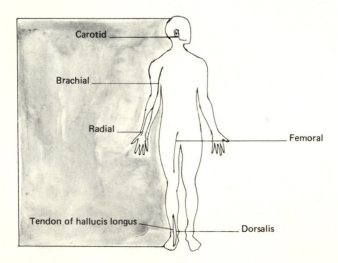

FIGURE 13.1   PULSE POINTS

Pulse

The pulse is a shock wave produced within the artery as the heart beats. It can be felt as an increase in the size of the artery each time the heart contracts. Thus, counting the pulse rate (beats per minute) is an indirect means of counting the heart rate. The pulse is present in every artery, but is counted at those points where a large artery passes close to the surface and can be easily palpated, or felt. (See Figure 13.1.)

For reasons of convenience and accessibility, the pulse is most commonly counted at the radial artery in the wrist. It may be counted at other points if information on circulation to a particular body part is needed. For example, femoral and popliteal pulses may be checked to assess the effectiveness of circulation to the leg. Heart rate may be counted directly over the apex of the heart by listening with a stethoscope placed over the space between the fifth and sixth ribs, directly below the arch of the left side of the clavicle. (See Figure 13.2.) This measurement is called the *apical pulse*. On occasion, some heartbeats are so weak that the waves they produce in the artery cannot be felt in the periphery. In such a case, the heart rate will be greater than the peripheral pulse. The difference between the apical and radial pulse rates, measured simultaneously, is called the *pulse deficit* and represents the number of weak, ineffective beats per minute.

Electronic pulse counters are now in limited use. Some function by sensing pulse in the earlobe, some in the tip of a finger.

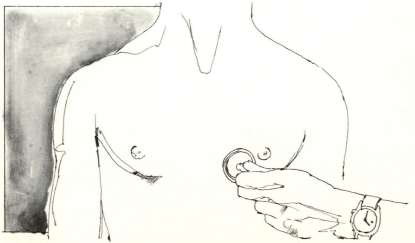

FIGURE 13.2   TAKING AN APICAL PULSE   Place the stethoscope between the fifth and sixth ribs, below the arch of the left clavicle.

These devices are very accurate, and make possible identification of even slight changes in pulse rate.

Pulse rates may vary greatly, and are affected by such factors as activity, eating, emotional tension, drugs, and illness. Mild to moderate activity usually raises the rate 20 to 30 beats per minute. In the healthy individual, the rate will return to normal within two minutes after discontinuing such activity. Age is also an important determinant of pulse rate: the infant's pulse rate is very rapid—120 to 140 per minute—and decreases throughout life to approximately 80 per minute in the adult.

Consistent strenuous exercise will cause the heart to enlarge and to beat more slowly and forcefully. Thus a normal resting pulse rate for an athlete may be 50 to 60 per minute.

An adult pulse rate below 60 per minute is referred to as *brady-cardia*, while a pulse rate that is above 100 is called *tachycardia*. Because these are relative terms, the heart rate itself is a more accurate way of characterizing heart function.

The length of time pulses should be counted has been variously recommended as fifteen, thirty, and sixty seconds. At least one study (Jones, 1967) found that the shortest duration was the most accurate for regular pulses, probably because it allows for fewer counting errors. Irregular pulses may need to be counted for sixty seconds in order to compensate for irregularities over time. Apical pulses are also usually counted for a full minute. Because all manually counted pulses deviate somewhat from direct readings taken by an ECG (electrocardiogram), the pulse rate should be considered approximate. If gross abnormalities are found, the pulse should be rechecked. An effort should be made to use a consistent technique so that trends and changes may be noted. It is advisable to check the policy of a facility when you begin working there so that your technique will be consistent with that of others who are checking a patient's pulse rate. One source of counting error can be avoided by beginning the count at 0 instead of 1, so that you are counting the beats that actually occur within a given period. For a patient whose condition is such that even small changes in rate and rhythm are serious, an electronic monitoring system is used.

It is also important to observe the *rhythm* of the pulse. A normal pulse has a regular beat. When the beat is irregular, the specific type of irregularity should be noted, since it may be of diagnostic significance. For example, double beats (bigeminy) may occur, either occasionally or at frequent regular intervals. The rate may vary from rapid to slow and back, or beats may be "skipped." Any such pattern needs to be recorded.

The *quality* of the pulse indicates the strength of the heart's contractions. It may be weak and "thready"—that is, the movement of the artery may be so slight that the artery feels threadlike—or strong and "bounding," which indicates that the blood is being propelled forcefully by the heart.

Blood pressure

The pressure of the circulating blood is a significant indication of the effectiveness of heart action and of the adequacy of the blood supply to the tissue. The term *blood pressure* usually refers to arterial pressure measured in millimeters of mercury. However, the pressure in the largest veins—central venous pressure (CVP)—is also an important indicator of circulatory efficiency.

An indirect measure of bood pressure using a sphygmomanometer (blood pressure cuff) and a stethoscope is commonly performed over the brachial artery at the elbow. It is also possible to measure blood pressure over the popliteal artery behind the knee, using a large cuff on the thigh. The principle underlying indirect measurement is that blood flowing through healthy arteries does not make sounds audible through a stethoscope. When the flow of blood in the artery is occluded by external pressure, and the pressure is then reduced until the heart is again able to pump blood through the artery past the point of occlusion, a sharp sound called a *Korotkoff sound* is produced with each contraction. The pressure at which the blood is first able to push past the point of occlusion and make a sound is equal to the *systolic* pressure, or the maximum pressure exerted by the heart during a contraction.

True *diastolic* pressure is the lowest pressure maintained in the artery between heart contractions. Indirect measurement of this pressure has been the subject of some difference of opinion. As the pressure applied by the blood pressure cuff continues to decrease after the first sounds are heard, a change or "muffling" of the sounds occurs. Then, as the pressure decreases more, the sound disappears entirely. Direct measures of blood pressure reveal that neither of these points, the muffling or the cessation of sound, is consistent with true diastolic pressure. In healthy arteries, the true diastolic pressure is usually 10 millimeters below the muffling and may coincide with the cessation of sound. However, in arteries diseased due to atherosclerosis, the sound may continue to be heard far below the true diastolic due to turbulence in the vessel. At present, the American Heart Association recommends that a blood pressure reading consist of three figures: (1) the first sounds heard, (2) the muffling of sound, and (3) the cessation of sound (even if this figure is zero). The

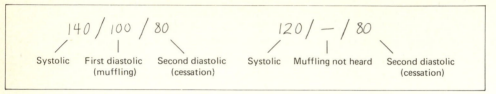

FIGURE 13.3   RECORDING BLOOD PRESSURE READINGS

A.H.A. labels these figures the systolic, the first diastolic, and the second diastolic. When a muffling is not detected, a dash may be drawn to indicate the lack of a figure. (See Figure 13.3.) If the facility where you are working records only two figures, be sure to check the policy to determine whether to measure the first or second diastolic. If only one is to be recorded, it is usually the second.

Blood pressure measurements are sometimes made by people with minimal training, and there are many possibilities of error in selection of cuff size, acuity of hearing, and reading of the instrument. When a gross abnormality is reported, it is wise for the nurse to recheck the measurement. .

Direct measurement of arterial blood pressure is ordinarily performed in special care units. A special catheter must be inserted into an artery, and equipment that permits direct readings of blood pressure is then attached. Various new electronic machines for the indirect measurement of blood pressure have been invented, but are not yet in general use.

Blood pressure is lowest in the newborn—approximately 40/20—and gradually increases to the adult level—approximately 120/80—during adolescence. Statistically, blood pressure rises as the individual grows older. However, recent evidence suggests that this phenomenon may be due not to aging but to decreasing physical activity. Those who maintain regular physical activity and do not gain excessive weight are less apt to experience increases in blood pressure with aging. As is true of all other body measures, there are wide individual variations in blood pressure. The "normal" range for adults is 110-140/60-90. Pressures above 160 systolic and/or 100 diastolic are are labeled *hypertensive*. A systolic pressure below 100 is labeled *hypotensive*. Such judgments must not be made, however, without gathering baseline data on the individual to determine whether the blood pressure reading represents the person's usual blood pressure or is an isolated instance.

Many factors affect blood pressure. Activity, drugs, anxiety, anger, joy, or any strong emotion can cause a sharp *rise* in blood pressure. Anything that dilates blood vessels or causes blood loss will result in a *fall* in blood pressure. The pattern of rising or falling blood pressure is important to the diagnosis of many pathological conditions.

Another important indicator is the difference between the systolic and the diastolic readings, which is called the *pulse pressure*. An increasing pulse pressure may indicate a serious problem, such as an increase in intracranial pressure.

When changes are noted in blood pressure and when medications are given to alter blood pressure, measurements may be taken at frequent intervals, in some cases as often as every five minutes. For other patients, such as those in rehabilitation, blood pressure may not be measured after an admission screening. The physician may make a decision on the frequency of blood pressure checks, but it is the nurse's responsibility to recognize any situation that demands closer monitoring and to act independently as necessary.

Central venous pressure is measured by a catheter inserted into a large peripheral vein and threaded into a large central vein. This catheter is kept open by an intravenous drip, and direct measurement of the pressure may be taken with a special manometer that can be attached. Measuring central venous pressure is an advanced technique, usually performed in special care units by nurses with additional training. More detailed information on the procedure is available in several of the references listed at the end of this chapter. Its use is increasing and may soon become widespread.

Respiration

There are two types of respiration. Internal respiration is the exchange of gases at the cell level. External respiration is the exchange of air between the environment and the lungs and the movement of gases from the lungs to the blood stream. The following discussion will concern external respiration.

Controlling respiration

Respiration is controlled by the respiratory center in the medulla of the brain. The primary stimulus to breathing is a rise in the carbon dioxide level of the blood. This mechanism is sensitive to minor changes, and keeps the blood level fairly stable by means of regular respiration. The respiratory center also responds to low blood levels of oxygen. However, this backup mechanism is less sensitive and, operating alone, produces irregular respirations and "peaks and valleys" of blood oxygen and carbon dioxide levels.

The autonomic nervous system can also affect respiratory rate, and is the mechanism responsible for the increasing respiratory rate that accompanies tension and anxiety. It also causes the body to change breathing patterns with changes in air temperature.

Respiration can also be voluntarily controlled. With thought and attention, a person can temporarily stop breathing or change the pattern of breathing. This control is secondary to the involuntary controls, and can only be maintained while the body is receiving adequate oxygen supplies. Thus an angry child may hold his breath until he loses consciousness, but involuntary control then causes him to resume breathing.

Assessing respiration

The first task in respiratory assessment is to check the *rate* of respiration. A single cycle of inspiration and expiration is counted as one respiration. It is usually easiest to count inspirations. Because it is difficult for a patient to maintain a normal breathing pattern

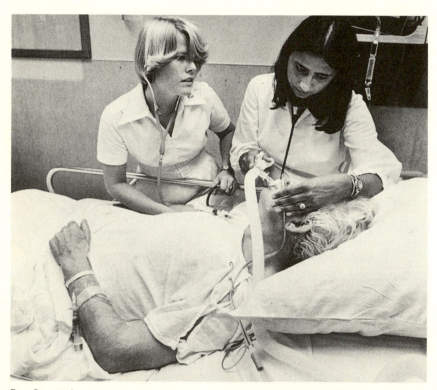

Dan Bernstein

knowing he or she is being watched, the nurse often counts by resting the patient's arm across the chest with the nurse's hand in place as if feeling for the pulse. The risings of the chest can thus be felt and counted. Beginning the count at zero will make for a more accurate count. Because only 14-20 respirations per minute are normal in the adult, counting for 30 seconds is preferable. If the respirations are irregular, however, counting for a full minute may be desirable. The respiratory rate is highest in the newborn—35-40 per minute—and gradually decreases, reaching the adult level in adolescence. Respiratory rate is increased by activity, fever, anxiety, and all the factors that affect the pulse rate. Many health problems create rises in respiratory rate, while others cause the rate to decrease. Very rapid respiration is called *tachypnea*. The absence of respiration is called *apnea*.

The extent to which the whole lung is involved in respiration is the *depth* of respiration. A shallow respiration is one characterized by minimal chest movement, and thus minimal air exchange. A deep respiration is one in which the rib cage is fully expanded and the diaphragm descends to create maximum lung capacity. Shallow respirations are not effective, even at a rapid rate, because they produce air movement in the physiologic dead space, where no gas exchange with the blood can take place, and inadequate air movement in the alveoli where gas exchange takes place. Sighing and yawning are automatic mechanisms to increase ventilation by forcing deep breaths. A pattern of shallow respiration is called *hypoventilation*. In addition to the lack of oxygen exchange, hypoventilation causes secretions to accumulate and alveoli to collapse. This problem, common to immobilized patients, can be combatted by encouraging movement, deep breathing, and coughing. Very deep respirations are called *hyperpnea*.

Healthy respirations have a regular *rhythm* characterized by expirations twice as long as inspirations. Irregularities in rhythm may indicate the presence of illness. Very deep, rapid respirations (tachypnea and hyperpnea), gradually tapering off to the point of cessation of respiration (apnea) and then gradually returning to hyperpnea and tachypnea, are called *Cheyne-Stokes* respirations and indicate that the patient is in very critical condition.

Normal breathing does not require thought and is free of discomfort. Pain on breathing is always a sign of something wrong. One of the first indications of pain on breathing is the patient's attempt to "splint" the painful area—that is, to hold it firmly to prevent movement. *Dyspnea* is breathing that requires conscious effort or work. It is normal after vigorous exercise, but abnormal in other situations.

Normal breathing is usually quiet, characterized only by the sound of air movement. Thus rattling, moistness, bubbling, *râles*—moist, crackling sounds in the small airways—or other sounds indicate a problem. Increasingly, nurses are using stethoscopes to listen for early symptoms of respiratory distress.

The cough is a protective mechanism for removing lung secretions and such foreign matter as dust, sprays, and the like from the respiratory tract. However, a cough may persist without raising any sputum and eventually exhaust the patient. Your concern should be aroused by any cough that produces large quantities of sputum or is prolonged or persistent. Normal sputum is a clear, semi-liquid mucus. Sputum that is thick, copious, colored, or flecked with other substances should be reported, and a sample should be saved for the physician to inspect or the laboratory to analyze.

Basic life support

In May 1973, the National Conference on Standards for Cardiopulmonary Resuscitation (CPR) and Emergency Cardiac Care recommended, among other things, that all medical and allied health personnel be trained in techniques of basic life support. These techniques include: (1) recognition of airway obstruction, (2) recognition

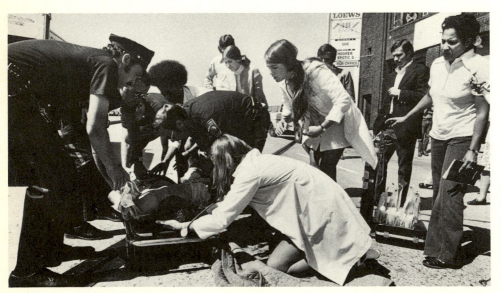

Dan Bernstein

of respiratory arrest and cardiac arrest, and (3) ability to perform cardiopulmonary resuscitation.

It is necessary for *all* health care personnel to be so prepared because resuscitation cannot wait for the arrival of special personnel. Resuscitation must begin as soon as the need is discovered. Special personnel or teams trained to perform more advanced life support measures can then be summoned to continue care. Some communities are even establishing extensive programs to teach basic life support skills to as many citizens as possible. These are not exclusively medical skills.

In an attempt to standardize techniques of CPR, the 1973 conference formulated and recommended "Standards for Cardiopulmonary Resuscitation (CPR) and Emergency Cardiac Care," which were published in a supplement to the *Journal of the American Medical Association* (see end-of-chapter references). No training in CPR is adequate unless it provides both a theoretical understanding of the process and mannikins on which to practice one's skills, but some basic concepts will be reviewed here.

Recognizing the need for life support

Because all basic life support measures have the potential to injure the victim, it is essential that a clear determination of need be made before undertaking them. The absence of breathing is determined by observing for chest movement and feeling for air movement through the mouth and nose. The use of a mirror or glass to check for moisture, and thus breath, has been recommended by some, but taking the time to find such an item could be inadvisable in an emergency. Sometimes chest movement can be felt when it cannot be seen.

The absence of heart action is determined by checking for pulse in the carotid arteries. Peripheral pulses are not checked because they may be too weak to be detected, though the heart is still beating. Checking for dilated pupils is sometimes recommended as a means of checking for circulation to the brain. Fixed and dilated pupils may indicate anoxia of the brain, but are not used as a criterion for the initiation of action.

Administering emergency life support

The actions that constitute emergency life support are most easily remembered as "the ABCs," or (1) Airway, (2) Breathing, and (3) Circulation.

The airway is checked and, if necessary, cleared, and positioned to maintain *patency* (open passage). Then rescue breathing

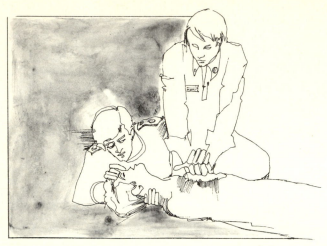

FIGURE 13.4   THE ABC OF CPR   Emergency life support can be administered most efficiently by a team of two rescuers. To start: check, clear, and position the *airway*. Second, restore *breathing* by mouth-to-mouth resuscitation. Third, restore *circulation* by massaging the heart.

(mouth-to-mouth resuscitation) is begun. After breathing has been established, circulation is restored by means of external cardiac massage. This process is performed most efficiently by two people (see Figure 13.4) but may be carried out by a single person.

Your school of nursing or the hospital where you have laboratory practice may train you in emergency life support. Alternatively, such training is available from some fire departments, the Red Cross, and local chapters of the Heart Association. It is your responsibility to see that you acquire these emergency skills and review them as often as necessary to maintain your proficiency.

Maintenance of body temperature

Body temperature is regulated by the hypothalamus in the brain, which balances heat production and heat loss. The human body's temperature must be maintained within very narrow limits for the optimal functioning of its various physiological processes. The normal temperature range is only 3.5-4.0°F (6-7°C), from 97°F (36.1°C) to 100.4°F (38°C). The "normal" body temperature is considered to be 98.6°F (37°C) when measured orally. Axillary temperature (temperature measured under the arm) is normally 1°F

(.6°C) lower, and rectal temperature is 1°F (.6°C) higher. Some researchers believe, however, that inadequate measuring techniques account for these differences.

Because it is subject to a twenty-four-hour cycle called its *circadian* rhythm, body temperature is highest from 4:00 to 8:00 p.m. and lowest in the early hours of the morning. Women also experience a temperature change cycle associated with the menstrual cycle: the body temperature increases .5-1°F at the time of ovulation and decreases again at the time of menstruation.

"Normal" temperature varies among individuals. The elderly often have relatively low normal temperatures, which is probably a function of their slower metabolisms. Infants' and young children's normal temperatures may be a full degree higher than adults'. For this reason, a single temperature reading provides only very general information unless it is considered in light of other data on the patient.

Heat production

Heat is produced by metabolism, and is therefore a by-product of all activities and processes within the body. The *specific dynamic action* of foods is the energy expended in the process of digestion and absorption. Because heat is always produced in this process, eating can produce an almost immediate increase in feelings of warmth. Muscular activity also produces considerable heat. Shivering is involuntary muscular activity that has the effect of increasing the body temperature. Infections and inflammations increase tissue metabolism, and thus increase tissue heat.

Heat loss

Heat is lost through four processes: radiation, conduction, convection, and evaporation. *Radiation*, the loss of heat to another object without contact, occurs constantly. *Conduction* is loss of heat through direct contact with another object. *Convection* is heat transfer caused by moving air, which carries heat away from the body surface to be replaced by cooler air. *Evaporation* also has a cooling effect, because the conversion of liquid to a gas requires heat energy. Evaporation of moisture occurs constantly from the surface cells, and more extensively through the secretion of perspiration from glands beneath the skin.

Heat loss is increased by the dilation of peripheral vessels, which transfers heat from the body core to the surface where heat loss can occur more readily. Increased perspiration also hastens heat loss by providing for more evaporation. The process of heat loss can be enhanced by using fans or a breeze to increase convection or by applying moisture to the body to bring about evaporative cooling. An automatic cooling blanket increases conduction of heat from the body by circulating cool water through tubing within the blanket. Such a blanket is usually equipped with a rectal thermometer and a means of regulating the temperature of the blanket.

Heat loss is minimized by the contraction of muscles in the hair follicles, causing "goose pimples," which in turn raises hairs on the body surface to provide an insulating layer and decrease convection. This process is most effective in individuals with large amounts of body hair. Vasoconstriction on the body surface decreases all forms of heat loss and preserves the heat of the body core. Adding layers of clothing or blankets decreases radiation and conduction, and also reduces convection losses by preventing air movement next to the skin. Because the blood vessels of the head do not constrict in response to cold, covering the head is particularly effective in preserving body heat.

Hypothermia

When body temperature drops so low that the metabolic processes are slowed to a point incompatible with life, a condition known as *hypothermia* occurs. Its initial symptoms are loss of judgment, confusion, and uncontrollable shivering. After a brief period this massive effort to generate body heat may exhaust the body's energy reserves. The body is then no longer able to maintain heat-producing activity, and temperature continues to drop until death ensues.

Hypothermia may occur accidentally due to exposure. Air temperatures need not be below freezing to cause fatal hypothermia. Winds that greatly increase convection cause "wind chill," whose effect is the same as that of a much lower temperature without wind. Getting wet can contribute to hypothermia by greatly increasing heat loss through evaporation and by providing a medium for conduction of heat away from the body. The combination of wetness and wind can cause hypothermia even when the air temperature is above 50°F. Treatment consists of providing hot drinks, food, and an external source of heat such as a fire or another person's body. Simply providing covering will not restore body heat, because the body has lost the ability to produce its own heat.

Hypothermia may also be purposefully induced to facilitate the performance of certain types of surgery. Because metabolism is slowed, tissues can be deprived of blood supply for a certain period of time without sustaining permanent damage. This technique has been particularly useful in certain heart and brain surgeries. The patient is anesthetized and given medications to prevent the body from exerting its heat-producing abilities, and then the body temperature is lowered to the desired level by means of hypothermia blankets and drugs. In the past, ice-water baths were used. When the surgery has been completed, the patient is either rewarmed with heating pads or allowed to recover his or her own heat-producing abilities. The body temperature must be closely monitored during the entire process to insure that it does not fall too low. Care must also be taken to see that upon return to normal, the body's heat-regulating mechanisms function correctly.

Fever

Fever, or *pyrexia*, is defined as a body temperature 1°F (0.6°C) or more higher than normal. It occurs when the body sets its temperature-regulating mechanism higher than usual because of infection, the presence of a toxin, or a disease of the endocrine or central nervous system. Because the body both increases heat production and initiates measures to prevent heat loss until the new temperature is attained, a fever is often preceded by "chilling." Shivering is thus a heat-producing mechanism. Withholding blankets and other aids to comfort will not prevent the development of a fever; it will simply increase the cost in energy of reaching the temperature level set by the hypothalamus.

Various terms are used to characterize fevers. In a *remittent* fever, the temperature is always elevated but may rise and fall considerably. An *intermittent* fever is one in which the temperature rises each day but sometime during each twenty-four-hour period returns to normal. A *constant* fever is one in which the temperature remains elevated at a constant level.

A high temperature is not always harmful. It is now recognized that some slight rises in temperature help the body to combat infections by increasing metabolic rates and providing a less favorable climate for some disease organisms. Often, however, the temperature rises so high that the body's energy stores are depleted and the temperature interferes with tissue functioning. For example, high temperatures may interfere with the functioning of the central nervous system and induce confusion, hallucinations, and even convulsions. Infants and children are especially susceptible to these effects.

FEVER REDUCTION   Temperatures above 114.8°F (46°C) are not compatible with life, and tissue damage may begin to occur at 105°F (40°C).
In order to maintain a margin of safety, then, measures to combat
fever are usually undertaken when the temperature reaches 101°F
(38.4°C). Measures to lower body temperature include antipyretic
medications such as aspirin and acetominophen; cooling baths of tepid water, ice water, or alcohol; the use of fans; and special cooling
or hypothemic blankets. There is some controversy over the use of
the various kinds of baths. All are cooling, but alcohol causes excessive dryness of the skin and ice water causes profound vasoconstriction in the skin. Both are extremely uncomfortable for the patient.
For these reasons, tepid baths may be preferred. In life-threatening
situations, enemas of cold water—or even ice water—may be used to
bring about rapid cooling of the body core. When a fever recedes, it
is said to have "broken." Profuse sweating occurs as the body resets
its temperature at a normal level.

ASSESSING FOR FEVER   A person with a fever commonly has a flushed
and dry skin that feels warm or even hot to the touch. The eyes lose
their luster. The person may report feeling listless and weak and may
complain of headache. Although the need for food is great because of
the high metabolic rate, lack of appetite and even nausea may be
present. "Fever blisters" on the lips are caused by the herpes simplex
virus, which may emerge due to the weakened resistance of the
body. The effect of elevated temperature on the central nervous system tends to cause irritability and anxiety. The body may lose quantities of water through perspiration, resulting in symptoms of dehydration (see Chapter 14).
       If all patients' temperatures are taken daily to screen for fevers,
doing so in the late afternoon or early evening, such as at 6:00 p.m.,
will be most likely to reveal low or intermittent fevers. The temperatures of patients with infections, those with special risk of infection
(new surgical patients, new mothers), and those whose temperature-
regulating mechanisms might not be functioning (the brain-injured,
young infants) are often measured every four hours.
       Whenever a patient "chills" or appears to have a fever, the
temperature should be taken as part of a complete assessment. Although health care facilities adopt policies on the frequency of
temperature-taking, such policies are not intended to substitute for
individual decision making. You should not hesitate to perform
this task more frequently if necessary. While a temperature is rising, and again when steps have been taken to reduce it, you may
check the temperature every 15-30 minutes.

INTERVENING IN FEVER   The physician must be notified of a fever so that it may be diagnosed and appropriate medical treatment may be ordered. If an infection is thought to be the cause of the fever, it may be necessary to culture wound drainage and to take steps to prevent the spread of infection to others (see Chapter 11).

In addition to medications or special baths the physician may order, many independent nursing actions may be taken for the patient with a fever. Comfort is a primary need. The skin may be dry and characterized by excessive salt deposits due to perspiration. Frequent bathing followed by the application of a lotion will promote a feeling of well-being and preserve the integrity of the skin. Because the skin of a feverish person is often very sensitive, bedding should be kept smooth and tight and should be changed as needed. Care should be taken to avoid bright lights and direct sunlight, to which the eyes may be sensitive. A cool, moist cloth placed over the forehead and eyes will often be welcomed. Petroleum jelly or another lubricant will prevent cracked or dry lips. The patient will be most comfortable if the hair is arranged off the forehead and neck.

Providing adequate nutrition can be very challenging. Liquids are of primary concern in order to prevent dehydration. Frequent offerings of cool liquids, especially slightly tart drinks such as fruit juice, may be welcomed. Foods ought to be light and simple. The prostration and weakness brought about by the fever may necessitate feeding the patient; otherwise the patient may fail to eat simply because the effort is too great.

Measuring temperature

In the United States, body temperature is usually measured in degrees Fahrenheit, but hospitals are increasingly adopting the Celsius (sometimes called *centigrade*) scale. Though Fahrenheit measurements are more familiar, Celsius measurements are more readily used in combination with other measurements, such as when calculations of calorie or fluid requirements must be made.

The most common instrument for temperature measurement is the glass thermometer containing mercury. Although careful attention is paid to quality control in their manufacture, some thermometers do exhibit errors in calibration or other aspects of manufacture. Whenever an extremely low or extremely high temperature reading is made on a glass thermometer, therefore, the temperature should be rechecked with a different thermometer.

To obtain an accurate measurement, the glass thermometer must be correctly positioned. For an oral temperature reading, it must be under the tongue, touching the tissue, with the lips closed. A rectal thermometer's bulb must be inserted one inch beyond the internal sphincter. The bulb of the axillary thermometer should be placed against dry skin of the axilla itself, not against the upper arm and chest.

The extent of time a thermometer is left in place may be the greatest contributory factor to errors in measurement. Oral thermometers must be in place ten minutes for children and eight minutes for adults to insure accurate readings. Only three minutes are required to obtain a maximum reading from a rectal thermometer. An axillary thermometer should be left in place ten minutes.

Although smoking two minutes before insertion of an oral thermometer does not significantly raise mouth temperature, the mouth temperature is lowered by drinking ice water and does not return to normal until five minutes later. There appears to be no significant change in oral temperature when a nasal oxygen catheter or nasogastric tube is in use. Therefore, rectal temperatures appear to be necessary only for persons who mouth-breathe and thus cannot keep their lips tightly closed.

Another instrument for measuring temperature is the electronic thermometer, which provides a much more rapid and accurate reading than does a glass thermometer. Its use also eliminates the hazards of broken glass and escaping mercury, and, because the probe covers are disposable, makes cleaning and sterilizing unnecessary. Furthermore, it is not necessary with some models for the patient to hold the mouth closed, because the reading is taken directly over a small artery under the tongue. However, these instruments are both very expensive and easily damaged if dropped or handled roughly. The method of use is specific to each brand, but in general, a temperature-sensitive probe is attached to an energy source and a measuring device. The temperature appears as lighted numerals or is indicated on a dial. Duration of use and placement are specified by the manufacturer.

Neurological function

The brain has been described as a computer for the body. Although there are dissimilarities, both the brain and the computer possess memory banks and circuitry, and need input from contact with the external environment; furthermore, neither performs physical tasks but both direct how such tasks will be done. In addition, the brain has unique capacities for synthesis (combining separate ideas for the first time), creativity, and evaluation not shared by computers.

Recognizing the indicators of brain function

A primary manifestation of brain function is "level of awareness," which is apparent in the type of external stimuli to which the person responds. A high level of awareness indicates alert functioning. A low level of awareness indicates diminished functioning, which is critical because a nonfunctioning brain is not compatible with life.

Levels of awareness are affected by a number of factors. Stimulants such as coffee, tea, and drugs may increase the level of awareness. Conversely, lack of oxygen and lack of glucose to the brain tissue diminish the level of awareness. Injury, tumor growth, shock, poisons, and infections can all diminish the level of awareness. The administration of anesthesia is a deliberate means of decreasing awareness.

Among other manifestations of brain function are muscle control, coordination, and strength; the functioning of reflexes; and the regulation of vital functions (pulse, blood pressure, temperature, and respiration). It is often up to the nurse to detect and report subtle changes in brain function—changes that may be observed and tested for while providing care.

The observations considered necessary for adequate assessment of the patient suffering neurological deficit are fairly uniform from one care facility to another. The six parameters generally specified—(1) blood pressure, (2) pulse, (3) respiration, (4) level of awareness, (5) pupillary response, and (6) muscular strength—will be discussed in more detail below.

Assessing neurological function

Levels of awareness are a continuum ranging from normal to total lack of awareness. When assessing, describing, and recording assessments of neurological function, you should train yourself to think in terms of *awareness*, not consciousness. Of what is the patient aware? Of what is he or she unaware? Such determinations provide the health care team a relatively clear idea of the patient's neurological status. Also, making the assessment as specific as possible renders changes in status more noticeable. For example, if a patient who did not previously appear aware of the lowering of a side rail begins to roll about when the rail is let down, you might conclude that the patient's level of awareness has risen and report this incident as a sign of improvement.

Specific testing is required to determine whether the level of consciousness or awareness is rising or diminishing. One technique is to observe the patient for signs of awareness of voices or noise. The patient may, for example, grimace or move about in bed. You may also call the patient's name to see if he or she responds. This technique is referred to as *name-call* and charted as such. A bit more sophisticated is the *command*: instruct the patient to do something, such as to "move your left leg" or "squeeze my hand," and observe the response. The only requirement is to command something the patient is reasonably capable of carrying out. A step neurologically beyond response to a command is *verbalization*. Depending on the patient's visual acuity, you might ask what color the ceiling or a bright cup is.

At a normal level of awareness the patient is alert and oriented, responsive to questions, and interested in the surroundings. By direct questioning or inference, you can determine whether the patient knows who he is, where he is, the date, and the approximate time of day. When recording, we generally use the term "person, place, and time," and the entry on the patient's record might read, "Patient is oriented to person, place, and time."

Let us consider four levels of decreased awareness in order of increasing severity. *Confusion* is a state characterized by some disturbance of awareness. Confused patients may not know their whereabouts, the date, or even their names. It is important to verify how confused a patient is by testing for this information. For example, a patient may know his name and where he is, but have no idea of the year; any variation is possible in a confused state. You must be cautious when gathering such information, for assertions that sound confused may not be so. For example, an elderly patient in an acute care facility stated that she was dictating a book about Indians in Montana. Though she was severely handicapped and had come to the facility from a nursing home where she had resided for some time, she had indeed been writing such a book. Another patient stated that he had walked to a town fifty miles away the night before, when the nurses knew he had been in bed: this was clear evidence of confusion.

Another state of decreased awareness, which may or may not coincide with confusion, is *delirium*. It is often characterized by great activity or hyperactivity. The patient may exhibit anxiety, see images that are not there (hallucinations), and be incoherent (not understandable) of speech. The delirious patient appears uninterested in the surroundings.

The patient in *stupor* may continue to be confused, but is even less responsive to the immediate surroundings. The stuperous patient is lethargic (drowsy) and responds only when stimulated. Methods of stimulating a response will be discussed shortly. Stupor invariably arouses concern that the patient is seriously ill and may be in danger of dying.

The most profound stage of unawareness is *coma*. In this state, the patient cannot be aroused. Neurological functioning is seriously compromised, and such other vital functions as respiration, heartbeat, and temperature regulation are often affected. The patient's subsequent recovery may be in some doubt. When the patient is in deep coma, it is important to know whether he or she responds to *painful* or *noxious stimuli* (either phrase may be used when charting). Nurses usually attempt to elicit a response by firmly pinching the chest or abdominal skin or the earlobe to the point of pain. Testing both sides of the body is essential.

As a nurse, you should be able to make accurate and complete assessments of neurological functioning. You need not be a specialist in neurological nursing to undertake the rather simple tests and observations that can provide the physician crucial information on which to base a diagnosis. We have already described how to assess for confusion by questioning the patient about person, place, and time. You should also look closely at the physical appearance of the patient. If the patient smiles, is the face symmetrical (even on both sides)? If not, a facial palsy may be present. Are there any visible twitches of the muscles? If so, where do they begin? Are they on both sides? How long do they last? Blood pressure and pulse are again important measurements. If the blood pressure rises and the pulse rate falls (just the opposite of shock), the patient could be suffering from increased intracranial pressure. Take these measurements carefully and frequently—as often as every fifteen minutes—for the neurologic patient. If the patient is less responsive than earlier, can he or she grip your hand? Is the grip of equal force with both hands?

The eyes are excellent indicators of neurological status. Does either eyelid droop; if so, which one or both? Does the patient blink? Are the pupils of equal size and active in response? To test activity, a flashlight beam is passed from the side of the patient's head over the curvature of the eye. The pupils should constrict in response to the light. In natural light, are the pupils dilated or constricted? Normal pupils are usually described as "equal and active"; in some facilities, the words "equal and brisk" or "equal and reactive" may be used.

The physician will often test a series of body reflexes. One reflex with which you may not be familiar is the *Babinski reflex*. Ordinarily, it is abnormal for the patient to have this reflex, though it is a normal finding in a newborn infant. The Babinski is elicited by stroking the sole of the foot, from heel to toe, with a sharp object. A broken tongue blade edge is commonly used by nurses. It is a positive or abnormal reaction for the toes to "flare"; if the toes fold under or downward, the response is negative or normal.

Muscular strength can be checked by asking the patient to

squeeze your hand. Check both hands to assess relative strength; note whether strength is equal in both hands.

Charting neurological function

Charting information about neurological function accurately is every bit as important as recording any vital sign. You should use the same terms employed by the other members of the health care team. The value of the nurse's assessment, description, and charting of neurological data cannot be overestimated. Such assessment can, in many cases, indicate whether or not a particular treatment is successful, and can guide revisions in the nursing and medical care of the patient.

Conclusion

Assessing basic vital functions is a key to thorough understanding of the patient's condition. As you acquire skill in making these assessments, you will become increasingly comfortable caring for very ill patients. You will become able to discern changes in the patient's status, and will have the foundation for skilled nursing intervention.

Study Terms

CIRCULATION

blood pressure
  diastolic
  systolic
bradycardia
hypertensive
hypotensive
Korotkoff sounds
pulse points
  apical
  brachial
  femoral
  popliteal
  radial
  temporal
tachycardia

RESPIRATION

airway
apnea
cardiopulmonary resuscitation
Cheyne-Stokes
depth
dyspnea
hyperpnea
hypoventilation
râles
rate
rhythm
sputum
tachypnea

BODY TEMPERATURE	NEUROLOGICAL FUNCTION
circadian rhythm	awareness
fever	Babinski reflex
constant	coma
intermittent	confusion
remittent	consciousness
heat loss	delirium
conduction	intracranial
convection	neurological signs
evaporation	noxious stimuli
radiation	painful stimuli
hypothermia	palsy
pyrexia	stupor
specific dynamic action	symmetrical

References

Bell, S. 1969. Early Morning Temperatures? *American Journal of Nursing* 69:4:764-766.

Beamont, E. 1975. Product Survey: Blood Pressure Equipment. *Nursing '75* 5:1:56-62.

Devney, A. M., and Kingsbury, B. A. 1972. Hypothermia in Fact and Fantasy. *American Journal of Nursing* 72:8:1424-1425.

Erickson, R., and Storlie, F. 1973. Taking Temperatures: Oral or Rectal and When? *Nursing '73* 3:4:51-53.

Gernert, C., and Swartz, S. 1973. Pulmonary Artery Catheterization. *American Journal of Nursing* 73:7:1182-1185.

Jones, M. 1967. Accuracy of Pulse Rate Counted for 15, 30, and 60 Seconds. M.A. thesis, University of Washington, Seattle.

Marcheondo, K. 1974. CVP: The Whys and Hows of Central Venous Pressure Monitoring. *Nursing '74* 4:1:21-24.

Nichols, G. A. 1972. Taking Adult Temperatures: Rectal Measurements. *American Journal of Nursing* 72:6:1090-1093.

Nichols, G. A., and Kucha, D. 1972. Taking Adult Temperatures: Oral Measurements. *American Journal of Nursing* 72:6:1090-1093.

Neilson, M. A. 1974. Intra-arterial Monitoring of Blood Pressure. *American Journal of Nursing* 74:1:48-53.

Palen, C. 1975. The Passage. *American Journal of Nursing* 75:2004-2005.

Purintum, L. R., and Bishop, B. E. 1969. How Accurate are Clinical Thermometers? *American Journal of Nursing* 69:1:99-100.

Standards for Cardio-Pulmonary Resuscitation (CPR) and Emergency Cardiac Care (ECC). 1974. *Journal of the American Medical Association* 227:7 (Feb. 18, 1974). Supplement.

14 Nutrition and Fluids

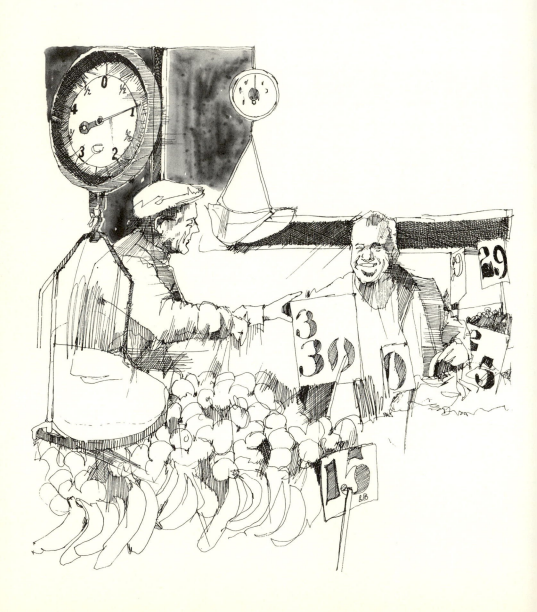

Objectives

After completing this chapter, you should be able to:

1 Discuss the meaning of "good nutrition," describing in detail how a diet can be evaluated.

2 Discuss the need for fluids and the many problems created by low fluid intake.

3 Assess the patient with regard to nutritional and fluid and electrolyte status.

4 Identify problems related to nutritional and fluid intake.

5 Plan nursing intervention to meet nutritional and fluid needs.

6 Evaluate the effectiveness of nursing intervention undertaken to satisfy food and fluid needs.

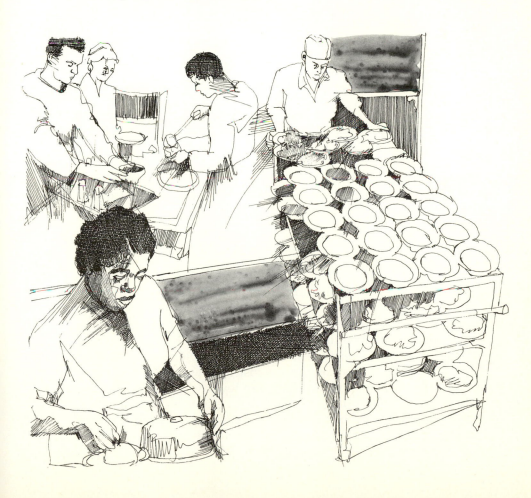

FOOD AND WATER are among human beings' most basic needs for survival. A person cannot be without water for more than a few days; then the body becomes unable to function. One can survive for a somewhat longer time without food, because the body can consume its own stores of fat and protein to provide for its most essential functions. But this supply is limited, and very soon the body cannot function.

Even those who nursed in antiquity, without education or understanding of disease processes, were aware of the value of nourishing food. Through trial and error, they had found some foods more helpful than others in restoring health. They also recognized that, in certain illnesses, some foods are better tolerated than others. Many nineteenth-century home nursing manuals focused mainly on the preparation of special broths and other foods for the sick person. Awareness of invalids' need for fluids is long-standing, and most foods were in liquid or semi-liquid form.

Basic nutrients

In the broadest sense, good nutrition consists of eating foods that provide all the nutrients needed by the body in amounts adequate for *energy, maintenance, repair, replacement* of tissue, and—in the young—*growth*. It also involves avoiding an excessive amount of any nutrient that can damage the body.

As our knowledge of body physiology and our understanding of foods have grown, the definition of good nutrition has expanded. We now recognize as essential a wide variety of nutrients and are beginning to ascertain the optimum amount of each that is needed for good health.

Carbohydrates

Carbohydrates are the starches and sugars in the diet. All fruits and vegetables have some carbohydrate content, but cereal grain products are the major source. Carbohydrates have approximately the same caloric value per unit of weight as proteins, but because they require less extensive metabolism they are available more quickly for energy. A majority of the calories in most diets are consumed in the form of carbohydrates, because they are low-cost, readily available foods. This is appropriate, because most primarily carbohydrate foods also contain needed vitamins, minerals, and even some plant proteins. The only exceptions are refined simple sugars, which do not have other food value. Providing additional carbohydrate is a way of increasing calorie level to meet the special requirements of growth or unusual activity. Carbohydrate intake exceeding current need is converted in limited amounts to glycogen (an animal starch) for storage in the liver. Carbohydrate in excess of that level is converted to fat for long-term storage.

Proteins

Proteins are the basic material for building and repairing body tissue. Amounts in excess of these needs are broken down into carbohydrates and nitrogen; the nitrogen is excreted and the carbohydrate is used just as is dietary carbohydrate. It is important to understand this process when advising people on their diets. Protein foods are usually the most expensive items in the diet, but large amounts are not necessary. Although protein needs may rise due to illness or injury, you will find that some people have exaggerated views of how much protein is required. It is quite satisfactory to consume only the necessary amount of protein, deriving additional calories from carbohydrate, when money is limited. Proteins do have an additional value when calorie control is necessary, in that their slow digestion and metabolism makes for long sustained calorie availability.

Fats

Fats are the most concentrated form of food energy. Though necessary to the diet because they serve as building-blocks for essential body components and as vehicles for the transport of certain fat-soluble vitamins, large amounts of fats can quickly raise the calorie value of the diet to an undesirable level. Excessive fats, especially saturated fats, are also receiving attention as contributing factors in coronary artery disease. Therefore, it is currently recommended that no more than 25 percent of the dietary calories be from fats.

Minerals

Minerals are present in a number of foods. Some, such as calcium and iron, are needed in fairly large amounts; of others, such as copper and zinc, only minute traces are needed. Excesses and deficiencies of these trace minerals are receiving increasing attention for their possible role in the origin of illness. The most common mineral deficiency is probably iron deficiency in women who are in the reproductive years and menstruating. The loss of menstrual blood increases the body's need for iron. The most effective means of supplying it is to consume adequate dietary iron.

Vitamins

Vitamins are minute organic substances essential to body processes. The list of vitamins is still growing, as more are discovered. Vitamins are found in a variety of foods. Fat-soluble vitamins are stored by the body, allowing for intake to fluctuate. The majority, however, are water-soluble, and must be ingested daily because amounts not currently needed are rapidly excreted.

Fiber

The need for nondigestible *fiber* in the diet recently began receiving increased attention. Fiber, or roughage, is composed mainly of cellulose and is found in fresh fruits and vegetables and in whole-grain cereal products, either raw or cooked. These fibers increase the bulk of the stool, making it pass along the bowel more easily, which helps to prevent constipation. Recent research has also demonstrated a higher incidence of certain diseases of the bowel in those who eat highly refined diets lacking in fiber or roughage. Though the exact relationship has not been determined, this finding enhances recognition of the need for a highly varied diet, restricted only when absolutely necessary. A wide range of foods makes probable an adequate intake of needed nutrients of which science is still ignorant.

Recommended diet

The Food and Nutrition Board of the National Research Council has established a standard called the *Recommended Dietary Allowance* (RDA) for most nutrients. Differing recommendations are made for different age levels and after age nine, for males and females. There are also special recommendations for pregnant women and nursing mothers. The exact recommendations may be found in a nutrition textbook. They are very generous, providing for considerable variance among individuals and for changes in needs due to minor illness. They do not, however, allow for needs caused by major illness or trauma. Recommendations are given for all nutrients on which there exist sufficient research data to establish need. Thus there are no recommendations for nutrients necessary in very small amounts, or those for which the exact need has not yet been established.

The RDA standard may not be attainable by low-income per-

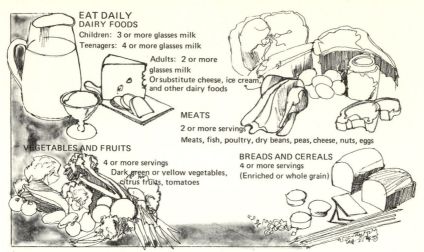

EAT DAILY
DAIRY FOODS
Children: 3 or more glasses milk
Teenagers: 4 or more glasses milk

Adults: 2 or more
glasses milk
Or substitute cheese, ice cream,
and other dairy foods

MEATS
2 or more servings
Meats, fish, poultry, dry beans, peas, cheese, nuts, eggs

VEGETABLES AND FRUITS
4 or more servings
Dark green or yellow vegetables,
citrus fruits, tomatoes

BREADS AND CEREALS
4 or more servings
(Enriched or whole grain)

FIGURE 14.1   THE FOUR BASIC FOOD GROUPS

sons or those who live in parts of the world where food supplies are
limited. Minimum daily requirements have been established by
some official groups, including the Canadian government. Because
these standards do not take individual variations into consideration,
they are of limited value. However, they may be useful in evaluating
diets to establish gross deficiency or malnutrition.

Nutritionists at the U.S. Department of Agriculture have devised a simple way to plan meals that supply the RDA, called the
Basic Four (see Figure 14.1). This approach is based on the most
common American dietary pattern, and other meal patterns may
be very nutritious and supply all the RDA without conforming to
the standards of the Basic Four. Thus it is much more accurate to
evaluate a diet in terms of the RDA than of the Basic Four.

Recent research reveals that variations in need among individuals may be much greater than was previously thought. The pre-
dominantly European background of most Americans has meant that
the value of milk for all persons has gone undisputed. Now we have
evidence that some persons, primarily of Asian and African origin,
do not have the digestive enzymes necessary to properly utilize milk
after the age of three or four years. For these persons, milk is not
merely of little value, but is actually harmful, causing gas, diarrhea,
and digestive upsets. Thus the concept of good nutrition must be
constantly modified in light of the latest knowledge.

Interest in vegetarian diets is currently widespread, for religious, economic, and philosophic reasons. A vegetarian diet can be
well balanced and supply the basic nutrients if it is very carefully

planned, incorporating a wide range of plants and plant products. It is easier to supply all nutrients if milk is included in the diet, known as a *lacto-vegetarian* diet. If eggs are also eaten—the *ovo-lacto-vegetarian* diet—it is still easier. The key is careful planning. Lifelong vegetarians have been found to have excellent health and longevity records. Certainly, the common American diet contains more meat than is needed, and one in no way jeopardizes health by decreasing meat intake.

Determinants of food intake

Hunger is a physical sensation of discomfort caused by an empty stomach. Hunger also seems to be affected by some poorly understood central nervous system mechanisms, and such factors as blood sugar level may play a part.

Appetite, the desire to eat, is affected by both physical and emotional factors. Appetite can be limited in focus to a specific food or group of foods, and may cause a person to eat far more than the body needs. Likewise *anorexia*, the loss of appetite, can prevent a person from eating even though the body requires more food.

Satiety is the feeling of having eaten a sufficient amount. Some foods, such as fats, promote satiety because they are digested slowly and thus remain in the digestive tract a relatively long time. Satiety may also be affected by central nervous system controls, blood sugar levels, and perhaps other unknown factors, as is hunger. Some persons do not seem to experience satiety even when the stomach is full, and thus tend consistently to overeat.

Sociocultural influences on diet

Culture

All societies impose values on food, making some foods more acceptable or desirable than others. Puréed foods are seen as infant foods in the United States, as is milk in some African nations. Other foods, such as champagne and cavier, are accorded prestige or status. Food that is familiar and typical of one's family or social group may arouse feelings of warmth and belonging. For example, the person from a traditional German background may derive feelings of security and comfort from dishes like sauerbraten and veal stew with dumplings because they are reminiscent of the comfort and security of the

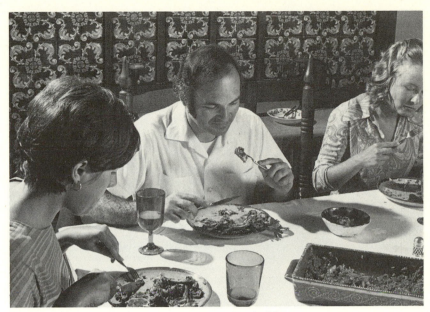

Culture has an influence on people's eating habits.
Top: *John Urban*; Bottom: *Peter Southwick / Stock, Boston*; Overleaf: *Owen Franken / Stock, Boston*

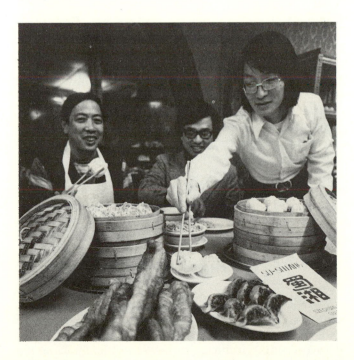

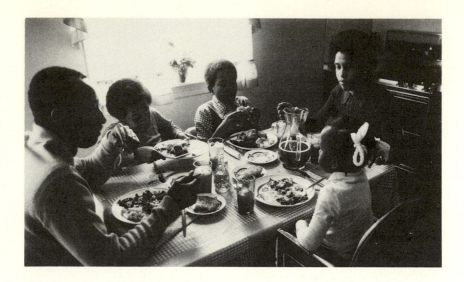

home. During illness, what is familiar may be a remedy in itself. For this reason, one person will prefer chicken soup when ill while another considers tea the perfect cure for all illness. The feelings associated with a given food may render it tolerable to the digestive system when nothing else is acceptable.

Some foods, though very nutritious, are simply not acceptable in certain cultures. In fact, cultural aversion to a food can be so great as to cause nausea and vomiting. Fish eyes elicit this response from many in Western cultures, although they are nutritious and considered a delicacy in Asia. The most extreme manifestation of cultural aversion is a food that is made taboo or forbidden.

The patterns of meals are also cultural in origin. American travelers to Europe find that breakfast is coffee and a bread-type roll in one country, and a large and hearty meal in another. The main meal is eaten at noon, at 6:00 p.m., or at 10:00 p.m. by different groups of people. In the United States we are accustomed to a pattern of three meals a day, while in England a fourth, small meal called "tea" is served in the late afternoon. People become used to a given meal pattern, and tend to become hungry at the usual time.

Religion

Some religions have dietary rules that are an aspect of their religious observance. Orthodox Jewish law, for example, requires that all foods be obtained, prepared, and served according to specific rules. For example, meat and milk products are kept completely separate, and pork, scaleless fish (like eels), shellfish, and other foods are not eaten. Food that conforms to Jewish dietary rules is called *kosher*. Hospitals in areas where there are many orthodox Jews may be equipped to provide kosher food. If you work in such a setting, you will need to be familiar with the rules for serving kosher food. If such food is not available, the orthodox Jew will usually eat nonkosher food as long as foods specifically prohibited by Jewish law are omitted. It should be expected that such a person may eat poorly while hospitalized because of emotional aversion to nonkosher food.

Some Christians omit certain foods from their diets during the Lenten (pre-Easter) season. Many Roman Catholics still omit meat on Friday, though it is no longer required by the Church. These customs may usually be set aside during periods of illness, but some persons prefer to maintain them regardless of circumstances. The individual's wishes are of primary significance, regardless of policy.

Adherents of many Eastern religions, such as Hinduism, are vegetarian. Eating flesh is so repugnant to such persons that even suggesting they do so may cause them to be ill.

Income

The income of a family largely determines its diet. Meat and fresh fruits and vegetables tend to be expensive, and those with limited finances eat more of such less expensive foods as bread, potatoes, and other starches. Such a diet might cause one to be overweight and undernourished. Severe economic deprivation usually restricts the quantity of food available, which could result in severe underweight and inadequate growth and development in children.

Personal preference

Everyone has likes and dislikes with regard to food. Given the variety of foods available in the United States, it should be possible to plan nutritionally adequate diets composed only of foods a person likes. When a person's likes and dislikes are taken into account in planning meals, the person is more likely to eat well. However, extreme and numerous dislikes may interfere with good nutrition, especially when a special diet is needed.

Emotional attitudes

In addition to culturally induced attitudes toward certain foods, food in general may evoke strong feelings. Food is often used as a reward for children, and the resulting attitudes persist into adulthood.

When food is withheld, for example, a person may feel punished. Or one may want to reward oneself for enduring illness by eating favorite foods, even when they are contraindicated. The person responsible for withholding desired foods may be seen as antagonistic and punishing.

Being fed, or having to eat what is considered baby food, may make a person feel dependent and inadequate, and may result in anger toward the person who provides such food. Recognizing the emotional importance of food will enable you to recognize these problems when they occur and to plan effective action. Intervention is based on skills of therapeutic interaction (see Chapter 7).

Nutrition and illness

Illness generally increases nutritional needs. Healing requires greater numbers of calories, more protein, and more vitamins and minerals than does maintenance of health. A fever raises the metabolic rate and increases the body's caloric requirements. And certain illnesses, such as hyperthyroidism, also increase metabolism and thus the calories needed by the body.

When a person is ill, appetite is often adversely affected. Food in general is less appealing, and fatigue may make eating an effort. Many illnesses cause unpleasant odors or tastes in the mouth, decreasing the desire for food. Furthermore, in some illnesses specific nutrients are not digested or metabolized in the normal way, making necessary special modifications of the diet.

The simplest such modification involves the *form* or *texture* of the food served. A general diet in which all foods are chopped is of special value to those without teeth, those whose dentures fit poorly and make chewing difficult, and those with very carious teeth. It is usually also possible to order all foods puréed for the person who cannot manage solid foods at all. The nurse often recognizes a need for such dietary modification and is generally free to order it. The physician may also order dietary changes. In facilities where only the physician may order dietary alterations, the nurse provides the relevant information to the physician and requests that an order for a change in form be written.

Other dietary modifications involve the *content* of the diet. Certain nutrients may be omitted or decreased, as in a low-sodium diet; nutrients may be carefully controlled as to type and time of serving, as in a diabetic diet; or nutrients may be added, as in a high-protein diet. Many other diets also restrict or increase nutrients in light of needs created by a specific illness or disease process. A nutrition text should be consulted for detailed information on the many special diets that may be ordered by the physician as part of the medical treatment plan. The nurse may not revise them at will.

Assessing the patient's nutritional status

The first step in assessing an individual's nutritional status is to closely observe his or her general appearance. Is the weight/height ratio appropriate, indicating neither too few nor too many calories for the person's needs? Is the skin color clear and the skin texture smooth? Many nutritional deficiencies are first evident in changes in the skin and mucous membranes. Is the hair thick and glossy? Are the lips and gums intact, or are they reddened, pale, or swollen? Many factors other than nutrition can affect a person's general appearance, but such observations may indicate a need for more complete investigation.

The patient's *dietary history*—information on the usual meal pattern, types of foods usually eaten, likes and dislikes, and allergies—is then gathered. This information will enable you to ascertain whether or not the patient maintains a sound diet at home. It will also assist you in planning a present and future diet that will involve the least disruption in the patient's pattern of living and be most acceptable. Information on the patient's sociocultural group and its attitudes and preferences with regard to food can also be helpful in diet planning.

Assessment of nutrition also involves consideration of current needs. Is the person growing? Are special needs created by tissue repair and healing? Is the person underweight and in need of weight gain, or overweight and in need of weight reduction?

The patient's physical ability to eat is especially important in nutritional assessment. A wide variety of factors, ranging from muscle strength and hand coordination to discomfort in the mouth, may affect ability to eat. Some common problems faced by hospitalized persons are immobilization in a position that does not allow easy eating or swallowing, restraint or immobilization of the dominant hand with an IV, and extreme physical fatigue and weakness. Paralysis of one hand and arm sometimes occurs in elderly patients who have suffered cerebrovascular accidents (strokes). After these basic aspects of nutritional status have been examined, special needs related to specific diseases—including information on the diet ordered by the physician—are considered.

Health teaching needs are always an important consideration. For some persons, health teaching will focus on normal nutritional needs, and consist of information on planning well-balanced meals and adapting general guidelines to personal preferences and patterns of eating. It may be necessary to teach family members about the patient's need and the foods that will meet the need. If the patient is to eat a special diet at home, such teaching is even more critical. The patient's understanding and acceptance of any dietary change ought to be explored, so that teaching may be planned in light of his or her readiness to learn (see Chapter 8).

Meeting the patient's nutritional needs

Positioning the patient

Persons who are ill often have special needs with regard to the eating process itself. Positioning is one factor that may make eating a problem. It is easiest to eat in a sitting position, with the food placed directly in front in one's line of vision. If this position can be maintained, it is important to position the patient before the meal. If this

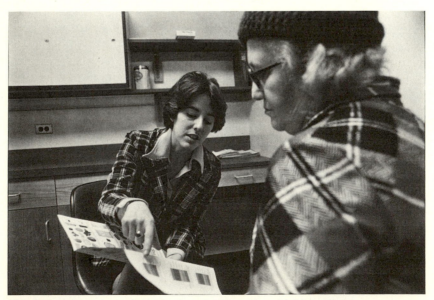

Health teaching is an important part of nutritional intervention.
Chris Maynard

position is impossible, the nearest approximation to it is made. The very weak or disabled person may need pillows or other supports on each side and under the arms to maintain correct posture for eating. If the patient is not permitted to sit up, a side-lying position may be used for meals.

People usually use both hands to feed themselves, the dominant hand performing the most skilled tasks. If only one hand is available, the person will have great difficulty with such tasks as opening a milk carton. If only the nondominant hand is available, even one-handed tasks may require more dexterity than that hand possesses. Planning ahead to place IVs and turning the patient so that the dominant hand is free for eating can avoid this problem. You may have to offer to perform some tasks, such as opening a milk carton or cutting meat. However, patients should always be asked whether they want help, the kind of help they want, and how such help is to be given. Independence in eating fosters self-esteem and should be encouraged.

Stimulating the patient's appetite

The environment for a meal is an important factor in promoting appetite. The control of odors and unpleasant sights in the hospital is often difficult, but any such steps that can be taken may help the patient retain a minimal appetite or regain a lost appetite. Removing soiled linen, opening a window, or using air freshener may be appropriate nursing actions in such a situation.

Personal comfort can promote appetite, and may be enhanced by bathing, washing the hands and face, straightening the bed, giving pain medications, or myriad other ways.

Stressful events tend to decrease appetite, and so should be avoided immediately before meals are served. Many pieces of equipment found in a hospital (such as those used for a venipuncture) are stress-producing to observe, and their removal from the patient's presence during meals will decrease anxiety.

Interaction with family and friends is typical of mealtimes for most people. If visitors can stay during the meal, or even order a tray and eat with the patient, a more suitable mealtime atmosphere is created. Sometimes several patients can sit together to visit during a meal, or a staff member might sit with a patient for a few minutes to make the meal a special event. Such company is especially helpful when the meal itself is less than tasty due to the omission of seasonings or salt: the interaction replaces the bland food as the focus of attention.

Assisting the patient to eat

Special feeding devices and methods are often used to help patients maintain independence in eating. The use of such equipment, which includes utensils with shaped handles, devices to keep a plate or dish in place, and special straws, needs to be carefully evaluated for each individual. One person may appreciate such an aid, while another prefers to eat more slowly and and with greater difficulty using conventional utensils.

Feeding a patient is sometimes necessary, because of muscle and joint disability that prevents movement; neurological involvement that prevents muscle function, or extreme weakness. Many patients are able partially to feed themselves if the nurse provides assistance with difficult tasks. Sometimes a patient can manage finger foods, such as bread and butter, but must be fed foods requiring more dexterity, such as soup. If weak vision is the problem, a description of the items on the tray, and their location, may enable the patient to eat without help. Because maximum independence increases the patients self-esteem, time and effort expended toward this end are well spent.

Alternative feeding methods

A nasogastric tube is a long flexible tube with a diameter narrow enough to pass through the nose to the nasopharynx, and then through the esophagus to the stomach. The nurse inserts such a tube only on the order of a physician. A nasogastric tube is frequently used to aspirate stomach contents, and may be attached to a low suction to remove gas and gastric contents in a number of circumstances. Here, however, we are concerned with its use to deposit food in a liquid form directly into the stomach.

Nasogastric tube feedings are performed for a variety of reasons, most frequently because the person is unable to swallow or lacks a gag reflex to prevent aspiration of food or fluids. A commercially prepared liquid formula may be used for the feeding. Such formulas vary in nutrient content and are ordered by the physician. Alternatively, a carefully planned combination of regular foods is liquefied in a blender, and liquid is added to achieve the appropriate consistency. The commercial preparations are easily controlled and convenient, but many persons suffer fewer digestive disturbances, such as diarrhea, when a blenderized formula is used. Additional water must always be given with tube feedings to meet the body's needs, and the exact amount may be ordered by the physician. Because tube feedings are meals, they should be served as such. If the patient is aware of the surroundings, a pleasant atmosphere will increase the flow of digestive juices and thus enhance digestion.

There are dangers in nasogastric tube feedings. If the tube is malpositioned, fluid could be deposited in the lungs or nasopharynx, allowing aspiration to occur. Excessive pressure may cause gastric irritation, gas, and reflex vomiting, and excessive rapidity may also precipitate vomiting. Allowing air into the tube will cause distention and discomfort, and may cause vomiting. Food is usually moderated in temperature in the mouth and esophagus, before it reaches the stomach. Temperature extremes can irritate the gastric mucosa, making it essential that the formula is of moderate temperature before instillation. Thus, any procedure for nasogastric tube feeding should take into consideration tube placement, prevention of air ingestion, the temperature of the fluid, and the force and speed of the fluid as it enters the stomach.

Persons receiving tube feedings frequently experience diarrhea. This phenomenon has been attributed to a variety of factors, including too concentrated a solution, inappropriate temperature, bacterial contamination of the feeding, and the unfamiliar consistency. Such diarrhea may decrease after a period of time. If care is taken with regard to the other possible causes of diarrhea, the patient usually adjusts to the consistency of the formula.

A surgically produced opening from the abdomen directly into the stomach is called a *gastrostomy*. A tube is inserted into the opening and a liquid feeding instilled, just as is done through a nasogastric tube.

Hyperalimentation is a recently developed means of providing nutrition to patients who cannot eat. Highly concentrated solutions containing refined carbohydrates, amino acids, and vitamins are administered with a catheter directly into a large vein, such as the subclavian. A major vein must be used because of the high concentration of the solution. This procedure requires very careful and skilled nursing supervision, because of the many complications that can occur.

Fluids and electrolytes

A minimum daily intake of water is needed by the body for the many processes involved in homeostasis. The optimal amount varies considerably with age, size, activity, and the environmental temperature. Approximately 2400 cc. of fluid daily will meet the needs of the average healthy adult.

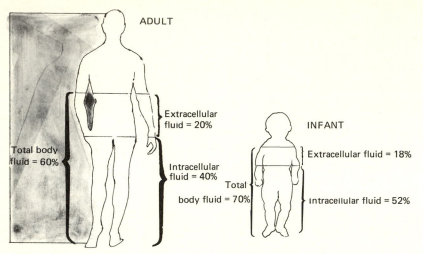

FIGURE 14.2   BODY WATER COMPARED TO TOTAL WEIGHT

Water is needed in the digestive tract itself to combine with starches to promote digestion and to prevent the fecal material from becoming hard and dry. It is needed by the kidneys to dissolve the waste products of the body so that they can be excreted. Water is also used by the body to regulate temperature through the evaporation of perspiration. And water is a component of all bodily secretions, such as mucus, tears, and digestive juices. Furthermore, the major component of every cell is water. If one considers this cellular water, the fluid of the blood, and the fluid that surrounds all the cells, it is not surprising that 50-65 percent of human body weight is water. (See Figure 14.2.)

The fluids of the body are generally divided into two *compartments*, the *intracellular* fluid within the cells and the *extracellular* fluid outside of the cells. The extracellular fluid is further subdivided into *interstitial* fluid, which lies between the cells, and *plasma*, which is the liquid component of the blood. Water moves easily between these various compartments by the process of *diffusion* or movement from an area characterized by lesser concentration of dissolved substances to an area of greater concentration.

Various chemicals are dissolved in the water of the body, where they separate into negatively charged particles (*anions*) and positively charged particles (*cations*) called *electrolytes*.

Electrolytes are measured in terms of their potential for activity, in units called *milli-equivalents*. Figure 14.3 shows the major electrolytes found in the body fluids. You will note that sodium

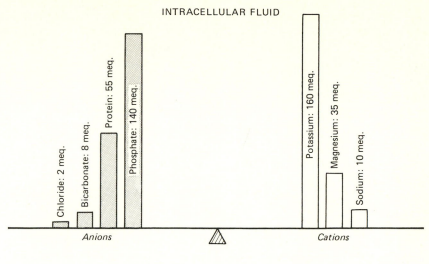

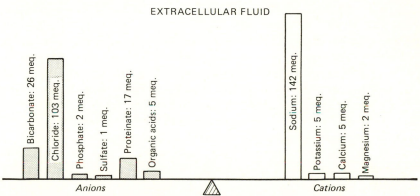

FIGURE 14.3   CHEMICAL COMPOSITION OF THE BODY FLUIDS   Both the intracellular fluid and extracellular fluid of the human body are composed of *anions* (negatively charged electrolytes) and *cations* (positively charged electrolytes). Note that the anions and cations balance each other when expressed in milli-equivalents.
Adapted from N. M. Matheny and W. D. Snively, Nurse's Handbook of Fluid Balance, 2nd ed. (Philadelphia: J. B. Lippincott, 1974), p. 5. Used with permission.

and chloride are the primary electrolytes in the extracellular fluid, and that potassium and phosphates are the primary electrolytes in the intracellular fluid.

Electrolytes also move between the various compartments of the body by the process of *osmosis*, or movement from areas of greater concentration to areas of lesser concentration. This process would be expected eventually to create equilibrium, in which all fluids have the same composition; however, cells also possess an active system that moves some electrolytes across the membranes separating the fluid compartments. These *active transport systems*, as they are called, result in different concentrations of electrolytes in different fluid compartments. These electrolyte concentrations are of critical significance.

A fluid in which the concentration of an electrolyte is the same as that of the body fluid is termed *isotonic*. One that has fewer electrolytes is called *hypotonic*, and one with more is called *hypertonic*.

Common problems of fluid and electrolyte status

Dehydration is loss of body water, which decreases the fluids available for all body processes. The term is often used interchangeably for two distinct situations. In true dehydration, *only* water is lost; thus the concentration of electrolytes in the remaining fluid is higher than desirable. However, the term is also used to describe the loss of both fluids and the electrolytes they contain, which causes the remaining body fluid to be of normal composition. Because dehydration decreases the fluids available for all body processes, it profoundly affects urinary elimination. The urine becomes dark, strong-smelling, and of small quantity, and its specific gravity is increased. If dehydration is severe the kidneys may be unable to excrete wastes, and their accumulation in the blood will have toxic effects on the body. The stool becomes hard and dry as the intestine atempts to recover all available water from the digestive tract; therefore the person becomes constipated or even impacted (see Chapter 15). Temperature regulation will be affected if the body is unable to produce enough perspiration for cooling. The skin loses its turgor and the eyes appear sunken and lusterless. Failure to drink adequate fluids is perhaps the simplest cause of dehydration.

Fluid retention causes an increase in the fluid of the interstitial areas, a condition known as *edema*. Manifested as swelling and puffiness of the tissues, edema may be generalized throughout the body or concentrated in dependent areas such as the lower extremities and the sacrum, as is common among patients on bedrest. Fluid retention occurs primarily in conjunction with circulatory and kidney disorders.

Electrolytes may be present in excessive or inadequate concentrations. The concentration of the various electrolytes in the body fluids is of critical significance to the body's functioning. Changes in electrolyte concentrations cause alterations in basic physical and chemical processes and, if severe, can cause death. Electrolyte disturbances are complex disorders, usually manifested as changes in such body functions as coordination, alertness, and muscle contraction and strength. A complete discussion of the complex processes involved in fluid and electrolyte balance may be found in a physiology text or advanced nursing text, but some general considerations are examined here.

Any situation that causes considerable water loss can also be expected to produce an electrolyte imbalance. Vomiting and diarrhea may draw off a large volume of fluid and concentrations of electrolytes in a short time. Excessive perspiration due to fever or extremely hot weather may rapidly expend the body's water and salt. Some disorders of fluid regulation may cause the body to excrete its water and electrolytes. Blood loss and drainage from wounds can deplete both fluid and electrolytes.

In the hospital, electrolytes are sometimes depleted by nursing procedures in which a hypotonic solution such as tap water or distilled water is used to irrigate a body organ, such as the stomach or bladder. Some electrolytes move across membranes to equalize the concentration on both sides of the membrane, and then pass off with the water. The very young and very old are most susceptible to this phenomenon because they are less able than others to tolerate changes in electrolyte concentrations. For this reason a normal saline solution, which is isotonic, is best used for irrigation.

Assessing the patient's fluid and electrolyte status

Measurement and comparison of fluid intake and output is perhaps the single best indicator of fluid balance. When the two amounts are approximately the same, the body is managing to satisfy its need.

Output greater than intake may indicate kidney damage, damage to regulatory mechanisms, or that the body is removing previously retained fluids. Intake greater than output may indicate dehydration or retention.

The appearance of the urine is another important clue. Dark urine with a strong odor may indicate that not enough fluid is being ingested to dilute waste products. Skin, hair, and eyes are examined for additional symptoms of dehydration. Signs of edema are checked for in dependent areas, where it is seen the earliest.

Assisting the patient with fluid intake

Increasing oral intake

Many ill persons need to consume large quantities of fluid to allow for excretion of excess waste products or to combat fever. The physician may order *force fluids*. This order means not that you literally force the patient to drink, but that you exert maximum effort to encourage the patient to consume fluids. Simply reminding the patient to drink frequently may be all that is needed.

Because patients are likely to consume more of fluids they enjoy, it is fruitful to take time to learn likes and dislikes and to order what the patient prefers. And because people are more likely to reach desired goals if they receive feedback on their progress, you might design a method of recording intake or graphing it on the wall. Furthermore, behaviors that are reinforced (rewarded) tend to be repeated. Thus praise or even marks on a chart for ingesting certain amounts of fluid may have the effect of increasing intake. Setting a specific goal for the twenty-four-hour period and ascertaining when fluid should be taken helps the nursing staff to organize its efforts. If the goal is 3000 cc. per twenty-four-hour period, a realistic plan acknowledges that the patient sleeps during the 11 p.m.-7 a.m. shift and therefore will usually take less than 200 cc. if offered fluids when awakened in the morning. If medications are given during the night, fluid intake at these times may be encouraged. The plan might provide for 2000 cc. to be taken from 7:00 a.m. to 3:00 p.m. That period of time includes two meals and two snacks, and if the patient also drinks fluids between meals, the goal can be reached. If the mechanics of drinking are a problem, special straws and cups are available to assist the patient.

Administering fluids intravenously

When patients are unable to take sufficient fluids orally, fluids may be given intravenously. A needle or plastic cannula is inserted into the vein, and very careful attention to sterile technique is essential to prevent infection. Cleansing with an iodine-base disinfectant before inserting the needle and when the dressing over the needle is changed has been shown to decrease the incidence of phlebitis (an inflammation of the vein). Sometimes an antibiotic ointment is used on the site to prevent infection. Every forty-eight hours the dressing is changed and a new sterile dressing is applied. New tubing is attached every twenty-four hours. No bottle is allowed to hang more

than twenty-four hours, to minimize the possibility of contamination of the fluids and equipment.

The physician usually orders the amount of fluid to be administered in a specified period of time. The nurse must then calculate the
number of drops per minute that will deliver this amount of fluid. The
drops per minute needed will vary depending on the brand of equipment in use: some equipment delivers ten drops per cc., some fifteen
drops per cc., and some sixty drops per cc. The following formula is
used to calculate rate of flow:

$$\frac{\substack{\text{drops per cc.} \\ \text{of equipment}} \times \substack{\text{number of ccs.} \\ \text{ordered}}}{\substack{\text{number of hours} \times \text{60 minutes} \\ \text{to run}}} = \text{drops/minute}$$

The rate of flow is important because is it is possible to give too little
to meet the patient's needs or so much so that the circulatory system
is overloaded. When electrolytes—especially potassium—have been
added, circulatory overload is of particular concern. Sometimes a
bottle of intravenous fluid is marked with the approximate level the
fluid should reach at specified times to provide the amount ordered.
This is a helpful aid in maintaining a general overview of fluid administration, but is unsatisfactory as the only method of checking
rate. If the IV is behind schedule, it may be tempting to increase the
rate to "catch up," without regard to how fast the fluid is being administered during the catch-up period. A general guideline is that 3
cc. per minute is an average flow rate for a healthy adult, two cc. per
minute is a slow rate, and 4 cc. per minute is a rapid rate. If you must
readjust an IV, consider the person's age, size, and cardiovascular
status to determine a safe speed.

The site where the needle enters the body should be inspected frequently for signs that the intravenous is not functioning. Swollen, hard tissue that is pale and cold at the site usually
indicates that the needle is out of the vein and the fluid is "infil-
trating" the subcutaneous tissue. Redness and pain associated
with swelling indicate phlebitis. Both of these conditions require
the removal of the intravenous. If the intravenous stops dripping,
blood may be clotted in the needle, the position of the arm may be
causing constriction of the vein, or the needle may be against the
wall of the vein. It may only be necessary to move the arm or the
needle slightly to re-establish the flow. Using a needle and syringe
to aspirate may remove a blockage. For many years nurses irrigat-
ed the needle with saline, a practice frowned on in texts because

of the possibility of liberating a clot, which might create serious problems. Recent investigations indicate that the pressure of 1-2 cc. of saline is not enough to loosen a large clot, and that the procedure is safe. Larger amounts, however, could create problems.

Because infection of the vein could lead to systemic septicemia, prevention of infection at the intravenous site is crucial. Contamination of the equipment and/or solution while setting up the intravenous is always a possibility. Therefore, changing fluid and tubing sets every twenty-four hours will insure that even if contamination does occur, the organisms will not multiply sufficiently to cause an infection.

When an intravenous is removed from the patient's vein, the primary concern is to prevent bleeding. A sterile cotton ball or sponge is placed over the site, and firm pressure is applied to it until bleeding has stopped. Some persons use an alcohol sponge to exert pressure, but the alcohol is irritating and causes discomfort.

Administering hypodermoclysis

When the patient's veins are unsuitable for an intravenous, a fluid may be introduced into the interstitial space by continuous drip. This process is called *hypodermoclysis*, or simply *clysis*. An enzyme (varidase) is frequently injected through the tubing into the site to increase the rate of absorption. The anterior aspects of the thighs or the subscapular areas of the back are most frequently used. The setup is similar to an intravenous infusion, but two tubings are connected. Each has a long two- to three-inch needle, which is inserted into the subcutaneous tissue at a 15-degree angle. Both thighs or both subscapular areas are used simultaneously. This procedure is becoming increasingly rare because of poor absorption and the discomfort caused the patient.

Limiting fluids

A physician may occasionally order that fluids be limited. This is very trying and difficult for the patient, and careful planning with the patient is needed to space the allowable intake throughout the day, and to provide for fluid to accompany oral medications. The patient will need support from others to tolerate fluid deprivation. When the limitation is very severe, close supervision may be necessary: it is difficult to maintain self-control when one's thirst is extreme. Ice chips must be considered as intake, but often serve to minimize the desire for fluid and provide greater relief than the same amount of water. Fluids are often withheld for short periods before procedures that require general anesthesia or slight dehydration. Allowing responsible patients to perform mouth care and to rinse the mouth may promote a feeling of well-being during this time. If a patient cannot be expected to refrain from drinking fluid while performing mouth care, you may moisten the lips and provide mouth care for the patient.

Conclusion

Providing food and fluids for patients is an emotional experience as well as a nursing task. Your role may seem pleasant when you are a provider, but when you must withhold or limit these essentials of life, it is difficult. Assisting the patient to understand and actively participate in this essential aspect of care and treatment requires skillful nursing.

Study terms

anion
Basic Four
cation
deficiency
dehydration
diet
  content
  form
edema
electrolytes
fiber
fluid balance
fluid compartments
  extracellular
    interstitial
    plasma
  intracellular

force fluids
gastric
kosher food
hyperalimentation
hypertonic
hypotonic
isotonic
minimum daily requirement
nasogastric tube feeding
normal saline
nutrition
Recommended Dietary
Allowances (RDA)
satiety
vegetarian
  lacto-vegetarian
  ovo-lacto-vegetarian

References

Colley, R., *et al.* 1973. Helping With Hyperalimentation. *Nursing '73* 3:7:6-17.

Dwyer, L. S., *et al.* 1974. Simplified Meal-Planning for Hard to Teach Patients. *American Journal of Nursing* 74:4:664-665.

Fenton, M. 1969. What to Do About Thirst. *American Journal of Nursing* 69:5:1014-1017.

Fleshman, R. P. 1973. Eating Rituals and Realities. *Nursing Clinics of North America* 8:1:91-104.

Gormican, A., *et al.* 1974. Nasogastric Tube Feedings: Practical Considerations in Prescription and Evaluation. *Nursing Digest* 2:1:59-63.

Grant, J. A. 1973. Patient Care in Hyperalimentation. *Nursing Clinics of North America* 8:1:165-181.

McCarter, D. 1973. Nourishing the Solute Sensitive Patient. *American Journal of Nursing* 73:11:1935-1936.

Nelson, A. H. 1972. Self-Recorded Diet Histories. *American Journal of Nursing* 72:9:1601.

Newton, M., and Falta, J. 1967. Hospital Food Can Help or Hinder Care. *American Journal of Nursing* 67:1:112-113.

Pederson, B. M. 1970. A Solution for Post-Infusion Thrombophlebitis. *American Journal of Nursing* 70:2:325.

15 Elimination

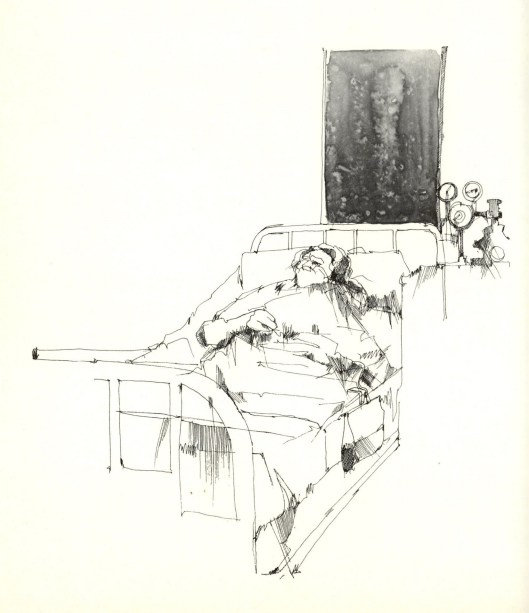

Objectives

After completing this chapter, you should be able to:

1 Describe normal urinary function and the properties of urine.

2 Define key terms relating to the urinary and intestinal systems.

3 Demonstrate a beginning ability to assess for urinary problems.

4 Demonstrate a beginning ability to assess for intestinal problems.

5 Describe specific nursing actions appropriate for the patient with urinary dysfunction.

6 Describe specific nursing actions appropriate for the patient with intestinal dysfunction.

7 List the nurse's responsibility with regard to the collection of urine and stool specimens.

8 Plan a bladder rehabilitation program.

9 Plan a bowel rehabilitation program.

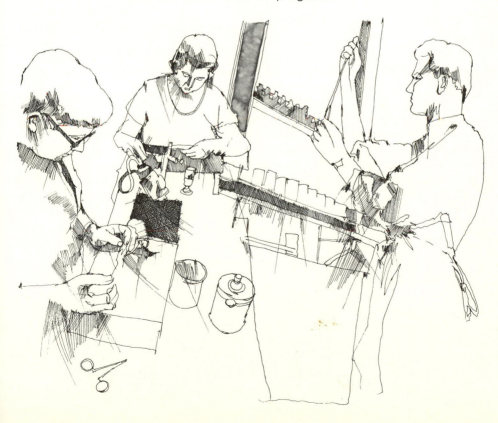

E LIMINATION IS TREATED as a taboo topic in our society. So-called "bathroom jokes" are more prevalent in American culture than in many others, and public rest rooms in the United States provide much more privacy than is characteristic in most countries. Although people treat the subject of elimination with some embarrassment, it engenders much interest. One need only listen to the radio or watch television to be reminded that "regularity" is a state much desired and "irregularity" is considered cause for concern.

Urinary or intestinal problems tend to be very upsetting to people, because they not only interfere with daily living but also arouse a sense of being unwell or suffering from a disturbance of the body's vital systems.

Fluids are eliminated from the body through the lungs and skin, as well as through the urinary system. Solid wastes are excreted exclusively through the intestines. In this chapter, we will consider the elimination processes of the urinary and intestinal tracts.

The urinary system

The organs of the urinary system are illustrated in Figure 15.1. The kidneys act as a rather complex filtration unit, selectively filtering out and eliminating water and certain substances not needed by the body. These substances, end-products of metabolism, are urea, creatinine, phosphates, sulfates, nitrates, uric acid, and phenols. The *nephrons*, after undergoing a distillation and reabsorption process, deposit urine in the pelvis of the kidney. Through the *ureter*, a small tube, the urine passes from each kidney to the bladder, where it is stored until micturition (emptying) takes place. The normal adult bladder can hold a maximum of 500 cc., though in some situations it may be stretched to accommodate as much as 3000 cc. From the bladder, the urine passes through the *urethra* and is excreted through the urethral meatus.

Micturition, sometimes called *voiding*, is both voluntary and involuntary. A full bladder activates the "stretch reflex," which causes the *internal sphincter* of the bladder to relax, allowing micturition. The *external sphincter*, or *meatus*, is controlled by the higher centers of the brain, which allows for voluntary control. Thus a person can postpone voiding for some time after the internal sphincter relaxes, although there may be some discomfort.

Normal urine is a sterile fluid, clear and pale amber or straw-

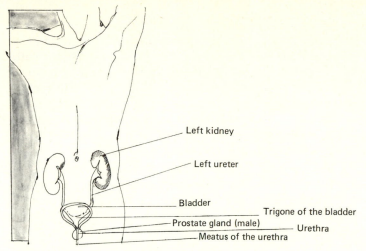

Left kidney

Left ureter

Bladder

Trigone of the bladder

Prostate gland (male)

Urethra

Meatus of the urethra

FIGURE 15.1   THE URINARY SYSTEM

colored. It may become cloudy upon standing. Urine has a pH of 4.5 to 7.5 (slightly acid) and a specific gravity of 1.010 to 1.025 (French, 1971, p. 22). There may be a faint odor. Abnormal substances sometimes detected in the urine include bacteria, parasites, calculi (stones), pus, casts, red blood cells, sugar, albumin, and acetone.

Collecting urine specimens

Urine may be collected for any of several reasons. It is routine to collect a voided specimen upon a patient's admission to the hospital, regardless of the diagnosis; this procedure is often referred to as a *UA* or *routine urinalysis*. If the physician wants a "clean-catch" or "clean-voided" specimen, the patient's external urethral meatus is cleansed and he or she is instructed to begin urinating, "catch" a portion of the flow in a sterile container, and finish voiding.

A "twenty-four-hour urine" specimen is one that contains all urine voided for a twenty-four-hour period. At the specified starting hour, the patient voids and discards the specimen. All subsequent urine is saved in a large container. At the end of twenty-four hours, the patient voids a last time into the container. In order to prevent chemical deterioration of the urine over the twenty-four-hour period, a preservative substance may be added to the container, or the container may be refrigerated or kept in a pan of ice.

If a sterile specimen of urine is ordered by the physician, a catheterization is performed: a small tube or catheter is inserted into the bladder and urine is withdrawn for the specimen. When a catheter is already in place, it should not be disconnected to secure a urine specimen, since each time the system is interrupted there is a chance of introducing pathogens that may cause a urinary tract infection. Instead, the nurse should clamp the distal (farthest from the body) portion of the catheter for twenty minutes to allow a small amount of urine to collect in the catheter. Then, after the surface of the catheter is cleansed with an alcohol sponge, the needle is inserted through the catheter wall and urine is withdrawn into the syringe. If the insertion is performed carefully and at an angle, the catheter will reseal. The insertion should be made between the end of the catheter and the tubing that connects to the catheter balloon, so as not to aspirate the sterile water in the balloon and cause the catheter to come out.

Whatever method is used to obtain a urine sample, it is the nurse's responsibility to see that the specimen is labeled properly, usually by attaching the appropriate laboratory slip. The urine should either be sent to the laboratory reasonably promptly or refrigerated to prevent the character of the urine from changing as it stands.

Recording intake and output

In assessing urinary function, the physician may order the patient to be placed on *intake and output*. Alternatively, the nurse may initiate the recording of intake and output. This procedure involves measuring and recording all fluids ingested orally or intravenously, including solidified fluids, such as jello and ice cream, and water. Data are usually recorded on an appropriate form and totalled every eight or twenty-four hours, depending on the policy of the facility. The intake sheet can also serve as a guide to the status of the patient's intake, enabling you to encourage or curtail fluids as the patient's condition requires. Output, the fluid lost from the body, is measured in conjunction with intake. If a very accurate measurement is necessary, emesis, blood loss, perspiration, and diarrheal stools are measured along with urine. Determining the amount of fluid that enters and leaves the body (water balance) allows urinary efficiency to be evaluated.

Common urinary problems

Urinary *retention* is the holding of urine within the bladder due to inability to void. This problem often occurs in the patient whose urinary system is obstructed, as well as in the postoperative patient as an effect of anesthesia or local trauma. If a patient who has consumed adequate fluid fails to void within eight hours of surgery, you should consult the physician, who may decide that catheterization is needed. Palpating with care over the bladder area will indicate the extent of retention.

Urinary *suppression* is the complete cessation of the production of urine by the kidneys. Another term for this condition is *anuria*, or absence of urine. No measurable output will be observed, and the patient will not feel distended because the bladder is not filled. The patient suffering from kidney failure will manifest this symptom.

Dysuria is difficult voiding or pain upon voiding. Patients sometimes use the expression "a burning sensation" to describe this condition. Obstruction and urinary infection are among the common causes.

Polyuria is an increased amount of urine. A patient who excretes more than 1500-1800 cc. in twenty-four hours might be said to have polyuria. Though often simply a result of high fluid intake, patients with hormonal disturbances—particularly diabetes—also display this symptom.

A decrease in the amount of urine produced in twenty-four hours to less than 50 cc. per hour is called *oliguria*. The many causes of this condition include dehydration and any disease or condition that causes the kidneys to produce less urine than is optimal for the patient.

Urinary *incontinence*, or involuntary micturition, is not a simple problem and has several variants: the inability to postpone micturition is called *urgency*; inability to hold urine in the bladder at all is called *complete incontinence*; *partial incontinence* is the inability to retain urine in the bladder on occasion or infrequently. If the patient is unable to hold urine in the bladder at all, a "dribbling" effect occurs that is particularly stressful. Incontinence is a symptom that calls for special nursing actions since it is not only distressing to the patient but also a hazard to skin integrity. Many incontinent patients could be continent if appropriate toileting devices or facilities were always near at hand.

The nurse must be familiar with the terms for abnormal substances found in the urine. *Hematuria*, the presence of blood in the urine, may give it a "smoky," slightly pink, bright red, or dark brown appearance, depending on the amount or character of bleeding. If the urine appears cloudy or whitish, pus or albumin may be present. Pus in the urine is called *pyuria*; albumin in the urine is called *albuminuria*. The presence of protein, in pure form or coagulated (casts), is *proteinuria*. And if glucose is found in urine, the patient is said to have *glycosuria*.

Causes of urinary problems

Because all the systems of the body are interrelated, disturbances of other systems can cause urinary problems. More localized problems can occur in specific parts of the urinary tract, such as the kidneys, ureters, bladder, or urethra.

As for localized factors, *obstruction* may occur anyplace within the system. Abnormal cell growth, benign or malignant, may occur in the kidney, ureters, bladder, or urethra. Stones (*calculi*) can also form, causing obstruction. Localized trauma may be evident in the form of bruising, hemorrhaging, or swelling of localized parts of the system. Because of the mucous membrane lining of the tract, the urinary system is particularly prone to infection, and infection travels readily throughout the system.

A considerable number of systemic factors can cause urinary problems. Heart disease and complications of the circulation cause urinary disturbances due to the decreased flow of blood to the kidney. Without sufficient blood to process, the body retains fluid and substances, and the kidney tissue may be damaged. The patient may show signs of electrolyte imbalance, such as muscle weakness, lassitude, and even confusion. Fluid is also retained in the tissue, resulting in edema, most commonly in the upper part of the buttocks and the ankles. Hormonal factors can also cause problems. Because certain hormones, such as aldosterone, have a regulatory effect upon the kidneys, a disturbance of the pituitary or adrenal glands that produce these hormones can cause urinary disturbance. This, then, is a systemic, not a localized, problem.

Severe dehydration, regardless of cause, may bring about serious kidney problems due to the decreased blood flow to the organs. Any overwhelming generalized trauma to the body has a systemic effect, causing kidney dysfunction. Generalized infection depletes body fluid due to elevated temperatures, affecting kidney function. Loss of muscle tone, often seen in the elderly and in pa-

tients suffering disease of the muscular system, may bring about
an inability to exercise muscular controls over urination. Conditions of the central nervous system and spinal cord may also directly influence urinary efficiency through interruption of innervation. The interplay between urinary function and other systems
can greatly complicate assessment.

The anatomical differences between males and females make
for some differences in the prevalence of specific problems. The female is more prone to infection because of the shortness of the urethra (1½-2 inches) relative to that of the male (6-9 inches). The male
may, however, be more susceptible to obstruction: because the *prostate* gland surrounds the male urethra, any hypertrophy, or swelling,
of this gland will cause some degree of obstruction. And of course
the male is more disposed to trauma of the urethra due to its external
position.

Assessing urinary function

Three general considerations are central to the assessment
process. First, it is important to know something about the patient's
condition and *diagnosis*. The female patient with an infection of the
vagina can readily develop an infection of the bladder as well, because of the close proximity of the organs. The male patient with an
enlarged prostate may have difficulty voiding. Any surgical patient
who is to spend a relatively long period under anesthesia should be
assessed for urinary retention.

Second, the patient's *subjective symptoms* are instructive to the
nurse. A patient who trusts the nurse is more likely to discuss his or
her urinary problems. If the patient does not volunteer such information, the nurse might without embarrassment ask one or two direct
questions. Patients often describe changes in the color or odor of
urine. A change in amount is sometimes mentioned, if the patient
becomes concerned. And the patient who experiences pain or burning on micturition will usually report it, since this symptom is very
disturbing.

The nurse also relies heavily on *objective observations*. The
patient may not want to talk about incontinence, since it is a very
sensitive subject, but sharp observation will reveal the degree and
frequency of this problem. Noting color and odor may point to
possible problems. Intake and output may be measured. You can
also perform some simple tests, such as measurement of specific
gravity and pH or assessment for the presence of sugar. The

equipment needed for these tests is available on the units of most hospitals. Various more sophisticated tests are done for renal function (see Chapter 10).

Nursing care for urinary problems

In cases of renal dysfunction resulting from a systemic condition, good general nursing care is important. Again, the close interrelationship of all body systems makes such supportive measures as adequate nutrition, rest, exercise, and hygiene essential. Let us examine several of the more specific measures that may be taken by nurses, in addition to collecting urine specimens and accurately measuring and recording intake and output.

Encouragement of voluntary micturition

It is very distressing to the patient to feel the need to void but be unable to do so. There are several ways the nurse can promote adequate emptying of the bladder. First, the patient needs privacy and benefits from an unhurried attitude on the part of the nurse. Adequate fluid intake is essential, since sufficient urine must be present before the bladder reflex is activated: only when the bladder contains at least 300 cc. is the desire to eliminate usually activated. Placing the patient's hands in a pan of warm water, pouring warm or very cold water over the perineum, running tap water within the patient's hearing, or putting pressure on one side of the urinary meatus may facilitate voiding. Manually exerting pressure on the bladder to force urine out, known as *crede*, should be avoided; this procedure does not allow the elasticity of the bladder wall to function and may cause damage to the sphincter. However, crede may be used appropriately in some rehabilitation settings, on the order of a physician, with the patient who has lost and is not expected to regain voluntary bladder control.

Bladder rehabilitation

Bladder rehabilitation, frequently called bladder training, is an important undertaking planned and carried out by the nurse for the patient suffering from urinary incontinence. Like any health teaching, it must be a cooperative effort on the part of both patient and nurse. The nurse should explain the program and its goals to the patient. Patients who fully understand that the goal is more normal functioning of the bladder usually become highly motivated. Sufficient fluid intake, usually from 2000 to 4000 cc. daily, is essential. The patient is encouraged to retain the urine as long as possible, not exceeding two hours. Use of the bathroom toilet to void is preferred; however, a commode or, if neither of the two is feasible, a bedpan (the patient in the upright position) may be used. Any of these approaches along with a provision for the male patient to stand, approximates normal voiding conditions. Positioning, of course, is contingent on the patient's physical condition. The voiding times are spaced increasingly far apart, from the duration that can initially be tolerated up to two hours. The stretching-relaxing sequence of this process reinstates bladder muscle tone, eventually affording the patient more voluntary control.

Although incontinence usually has a physiological basis, it also has overtones of dependency. With older patients, it has been demonstrated that getting up out of bed, dressing in their own clothing, and being offered bathroom accommodations on a regular schedule can often reverse a trend toward incontinence.

Whether the patient has difficulty voiding or controlling voiding, the nurse's attitude is crucial. It is understandable for the patient to be noticeably embarrassed and upset over such a situation, and the nurse should exhibit an understanding attitude.

Catheterization

A physician orders catheterization either to secure a sterile specimen or to relieve the distended patient. Following the procedure checklist in Chapter 10, equipment is assembled and a sterile procedure is performed: the urinary catheter is inserted into the bladder and the urine drained into a collection container of some type. Very large amounts of urine should not be withdrawn all at once, since doing so can cause local trauma to the bladder or cause a mild-to-severe systemic reaction characterized by symptoms of shock. This outcome is due to pressure changes in the abdomen as a result of autonomic nervous system reactions. The patient may be catheterized with a "straight" catheter, which is removed from the bladder at the end of the procedure, or, in cases of incontinence, a catheter that remains in the bladder. It stays in place due to the inflation of a 5-20 cc. balloon filled with sterile water (also in the bladder). Such a catheter is called an *indwelling*, *Foley*, or *continuous drainage catheter*, depending on the facility. For specific aspects of the skill of catheterization, a skill module should be consulted.

When the patient has an indwelling catheter, a bladder rehabilitation program can be initiated. A physician may order a "clamp and release" routine before the catheter is removed, which means that the catheter is clamped for a period of time and then released so that the bladder empties. The alternate stretching and relaxing of the bladder walls simulates normal bladder wall functioning, and helps maintain or restore tone. At first, the conscious patient may be able to tolerate clamping only as long as thirty minutes at a time. The duration of clamping is gradually increased until the patient can tolerate it two hours. After removal of the catheter, the bladder rehabilitation program continues as described above. The unconscious patient who has an indwelling catheter should also be placed on such a program. One word of caution: if the patient is unconscious, and cannot voice discomfort, the nurse must be scrupulously conscientious about releasing the catheter clamp at the designated time. Serious injury can occur to the bladder if proper drainage does not take place.

Catheter removal and health teaching

The patient who has had an indwelling catheter is in need of health teaching when it is removed. It is unusual for a patient who has an indwelling catheter for a long time to be completely free of urinary tract infection. For this reason, the importance of consuming large amounts of fluid is stressed before, during, and after the insertion of an indwelling catheter. A high fluid intake "flushes" the system and prevents the pooling of urine in the bladder. It is sometimes recommended that the patient drink cranberry juice, which tends to render the urine acid, discouraging the growth of pathogens. The patient may be warned that a mild burning sensation might occur initially upon urination. Very frequent urination may also be necessary for a short time at first. To help the nurse observe, assess, and plan care relative to urinary problems, the patient should be asked to tell the nurse when voiding occurs, the amount voided, and whether discomfort arises.

Replacements for the kidney function

When complete *renal* failure, or kidney failure, occurs, there are a number of procedures for replicating the kidney function, referred to as *dialysis* procedures. Some employ elaborate machinery outside the body ("artificial kidneys"), while some use peritoneal tissue or bowel tissue. These procedures are studied in advanced nursing courses.

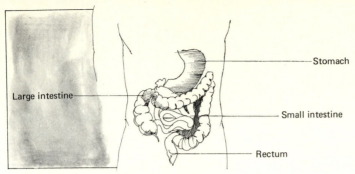

Large intestine

Stomach

Small intestine

Rectum

FIGURE 15.2   THE INTESTINAL SYSTEM

The intestinal system

The intestinal system is illustrated in Figure 15.2. After the essential nutritional components have been removed from the ingested food, the solid wastes are eliminated from the body through the large intestine. The waste products are propelled along by wave-like motions of the intestines called *peristalsis*. As is true of urination, *defecation*, or the passing of stool, is both voluntary and involuntary. The parasympathetic nervous system carries the rectal sensation of fullness to the sacral area of the spinal cord and stimulates peristalsis and muscle tone. The *sympathetic nervous system* has the opposing effect. The alternating effects of these two systems allow the rectal sphincter to relax and the fecal contents of the rectum and large bowel to pass. Voluntary control can also be exerted to delay defecation.

The frequency of stools varies a great deal from individual to individual. Some persons defecate regularly on a daily basis, while others have bowel movements as infrequently as every three to four days. Each pattern is normal for a given individual. Thus it is prudent to talk in terms not of "normal" frequency but of what is usual for the person in question.

Common defecation problems

Constipation, the retention of fecal material within the rectum, is a common problem. Many older people grew up at a time when it was thought appropriate for parents to give their youngsters strong laxatives on a daily basis, whether or not a laxative was warranted. These children gradually lost the ability to defecate unaided by the stimulus of a laxative, and as adults they have severe problems with constipation. Patients who must take drugs that are constipating often have orders to take a stool-softener in conjunction with the primary medication to relieve constipation. *Hemorrhoids*, which are distended veins either immediately inside or outside the rectum, may predispose to constipation by causing pain when the individual defecates. If the patient with hemorrhoids postpones passing stool to avoid pain, the fecal matter becomes hardened and even more difficult to pass.

Impaction is a different and more severe condition than constipation. A bolus, or rounded stone-hard stool, becomes lodged in the lower bowel and cannot pass. The presence of such a condition can be ascertained by digital examination of the lower intestinal tract, for which a clean glove and the middle finger are used. The patient may pass very small amounts of liquid stool at frequent intervals. The bowel can become very irritated and produce this liquified stool, which can flow around the impaction.

Diarrhea is the frequent passage of unformed or liquid stool, which can become so profuse as to make defecation involuntary.

Causes of defecation problems

As is true of urination, there are numerous factors that can cause bowel problems. Because of the innervation of the tract by both sympathetic and parasympathetic nerve pathways, emotions can play a direct part in bowel disturbance. The effect of emotions on intestinal function is not simple, but it has been suggested that over-stimulation of the parasympathetic nervous system due to emotional stress results in diarrhea, and that excessive stimulation of the sympathetic nervous system results in constipation.

Fecal elimination is directly related to diet. Lack of roughage, which characterizes bland or liquid diets, usually causes diarrhea, because such substances pass through the intestinal tract very rapidly. After a short time, the patient develops constipation due to stagnation of the diet in the tract. A certain amount of roughage seems essential to maintain regularity.

Because increasing the water in the intestine causes the stool to soften, drinking sufficient fluid is an important part of avoiding constipation. Many physicians recommend at least 2800-3000 cc. of fluid per day. Conversely, dehydration causes constipation; in an effort to provide itself with water, the body reabsorbs fluid from the bowel, leaving hard, dry feces that are difficult to expel.

The effects of drugs on ability to defecate and stool consistency have long been known. The *psychotropic drugs*, iron preparations, and some medications for pain, such as morphine, cause constipation. Iron turns the stool black.

Structural conditions such as loss of tone in the intestinal wall and partial or complete obstruction interfere with the passage of solid waste products. Inflammatory or infectious conditions, various types of colitis, and the presence of parasites can alter intestinal function. Damage to the brain or spinal cord can interrupt nerve impulses, causing either fecal retention or fecal incontinence.

Assessing for defecation problems

Several factors should be considered in an assessment. The patient's *condition* is important in that a patient who is immobilized or on bedrest is prone to constipation. Lack of exercise decreases tone within the intestinal wall. Abdominal or pelvic surgery has a direct effect on defecation, because of the mechanical manipulation of the intestinal structures. The *diagnosis* is crucial to assessment. For example, the patient with ulcerative colitis is observed and assessed for the frequency and character of stools and for intestinal bleeding. What the patient tells the nurse about bowel problems or habits, or *subjective data*, enhances assessment. Such information is usually requested when a nursing history is taken on admission to the hospital.

An accurate record of the frequency and character of the patient's stools is necessary to plan care. Very often patients in hospitals have standing orders for a laxative or antidiarrheal drug to be provided at the discretion of the nurse. Such a record helps the nurse to gauge the administration of such drugs and to promote a regular pattern of defecation. Stools are usually described as small, moderate or medium, or large, though you may wish to be more explicit in unusual cases. To describe consistency, terms such as "formed," "semiformed," and "liquid" are employed. Unusual color or odor, such as "green," "yellow," or "clay-colored" should also be noted. Occasionally, a stool may be observed that requires such special terms as "frothy" or "mucoid."

It is also important to look for unusual or foreign substances in the stool. If frank, bright-red blood is present, it should be so described. Some foods and drugs may turn the stools reddish, but this phenomenon does not resemble fresh blood. Tests must be performed to identify the substance. Black tarry stools are caused by blood that has been passed through the stomach and small intestine and been digested.

Examination of stool specimens in the laboratory is an adjunct to diagnosis and measurement of a patient's progress. Some tests for the presence of *occult blood* (hidden or invisible blood) in the stool, such as the *guiac* test, are usually performed in the laboratory. Another test for blood in the stool is the "Hematest," for which the directions on the package should be consulted. Tests for parasites require that the stool specimens be sent to the laboratory promptly or kept warm, so that any parasites present will be viable and observable. Stool cultures reveal the presence or absence of bacteria. It is the nurse's responsibility to see that specimens are collected and cared for properly.

Nursing care for defecation problems

An *enema* is a procedure whereby a fluid is injected or instilled into the colon through the rectum. It is usually done for cleansing purposes, either to allow for the passage of hard stool or in preparation for tests. Medications are also occasionally delivered by means of an enema, using a small amount of fluid. An enema is a clean but not sterile procedure, relatively free of discomfort if good technique is observed. A physician's order is needed. Many physicians leave standing orders for bowel care, allowing the nurse to exercise independent judgment as to a particular patient's needs.

It is not uncommon for a patient to experience alternate periods of constipation and diarrhea during an illness. The nurse must thus vary the nursing actions in response to the immediate situation.

Unless specially prescribed by the physician, laxatives should be avoided as the principal treatment for constipation because of their habit-forming and irritating characteristics. It is better to increase fluid intake, supply adequate roughage in the diet, and provide sufficient exercise if the patient's condition warrants. Private toilet facilities and the provision of sufficient time to relax are a great help to the patient, who is too often hurried because of care or procedures to be performed. If the patient is made anxious by the busy hospital environment, defecation becomes difficult.

The patient with diarrhea has multiple problems. Within a very short time, profuse diarrhea can cause dehydration. The patient soon becomes debilitated and exhausted, and adequate rest must be allowed for. Losing liquid stool can cause disturbances in the electrolyte and acid-base balance, with dire consequences for the very young and very old. Skin care becomes a major concern, due to excoriation of the skin in the rectal area. Encouraging fluids prevents the effects of dehydration, and good skin care and the application of protective emollients restore the skin.

Abdominal pain and cramping can occur in conjunction with both constipation and diarrhea. The application of heat and medications ordered by the physician are often used to relieve such symptoms.

Although impaction happens most frequently to the elderly patient, it can occur at any age, particularly in cases of immobilization. An oil-retention enema is frequently administered to soften the impaction and lubricate the intestinal wall, facilitating passage of the impaction. After the oil-retention enema, a cleansing enema may be ordered. If this procedure is not successful, the impaction may need to be broken up and removed with the gloved hand. Good general nursing care supportive of all body systems is essential to the patient with intestinal dysfunction of any type.

Although urinary incontinence is a more common problem than bowel incontinence, involuntary defecation may characterize patients suffering from chronic illness, particularly of a neurologic nature. The paraplegic patient—who is capable of little or no sensation and/or movement in the lower portion of the body—can often neither feel nor control bowel movements. However, bowel rehabilitation, sometimes called bowel training, is usually successful. As is true of bladder rehabilitation, the patient's understanding and cooperation are essential even though the program is initiated by the nurse, usually on the order of the physician. The patient is given extra fluids, often prune juice, with the morning meal. Approximately thirty minutes after breakfast, a glycerine *suppository* is inserted into the rectum. The action of the medication causes peristalsis to begin shortly thereafter, and the patient is placed on the commode or bedpan to defecate. Bowel rehabilitation sometimes also employs the technique of digital stimulation: shortly after the suppository is inserted and before defecation takes place, the nurse, wearing a clean glove, inserts the middle finger into the rectum to stimulate peristalsis. Another method is to give a small cleansing enema after the morning meal. The amount of solution used is gradually decreased each morning until the enema is no longer needed. Regardless of the method used, the goal of causing the bowel to empty of its own volition at approximately the same time each day is usually attained.

Conclusion

The processes of elimination are important, both physically and psychologically, throughout our lives. Development of the ability to control the elimination of waste products provides infants and young children a feeling of independence and a degree of power. Even the adult in full control of such mechanisms recognizes the relationship of healthy functioning to the sense of well-being. In later life, some compromise is usually necessary, and older people may feel they are once again becoming dependent. Knowledge and understanding of the impact and connotations of elimination on individuals of various ages helps us to afford maximum comfort to patients.

Study terms

URINARY SYSTEM

albuminuria
anuria
calculi
catheterization
casts
dialysis
dysuria
emesis
glycosuria
hematuria
incontinence
lassitude
meatus
micturition

nephron
oliguria
polyuria
proteinuria
prostate
pyuria
renal
retention
sphincter
suppression
ureter
urethra
urgency

INTESTINAL SYSTEM

constipation
defecation
dehydration
diarrhea
enema
feces
guiac
hemorrhoid

impaction
occult blood
parasympathetic nervous system
peristalsis
psychotropic drugs
suppository
sympathetic nervous system

References

Beaumont, E. 1974. Urinary Drainage Systems. *Nursing '74* 4:1:52-60.

Broad, J. N. 1972. Urinary Incontinency—A New Method of Control. *Nursing Times* 68:9:1212-1213.

Caldwell, K. P. S. 1973. Sphincter Stimulators to Prevent Incontinency. *Nursing Times* 69:11:1524-1525.

DeGroot, J., and Kunin, C. M. 1975. Indwelling Catheters. *American Journal of Nursing* 75:3:448-449.

French, R. M. 1971. *The Nurse's Guide to Diagnostic Procedures,* 3rd ed. New York: McGraw-Hill.

Garner, J. S. 1974. Urinary Catheter Care: Doing It Better. *Nursing '74* 4:2:54-56.

Khan, A. J., *et al*. 1973. Urinary Tract Infection in Children. *American Journal of Nursing* 73:8:134-136.

Langford, T. L. 1972. Nursing Problem: Bacteriuria and the Indwelling Catheter. *American Journal of Nursing* 72:1:113-115.

Nickerson, D., *et al*. 1972. Two drop and one-drop test for Glycosuria. *American Journal of Nursing* 72:5:939.

The Safe Approach to Laxatives. 1975. *Consumer Reports* 40:8:508-510.

Tudor, L. L. 1970. Bladder and Bowel Retraining. *American Journal of Nursing* 70:11:2391-2394.

Wilson, M. F. 1975. Bladder Training for the Chronically Ill. *RN* 38:6:36-37.

16 Activity and Rest

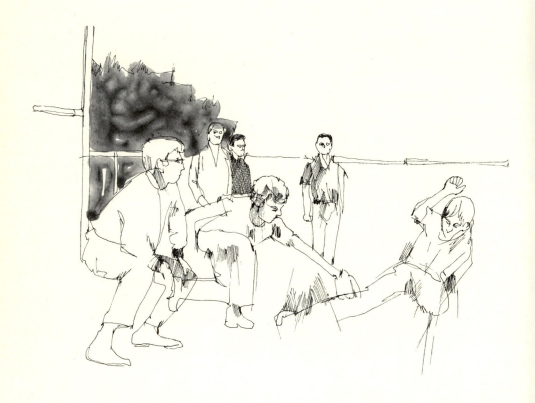

Objectives

After completing this chapter, you should be able to:

    1 Discuss the relationship of activity and rest to optimum health.

    2 Plan appropriate activity in light of a complete assessment of the patient's activity and rest status.

    3 Assess your own and a patient's posture and body mechanics and alter either, if incorrect.

    4 Identify the problems resulting from immobility.

    5 Plan nursing intervention to prevent problems caused by immobility.

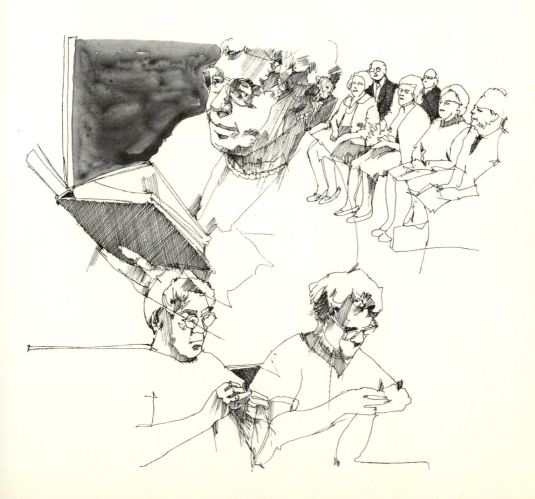

CTIVITY IS A BASIC need for all persons. Research indicates that activity is essential from birth on for optimum development. Without physical activity, a child's muscles, joints, and bone will not develop to maximum size and strength; the circulatory system will fail to develop the extensive network of small vessels that provides for additional circulation to meet stressful situations; and the respiratory system will not develop additional lung capacity. Insufficient physical activity causes muscles to atrophy, joints to become stiff, and internal organs to function less effectively. And the loss in strength of atrophied muscles undermines the systems they support. For example, weakened back muscles make the spine more liable to injury; weak abdominal muscles cause the bowel to function less effectively.

Physical activity enhances the functioning of the gastrointestinal system, increasing appetite and promoting elimination. The metabolic rate increases during activity, exercising the temperature-regulating mechanisms and a wide variety of other physiologic processes.

Activity seems to enhance the ability to think clearly by increasing circulation and promoting optimum ventilation. Activity also serves as an outlet for tension and anxiety. A game of tennis or a long walk may reduce tension and anxiety to manageable levels and permit one's energy to be focused on problem-solving. Even asleep we are physically active. We move our extremities, turn from side to side, and change position repeatedly.

Rest, the nonuse of a body part, can be thought of as the opposite of activity. It is not the same thing as sleep (see Chapter 17). All body parts need regular rest, just as they need activity. Overused muscles are unable to rid themselves of all waste products and become painful and nonfunctioning. If required to do close work for long hours, the eyes may ache and vision may be impaired.

Thus, it is apparent that a balance between activity and rest is necessary for optimum health. Though there is no simple way to determine what constitutes such a balance, one guideline is that all body parts should be used daily. If possible, they should be forced, at least briefly, to near-maximum functioning. This is especially true of muscle tissue, including the heart. Rest should be interspersed with activity so that the various body parts are allowed to recover completely.

In some situations, more extended or more complete rest of a body part is needed to allow for recovery from illness or the healing of damaged tissue. For example, a sprained ankle is supported by elastic bandages and walking is curtailed to allow the ankle to rest. During this rest period, the body has the opportunity to use all its resources to repair damaged cells, remove excess fluids, and restore function to the tissues. If rest is not provided for, healing is slowed or prevented.

If rest has been prescribed as part of the medical plan of care, it is important to distinguish between rest of a specific body part and rest of the entire body. The patient on bed rest for a broken leg is still able to move the arms and the other leg; indeed, he or she should be encouraged to do so. However, the patient on bed rest to rest the heart after a heart attack is discouraged from moving other body parts, because all activity requires increased heart activity. Clarifying the exact meaning of a prescription for rest is the responsibility of the nurse. The meaning of any prescription for activity or rest is carefully explained to the patient, and arrangements are made for the support and assistance necessary to carry out the prescription.

The effects of immobility on the body

Since both activity and rest are basic needs, restricting mobility has profound and far-reaching effects. Mobility may be restricted only slightly or so fully as to allow no movement at all. Immobilization causes changes and deterioration in even a healthy person; the axiom "that which is not used is lost" is appropriate. However, nursing measures can help prevent such deterioration. Common problems resulting from immobility will be discussed in terms of the various body systems. It is important to remember that no system is affected independently, and that preventive measures addressed to one body system may also help prevent problems in others.

The musculo-skeletal system

Muscle *atrophy* due to lack of exercise causes the muscles to become weaker, smaller, and even shorter. If this situation persists for a long enough period of time (variable from person to person), it can limit the joint's range of motion and eventually cause a contracture of the joint. A *contracture* is a permanently flexed joint, incapable of extension due to soft tissue changes. If these changes in the soft tissue are allowed to persist and the joint is not moved, changes will eventually occur in the bony structure of the joint itself.

When the stresses and strains on the bone imposed by normal movement and weight-bearing are suspended, the body begins to reabsorb calcium and *osteoporosis*—weak and porous bone—occurs. This condition may cause pain on stress and can result in easily fractured bones.

The integumentary system

The skin and subcutaneous tissue are not equipped to tolerate continued pressure in one area. Small blood vessels become occluded by the pressure, and cells begin to suffer from *ischemia* (lack of blood supply to a tissue). When pressure is removed, blood supply is restored and the cells recover; however, if the blood supply is interrupted too long, cells are unable to recover and *necrosis* (cell death) begins. This situation is the origin of most *pressure ulcers* or bedsores, as they are commonly called. Sometimes the term *decubitus ulcer* is used to refer to any pressure ulcer; but, correctly speaking, a decubitus ulcer is one that results from the decubitus, or lying-down, position. Pressure ulcers may occur on any body surface as a result of any position maintained for too long.

A pressure ulcer usually begins as an area of reddened skin. If it disappears when massaged, permanent tissue damage has not yet occurred. If the redness does not disappear, an *incipient pressure ulcer* is present. Further breakdown may be prevented by aggressive nursing care, but damage to deeper tissues may have already occurred. If so, surface tissue may continue to break down in spite of intensive nursing action.

Other factors that contribute to the formation of pressure ulcers are the presence of moisture, which tends to macerate the skin, decreasing its resistance; shearing forces, which catch the soft tissue between bone and another surface (such as a sheet) and tear or bruise the underlying tissue; and chemical irritation from stool and urine, which tends to break down the skin. Friction may cause abrasion of the skin and begin the breakdown process.

Persons with decreased awareness of peripheral sensation, including diabetics and those who have suffered strokes, have a high risk of pressure ulcers. Unable to perceive discomfort in the tissue, such individuals do not respond to it by correcting its cause. Those with impaired circulation also develop pressure ulcers rapidly, because the cells cannot recover from minor damage.

Pressure ulcers are most common over bony prominences, such as the coccyx, trochanters, scapulae, ankles, and elbows. An ulcer may occur over ischial spines due to prolonged sitting, or on the ankle bone due to a prolonged side-lying position. Ulcers are less likely to occur when there is adequate soft subcutaneous tissue to pad the bone, and more likely when the person is thin. Adequate nutrition, especially enough protein and fluids, assists in prevention by providing the means for cells to repair themselves.

Treatment of a decubitus ulcer is a serious medical problem. A culture is usually taken if infection is suspected; preventing and treating infection is a primary concern. A variety of agents, ranging from antacids and sugar to topical insulin, have been used in treatment. Enzymatic ointments are often used to remove dead tissue, and direct exposure to oxygen has been used in some areas of the country. Heat lamps have been employed to dry the surface of the ulcer and increase circulation. In extreme cases, surgical debridement and skin grafting may be needed. All the preventive measures discussed on pages 297-299 are also used in treatment.

The urinary system

Some persons' ability to void is impaired by lying down. This is especially true of men, who are accustomed to standing in order to urinate. If a person cannot maintain a normal position to urinate, the bladder may not empty completely and catheterization may be necessary. The overdistended bladder may also overflow, causing incontinence. Both of these situations may predispose to infection (see Chapter 11).

Normal kidney drainage is maintained by gravitational flow. If a person must remain prone, urine may pool in the kidney pelvis, creating a climate for infection. Furthermore, the stagnant urine may be a source of kidney stones, which are minerals precipitated out of the urine. This problem is aggravated by the excess calcium excreted when the body is reabsorbing it from inactive bone.

The gastrointestinal system

The progress of food through the digestive system is also facilitated by gravity and the normal movement of abdominal muscles. When these forces are not functioning, the entire digestive process may be slowed. This situation can result in increased gas formation and the retention of stool for such a long time that excess fluid is reabsorbed, making the stool dry and hard. If a patient is required to use a bedpan, the normal position for defecation cannot be achieved. Lack of privacy also inhibits bowel function. Together, these factors often lead to constipation and even impaction (see Chapter 15).

The respiratory system

Secretions in the lungs are usually moved from the alveoli by changes in gravity due to position change and the pressure of moving air. Once the secretions are in the bronchioles, cilia move them upward and out of the respiratory passages. When movement and position changes are minimal, secretions tend to pool in the dependent sections of the lungs, causing *hypostatic pneumonia*.

The circulatory system

Although the heart pumps blood through the arterial system to the tissue, there is no pump to return blood to the heart. Thus return blood flow depends greatly on movement and pressure from muscles surrounding the veins, aided by a system of valves that maintains one-way flow. When muscle movement is decreased, blood moves sluggishly in the large veins, predisposing to *thrombus* (clot) formation and *phlebitis* (inflammation of the vein). Clots dislodged by rubbing the muscles become *emboli* (moving particles in the blood stream), which can move through the circulatory system to the heart and out into pulmonary arteries, where they lodge in the small vessels and block circulation. Called *pulmonary embolism*, this situation is a serious threat to lung function and possibly to life.

Ordinarily, the body compensates for changes in position, and the resulting changes in the effect of gravity on circulation, by constricting and dilating vessels as necessary to maintain constant blood flow. After a period of bed rest, during which these mechanisms are not used, they do not function as effectively. Thus, if the circulation is unable to make the rapid adjustment to first arising, blood pools in the lower extremities, causing hypotension, diminished blood flow to the brain, and dizziness or even fainting. Low blood pressure caused by position change is called *postural hypotension*.

Assessing the patient's activity and rest

In assessing a patient's activity and rest status, the following aspects of the patient's musculo-skeletal system and its condition should be considered: posture; muscle tone; joint mobility; body mechanics; and actual ability to perform such activities as turning, sitting, standing, and walking. Attention should be paid to the relation between activity and need for rest, and to the patient's usual means of recognizing the need for rest.

In order to plan effective action, it is important to gather basic data on the patient's activity and rest status. Your efforts will usually be directed at maintaining an activity level as near to normal as possible. Thus you need to think in terms of a time span encompassing past, present, and future, and to consider both what the patient was able to do and what he or she actually did. Previous level of activity will affect the patient's physical condition, as well as feelings and attitudes about activity. Knowledge of the patient's prognosis will help you to plan with the patient for the future and to take into account any adaptations that must be made. Current activity level will govern your current nursing actions.

The physician's current prescription for activity and rest is a major determinant of what the patient should be encouraged to do. Sometimes this prescription is very specific, such as "Up in chair twice a day." In other cases, a prescription is very general: "Activity as tolerated." Whatever the prescription, the nurse is responsible for thorough observation of the patient's response to whatever activity is undertaken. Measuring vital signs before and after activity may yield important information on the patient's response or tolerance. If pulse, respiration, or blood pressure rises considerably and does not return to the preactivity level within a few minutes, the activity may have been too strenuous. Excessive dizziness may indicate that the activity was undertaken too rapidly. If severe fatigue occurrs, you may be increasing the amount of activity too rapidly. Your evaluation of the patient's response will enable you to replan your nursing actions.

When the goal is to increase activity progressively, a gradual approach is used. The first step may be *dangling*—that is, sitting with the legs over the edge of the bed. Simply standing at the bedside, which requires balance and increased strength, may be undertaken next. Then, ambulation can begin, increasing only a few steps each time until the patient has achieved an optimal level of activity. Sometimes patients need to remain at one level of activity for a while before proceeding further, or to regress temporarily due to other problems associated with their illnesses. Helping the patient to remain motivated to increase activity and not be discouraged by the slow pace of progress is a very challenging task. A patient who is responding well to treatment, such as a person recovering from gastroenteritis, may be able to make advances in activity at four-hour intervals during the day.

Observations are essential at each step, so that the effectiveness of the plan for the patient's activity can be evaluated, and revised as needed.

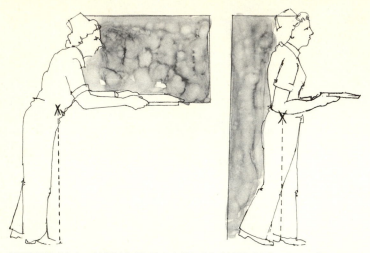

FIGURE 16.1   USING THE BASE OF SUPPORT   *Left:* Center of gravity (*X*) not over base of support (incorrect). *Right:* Center of gravity (*X*) over base of support (correct).

Posture and body mechanics for the nurse

The position of the body and the relationship of its parts to one another is called *posture*. The human body is constructed so that it functions best and is healthiest when its parts are in correct anatomical alignment. *Body mechanics* is the manner in which the body is moved.

The spine is basically a shallow S-curve that balances the body's weight evenly over its *base of support*. When the spine is not balanced vertically, an undue strain is placed on the muscles by the task of supporting the body's weight. Weight is balanced best when the *center of gravity* (a point approximately at the level of the pelvis) is directly above the base provided by the feet (see Figure 16.1). This relationship may be preserved when moving by bending from the knees, rather than the waist, or by placing the feet far apart in order to enlarge the base of support.

Twisting or *torsion* of the spine also lessens its ability to function effectively and makes it more susceptible to injury. Rather than maintaining a twisted position, the entire body should be turned in one plane as shown in Figure 16.2.

The broad, flat muscles of the back are weakest when stretched and flattened, and are susceptible to injury when lifting heavy objects. The large, thick muscles of the legs are better able to

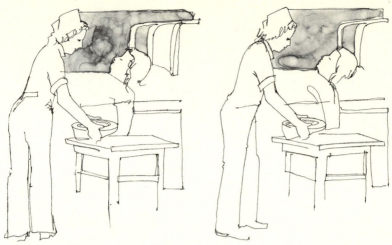

FIGURE 16.2   AVOIDING TORSION OF THE SPINE   *Left:* Nurse twisting to lift basin from bed to table (incorrect). *Right:* Nurse turning whole body to lift basin from bed to table (correct).

tolerate heavy loads. Therefore, lifting is better undertaken by bending the legs and using leg muscles than by using the back muscles. By lifting excess weight or bending from the waist, it is possible to injure not only the back muscles but also the spine itself, which can cause life-long disability.

Before moving an object or a patient, consider whether the weight might be pulled or slid, rather than lifted, to the new position. Both alternatives require less strength. Sliding is resisted by friction of the surface under the object or person, and can be minimized by providing a smooth surface (such as tight bedsheets) and/or a lubricating substance (such as talcum powder). A turning sheet placed under a patient is an effective aid, since there is less friction between the two dry sheets than between the bottom sheet and the patient's skin, which is moist. Because movement against the force of gravity requires more strength than horizontal movement, it will be less difficult to reposition a patient if the bed is first returned to a flat position.

All muscles are strongest when contracted. The closer you can position yourself to the object to be moved, the more your muscles can be shortened and strengthened. At a distance from the object, the muscles are stretched and therefore weak.

Undue strain on the abdominal muscles when lifting can tear the muscle along a weakened point, causing a hernia. This outcome

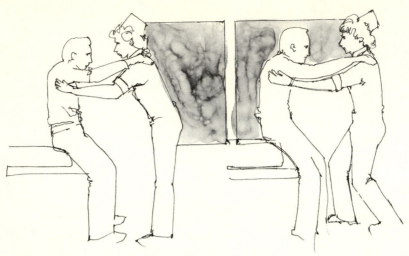

FIGURE 16.3   LIFTING WITH THE LEG MUSCLES   *Left:* Nurse assisting the patient to stand, hands under patient's arms, body bent over from waist (incorrect). *Right:* Nurse assisting patient to stand, hands under patient's arms, knees bent (correct).

can be avoided by contracting the abdominal muscles before undertaking any effort. Such tightening of the abdominal muscles has been likened to wearing an *internal girdle*.

Your weight and that of the object or person to be moved may be used to assist movement. This is accomplished when you hold your body in a solid position and then rock back, using your entire weight, rather than simply your muscular strength, as a counter-balance to assist the patient to a standing position. This procedure is illustrated in Figure 16.3. To turn a patient from back to side, bend the knees up. Then the weight of the legs turning to the side will help pull the entire body over.

Keep in mind that no one has unlimited strength. If you cannot move a patient by yourself, do not hesitate to seek assistance. In doing so, you may avoid permanent injury.

Posture and body mechanics for the patient

The nurse must take the responsibility for maintaining correct body alignment in the patient confined to bed. In order to approximate the optimal erect body posture when prone, it is necessary to use pillows, sandbags, and other supportive devices. The spine is positioned in its optimal S-curve without twisting or torsion. The shoulders and hips must be squarely aligned, and arms and legs should be supported parallel to the spine. This may be accomplished in a variety of positions: back-lying, side-lying, or on the abdomen.

Sitting posture is also important for the ill person. The back muscles need to be well supported and the body should be flexed at the hips, not slumped along the spine. The patient's feet should have a firm support, either the floor or a footstool, to prevent excess pressure behind the knees and to allow them to remain in a functional position. Arms need support so that their weight does not pull on the shoulders. The head must be either positioned vertically over the neck or supported, because neck muscles are not strong enough to support the head adequately against the pull of gravity.

Patients often need to be taught how to move safely and effectively. Though this is especially true of those with disorders of the musculo-skeletal system, it is necessary for all. The nurse can promote proper body mechanics by such acts as placing the bedside stand in a position that does not require twisting and by demonstrating correct techniques for moving in bed and for getting in and out of bed.

Exercise for the patient

Normal living usually provides the healthy individual enough exercise to insure optimal functioning of the musculo-skeletal, circulatory, and respiratory systems. But when a person is immobilized and unable to perform the usual activities, special attention needs to be given to exercise.

The range of motion

The full extent to which a joint can move in any direction is called its *range of motion*. Types of joint movement are illustrated in Figure 16.4. Maintaining the flexibility and full range of motion of the bed-ridden patient's joints is a nursing responsibility. If range of motion has already been impaired, a physical therapist is usually responsible for planning an exercise regime, although some exercises may be delegated to others.

Because the purpose of range-of-motion exercises performed by the nurse is to maintain existing function and flexibility, the joints must be subjected to all types of movement to the point at which resistance is felt. Joints should not be pushed to the point of pain, but may gradually be moved more as they become more relaxed due to preliminary exercises. Each maneuver is performed eight to ten times, usually at least once a day but possibly several

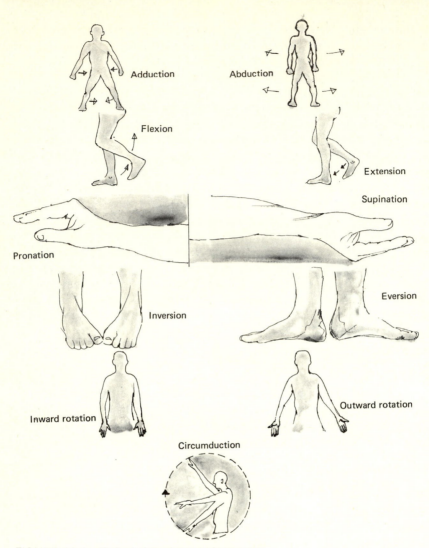

FIGURE 16.4   TYPES OF JOINT MOVEMENT

times a day, depending on the individual needs of the patient. Range-of-motion exercises need to be done frequently to maintain joint flexibility.

Active exercise

Many patients may be encouraged to perform range-of-motion exercises independently in the course of their daily self-care. The arms may be exercised by brushing the hair and by reaching to bathe arms and legs. The legs may be exercised by lifting them to put on pajama bottoms or by changing position in bed. Specific exercises may be prescribed by the physician or physical therapist, or the nurse may direct simple range-of-motion exercises. Exercises in which body parts are actively moved are called *isotonic*. When performed vigorously, isotonic exercises increase circulation and respiratory rate and have beneficial effects on the entire body. However, some individuals are unable to tolerate such increases in activity. For them, *isometric* exercise—tightening or tensing of the muscles without moving body parts—may be prescribed. Although isometric exercises can also be done very vigorously, it is possible to perform them without increasing the heart and respiratory rate. This type of exercise does not contribute to flexibility of the joints, but does promote circulatory function in the muscles exercised and increases muscle tone. Both isotonic and isometric exercises can prevent atrophy of muscles from disuse and combat osteoporosis.

Passive exercise

For patients less able to move, you must assume full responsibility for maintaining joint and muscle function. Joints may be moved as the limbs are bathed and as the patient is moved in bed. Often more specific attention must be given to exercising each and every joint. For the paralyzed patient, these exercises may need to be performed several times during the day to enhance circulation and flexibility. For the patient capable of some independent movement, daily exercises may be sufficient. Passive exercise is less effective than active exercise in combating disuse problems.

Ambulation

Exercise may be provided for by scheduling regular *ambulation*, or walking with assistance. When ambulation is ordered, the first step is to assess the patient's ability and present activity level. The longer it has been since the patient last walked, the more assistance you can expect to give. The distance to be walked and the need for assistive devices such as a walker or crutches must also be considered.

The nurse serves as the planner and decision maker regarding ambulation, and as a provider of balance to the patient while he or she walks. The nurse does not try to support the weight of the patient; if the patient cannot support his or her own weight, a walker will allow part of the weight to be supported by the patient's arms. If the patient is still unable to support his or her own weight, two persons may assist with weight-bearing, but ambulation should be reconsidered. Attempting to bear the patient's weight can cause injury to the nurse.

It is most helpful to the patient to stay on his or her strongest side, which allows the patient to lean toward that side. Your own position should be such that the patient will not pull you to the floor if he or she falls. This may happen if the patient's arm is around your shoulders: if the patient falls from that position, a twisting pressure may be applied to your back. This is a common cause of back injury in nurses. One of the best ways of giving support is for the patient to wear a safety belt around the waist, and the nurse to hold it at the

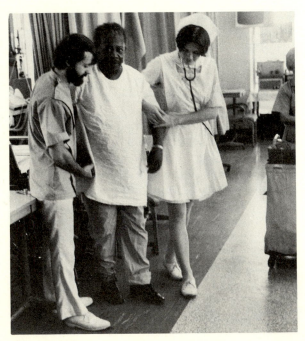

Elizabeth Wilcox

center back. Another method is for the nurse to bend an arm at the elbow and allow the patient to hold and lean on the arm. Either of these positions provides balance and a feeling of security to the patient without endangering you.

If the patient should begin to fall while being ambulated, simply assist him or her to the floor, avoiding protruding corners and protecting the head. It is the policy of some health care facilities for a physician to examine the patient who has fallen before he or she is moved. In other facilities, the patient is initially examined by a nurse, who takes responsibility for deciding whether the patient can be moved back to bed and examined by a physician later or whether immediate care by a physician is needed. In either case, the patient will need constant attention and reassurance until he or she is returned to bed.

Position changes

Position changes—from one side to the other, to the back, and from prone to raised head—combat immobility by enhancing drainage of the kidney, encouraging movement of respiratory secretions, stimulating circulation, and relieving pressure on skin and subcutaneous tissues. Immobilized patients have traditionally been placed on a two-hour turning schedule, but the patient is served best if the schedule is individualized. For some persons, more frequent turning is necessary. A guide is the appearance of the patient's skin. If the reddened pressure areas begin to blanch when rubbed, and there is no residual reddening at the next turning, the tissue is recovering. If the tissue does not blanch or the reddened areas are still present when it is time to resume pressure on them, the length of time in one position needs to be reduced. Positon changes are as critical for the person immobilized in a wheelchair as for the person in bed. Even very slight movement can change the focus of pressure. Whenever position is changed, massage of the pressured area will help restore the tissue more rapidly.

Additional measures for combating the effects of immobility

A host of devices are manufactured to help prevent pressure sores. An alternating pressure mattress is a plastic air mattress whose air-filled tubes are attached to a motor that automatically inflates and deflates the mattress. Alternating tubes are connected to different outlets, with the result that one set of tubes is inflated while the other set is deflated and the pressured areas constantly change. The effectiveness of the mattress is diminished if there is more than one layer of bedding between it and the patient, because fabric packs into the spaces left by the deflated tubes and equalizes pressure. Sheets pulled tightly across the surface of the mattress have the same effect.

Silicone gel pads are used most frequently under the buttocks. These devices, very similar in density to body fat, provide padding and distribute pressure across the entire body surface, preventing its concentration on any one point. They must usually be rotated regularly to prevent premanent ridges from occurring on their surfaces. Such pads are encased in easily cleaned plastic, and may be covered with protective padding.

Soft foam-rubber pads characterized by many small fingerlike projections serve a very similar purpose. The irregular surface allows air to circulate near the skin, helping to alleviate skin maceration due to perspiration. Pads are produced in small sizes to fit under the buttocks or in wheelchairs and in large sizes to cover entire beds.

Sheepskins, both natural and synthetic, have been used under bony prominences to provide a soft surface that does not abrade the skin. The furry surface also allows for air circulation and the distribution of weight. Natural sheepskins have the added advantage of surface lanolin, which softens and protects the skin; however, they are difficult to clean and quite expensive. Artificial sheepskins are completely washable. Both kinds are effective only in direct contact with the patient's skin.

Water beds have been used successfully for persons who need to be immobilized for prolonged periods. Because the patient literally floats on the surface of the bed, pressure is distributed evenly over the entire body.

Other special beds (Stryker, Foster, or Bradford frames; Circolectric beds) are sometimes used to facilitate position changes for immobilized patients.

All of these devices have demonstrated value in the prevention of pressure sores. They are used in conjunction with a regular program of skin care that provides for position changes, massage, and cleanliness, and by no means replace regular care.

Coughing and deep breathing can be effective in preventing hypostatic pneumonia. Though the patient may not feel a need to cough, coughing expands the lungs fully and helps move secretions.

A high fluid intake—3000 cc. or more—if feasible in light of the patient's condition, will help keep minerals in suspension and guard against stones in the urinary tract. Also, a dilute urine helps protect against infection, and ample fluid intake keeps the skin and mucous membranes moist and lessens the risk of their breaking down. High fluid intake also combats the tendency toward constipation and enhances bowel function.

A *well-balanced diet* provides the nutrients necessary for the body to repair and maintain tissue, especially the integument. Particular care should be taken to provide fruits and roughage, which tend to combat constipation. If the patient is troubled by digestive upset and gas, foods that cause gas or increase digestive problems should be eliminated.

Conclusion

Activity and rest may be profoundly affected by any illness. Often the patient experiences some degree of immobility, and the nurse must assume a major role in maintaining the patient's ability and functioning. As you assess the patient's activity and rest status, identify particular problems and needs, and undertake those nursing actions that will be most supportive, keep in mind that your goal is the optimal activity level for the patient.

Study terms

ambulation
atrophy
base of support
body mechanics
center of gravity
contracture
dangling
decubitus ulcer
emboli
exercise
  active
  isometric
  isotonic
  passive
hypostatic pneumonia

immobility
incipient pressure ulcer
internal girdle
ischemia
necrosis
osteoporosis
phlebitis
posture
postural hypotension
pressure ulcer
pulmonary embolism
range of motion
thrombus
torsion

References

Brower, P., and Hicks, D. 1972. Maintaining Muscle Function in Patients on Bed Rest. *American Journal of Nursing* 72:1250-1253.

Browse, N. L. 1965. *The Physiology and Pathology of Bed Rest*. Springfield, Ill.: Charles C. Thomas, 1965.

Carnavali, D., and Brueckner, S. 1970. Immobilization: Reassessment of a Concept. *American Journal of Nursing* 70:1502-1507.

Drapeau, J. 1975. Getting Back into Good Posture: How to Erase Your Lumbar Aches. *Nursing '75* 5:9:63-65.

Foss, G. 1973. Body Mechanics: Use Your Head and Save Your Back. *Nursing '73* 3:5:25-32.

————. 1973. Breaking Architectural Barriers with Crutches, Wheelchairs, Walkers. *Nursing '73* 3:10:16-31.

Gordon, M. 1976. Assessing Activity Tolerance. *American Journal of Nursing* 76:72-75.

Hoover, S. A. 1973. Job Related Back Injuries in a Hospital. *American Journal of Nursing* 71:2078-2079.

Jordan, H. S., and Kauchak, M. A. Transfer Techniques. *Nursing '73* 3:3:19-22.

Kamentetz, H. L. 1972. Exercise for the Elderly. *American Journal of Nursing* 72:1401.

Olson, E. V., ed. 1967. The Hazards of Immobility. *American Journal of Nursing* 67:779-797. Supplement.

Works, R. F. 1972. Hints on Lifting and Pulling. *American Journal of Nursing* 72:260-261.

17 Sleep

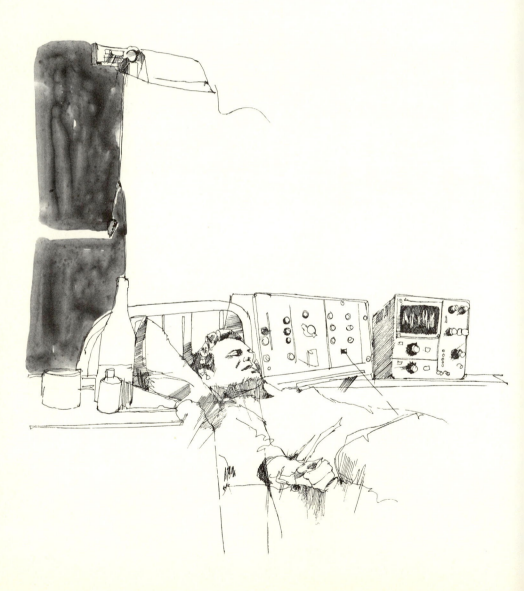

Objectives

After completing this chapter, you should be able to:

1 Define the term *circadian rhythm* and describe the general level of functioning of both body and mind throughout the cycle.

2 List the five stages of sleep in sequence and briefly describe each stage.

3 Discuss common causes of sleep deprivation and its effects on the individual.

4 Describe the effects of hypnotics and amphetamines on sleep.

5 Outline appropriate nursing measures for the patient experiencing sleep disturbance.

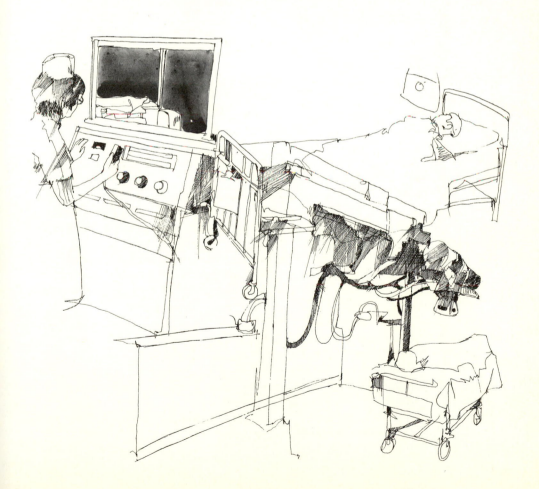

S LEEP AND REST are neither identical nor interchangeable. Rest certainly promotes muscular relaxation, which may or may not be accompanied by a reduction in psychic tension. But rest is not characterized by the pronounced muscular relaxation, decreased body functioning, and psychic fluctuations that occur during sleep.

The subject of sleep has long been ignored in the nursing literature, which is odd in view of the fact that sleep is a basic need and sleep management an integral aspect of nursing care. The medical literature, meanwhile, has focused considerable attention on sleep, and some of its conclusions are highly relevant to nursing care. It is distressing for a night nurse to chart that the patient slept well, only to discover the following night that the patient complained of fatigue and irritability during the day. As we shall see, this situation usually has a scientific basis that resides in the answers to certain basic questions. What is adequate sleep for a given patient? Is all sleep alike? Most important, how can the nurse promote and provide for adequate sleep when planning care?

Circadian rhythm

Like plants and animals, human beings are cyclic; that is, they experience sequentially patterned periods of activity and inactivity. Each day of life is composed of a period of awareness and a period of relative unawareness (sleep), a pattern characteristic of all human beings and known as the *circadian rhythm*. This term, derived from Latin, means "approximately a day." Most of us identify ourselves as "day people" or "night people"—more alert and productive in the morning or in the evening. Despite such differences, however, the twenty-four-hour circadian cycle is very uniform in humans. A French man set a record by remaining in isolation in a Texas cave 205 days without time-measuring devices of any type. Within a very short time, he had established a circadian rhythm of just under twenty-six hours, thus approximating the twenty-four-hour day.

It is useful to consider sleep as one end of a continuum whose other extreme is wakefulness. As Figure 17.1 shows, wakefulness is characterized by maximal functioning of the body systems. Muscular activity stimulates the respiratory system, food intake arouses the production of gastric and intestinal secretions, and the processes of elimination function forcefully. Furthermore, mental awareness is heightened, and the reflexes are active and prepared for a threat response.

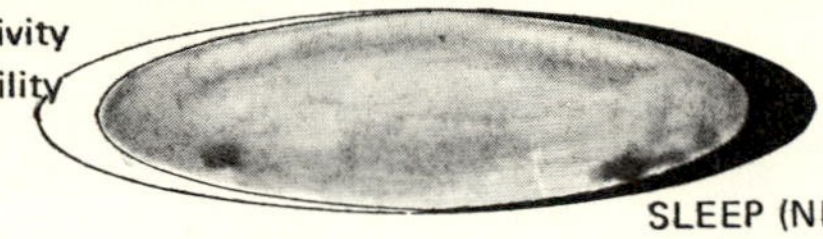

WAKEFULNESS (DAY)
Consciousness
Increased physiological functioning
Increased reflex activity
Decision-making ability
Muscular tonus

SLEEP (NIGHT)
Unconsciousness
Decreased physiological functioning
Decreased reflex activity
Increased muscular relaxation

FIGURE 17.1   PHYSIOLOGICAL AND PSYCHOLOGICAL RESPONSES DUR-
ING CIRCADIAN RHYTHM

Although sleep is a less active state than wakefulness, it is
not—as was once believed—inactive. Blood pressure, temperature,
pulse, and respirations decrease; digestive juices subside to some
degree; and the kidneys become less productive. The BMR (basal
metabolism rate) decreases as muscle relaxation increases. Most of
the reflexes weaken or disappear entirely, with the important exception of the cough reflex. And the psychological self focuses during
sleep on the internal environment of the mind. The activities of the
mind during sleep will be considered in detail shortly.

The causes of sleep

Precisely what causes or induces sleep is currently unknown.
Chemical theories propose the increased carbon dioxide in the
blood immediately before and during sleep as the causative agent.
However, decreased physical activity could account for the increase in carbon dioxide. Although it is a common experience for
drowsiness to occur in inadequately oxygenated surroundings, the
chemical theory has proved questionable in explaining the more
complex findings about sleep.

The *vascular* theory rests on the assumption that the fall in
blood pressure that occurs during sleep decreases the flow of blood
within the brain, sustaining the state of unconsciousness. Current
studies clearly show, however, that the opposite is the case: cerebrovascular blood flow increases during sleep.

It has long been thought that the *pituitary* is a sleep regulator,
if not its primary activator. Nevertheless, persons whose pituitary

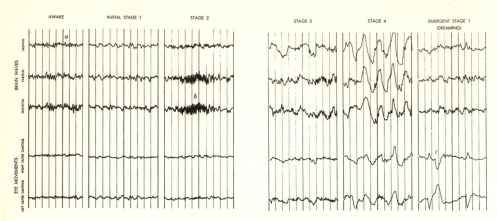

FIGURE 17.2 ELECTROENCEPHALOGRAPHIC TRACINGS OF SLEEP STAGES

From Nathaniel Kleitman, "Patterns of Dreaming," Scientific American, November 1960, pp. 46-47. Courtesy of William Dement, Stanford University School of Medicine.

glands are removed surgically do not experience great changes in their sleep patterns.

Neurophysiologists, working on the *neurohormonal* theory, have singled out the neurohormone serotonin as a possible causative agent of sleep. When this substance is injected directly into the cerebral vascular system of an animal, sleep immediately ensues.

One of the most promising theories to date—and a very complicated one—is the *feedback* theory, which proposes that, after a period of neuronal activity during which electrical impulses are relayed throughout the system, fatigue takes place at the synapses and brings on sleep.

Finally, some dismiss the entire controversy by stating plainly that sleep is *instinctual*.

The stages of sleep

To the person who awakens in the morning feeling fairly well rested, sleep may seem to be no more or less than a period of unawareness and quiescence, highlighted only by an occasional dream or the sensation of turning. However, several well-known authorities in the field of sleep research have demonstrated that the nature of sleep is far more active and complicated than has been supposed. Dement, Kleitman, and Oswald, three prominent researchers work-

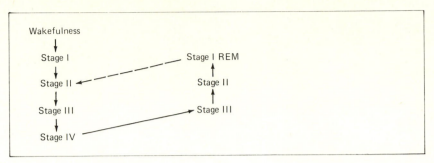

FIGURE 17.3   THE SLEEP CYCLE

ing separately, have found that the character of sleep changes during
a given sleeping period, progressing through sequential stages.
Their findings are based on the use of the *electroencephalograph*
(EEG), a machine that measures and records the electrical energy
produced by the cortex of the brain. The recording is called an *electroencephalogram* or tracing. (See Figure 17.2.)

According to Dement, Kleitman, and Oswald, the period of
sleep for most individuals consists of from four to six complete cycles, each of which is composed of five stages. Each of the five stages
has its own special characteristics. The sleep cycle is illustrated in
Figure 17.3.

Stage I most closely resembles wakefulness, and produces a
recording of brain activity similar to that of a person who is awake,
except for a few slow waves on the tracing. Muscles retain their tone
(tonus), although a slow rolling of the eyes takes place. If aroused in
this stage, a person will often deny having slept, saying that he or
she was "just drifting off"—though sleep had actually begun.

Stage II marks the beginning of muscle relaxation. The EEG
waves become more regular and the person appears to be asleep.

Stage III consists of deeper sleep, manifested in still more
slowing of the EEG tracing and loss of muscle tone. Some reflexes diminish at this point, and snoring may occur.

Stage IV, the period of deepest sleep, is characterized by very
large, slow waves on the electroencephalograph. The muscles are in a
state of relaxation, the most relaxed since the onset of sleep. The
dreams that often occur during this stage have a conventional, every-
day quality. These dreams may be extensions or revisions of the previous day's events or of familiar experiences.

Some twenty to thirty minutes elapse between falling asleep
and Stage IV. At this point the process is reversed, and the sleeper
begins an ascent from Stage IV through Stages III and II.

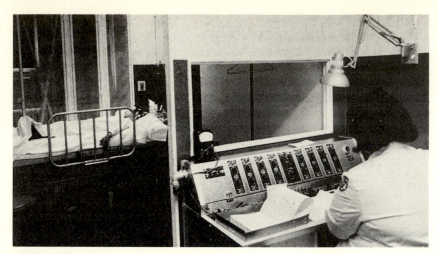

Elizabeth Wilcox

Then begins another stage called *rapid eye movement sleep* or *Stage I REM*. This stage, which we shall refer to as REM, should not be confused with Stage I; it is a distinct phenomenon, and its characteristics are dramatic. Both eyes move rapidly back and forth horizontally. One observer has reported occasional twitching of the ears, and body twitching is not uncommon. With the exception of the eyes, the muscles are almost totally relaxed. Reflexes are even more diminished than in Stage IV. However, both blood pressure and respirations increase. Although the muscles are completely relaxed, cortical activity is high. The tracing is varied and quite active, not unlike that of waking. The dreams that frequently take place during REM sleep are much more vividly detailed than those of Stage IV, and may be colorful, violent, or erotic. The contradiction between the relaxation of the muscles and the extreme activity of the brain leads some to refer to REM sleep as *paradoxic sleep*. This term is used interchangeably with REM and Stage I REM.

With the end of REM sleep, one sleep cycle has been completed. This process usually takes about ninety minutes. The next cycle begins with the entry into Stage II sleep. As the night progresses, Stages III and IV decrease in length and REM increases. Though scientists are disputing the precise purpose of REM sleep, they seem to agree that it is essential.

Some of the important findings of sleep research may well have significance for nurses in the future. First, persons suffering from schizophrenia experience much less REM sleep than do normally functioning persons. Second, a recent exploration into the cause of SID (sudden infant death or "crib death") has led one authority to hypothesize that the combination of a mild respiratory infection and a malfunction of the autonomic nervous system during REM sleep brings about laryngospasm and silent death.

Sleep deprivation studies appear to demonstrate that the duration of REM sleep is even more important than the total hours of sleep. Whether REM sleep serves as a psychic outlet for stress and tension accrued during the waking hours or as a data-processing mechanism that establishes new neural pathways is an interesting question. However, these conjectures are less important to you as a nurse than is understanding that both Stage IV and REM sleep are essential to human functioning in some manner that is not fully understood.

Insomnia

Insomnia, or inability to sleep, is a relatively common condition. It is said that the United States has more insomniacs than any other country in the world. One type of insomnia is caused by such contributing factors as pain, emotional upset, and poor sleeping conditions. Eliminating the cause of such sleeplessness usually brings about relief. However, as much as 10-15 percent of the population suffers from chronic insomnia, a more troublesome phenomenon whose cause is not so evident. It is often a longstanding sleep pattern on the part of the individual. The resulting fear of being unable to sleep only intensifies the problem. Medical intervention, including drugs, may be necessary until new patterns are established.

Age and sleep

Almost as if resting in preparation for life's journey, the infant spends many more hours of the day sleeping than does the adult. Of this time, approximately 50 percent is spent in REM sleep. During the REM stages, grimacing, twitching, and sucking movements are frequent.

The adult, on the other hand, experiences four to six sleep cycles per night, averaging a total of 7.9 hours of sleep. Of this time, 23 percent is REM sleep. There are no appreciable differences between males and females with regard to sleep.

Elderly persons experience less Stage III and IV sleep, as well as less REM, than do infants and adults. As little as 15 to 18 percent of total sleep may be REM. Nurses should keep in mind that, though the aged may appear to sleep a great deal, they experience less total sleep than younger people due to frequent awakenings. The discomforts associated with many degenerative conditions are not conducive to sleep. Arthritic pain can cause frequent interruption in the sleep pattern. The patient with respiratory problems is often forced to sleep in an almost upright position, which interferes with sleep. And urinary urgency in the elderly also interrupts sleep.

Sleep deprivation

Sleep deprivation studies have been undertaken by paying a willing subject to sleep in a laboratory. When the EEG indicates that dreaming is occurring, usually during Stage IV or REM, the subject is awakened, tested, and allowed to return to sleep. This arousal upon dreaming is repeated over and over until certain signs and behaviors indicate that the subject is experiencing sleep deprivation. Some studies do not allow the subject to sleep at all for long periods of time.

Initially, sleep deprivation causes a decrease in attention span, irritability, slowed reactions, and heightened sensitivity to pain or a lowered pain threshold. These reactions are significant for nurses responsible for alleviating the pain of their patients. Sleep deprivation also results in an inability to perform repetitive tasks. As the deprivation becomes more pronounced, the behavioral and physiological signs intensify. The subject may enter a state of confusion, and even manifest disorientation and psychosis. Hallucinations have been reported to characterize extended periods of sleeplessness. Persons with seizure disorders, such as epilepsy, may have convulsions.

Studies have shown that prolonged sleep deprivation lowers the seizure threshold, as well as the pain threshold. Thus nurses who undertake health teaching caution epileptic patients against undue sleep loss or jobs that require frequent changes in schedule. It is an interesting peripheral fact that persons who have had seizures appear to experience much less REM sleep than is usual for several days after such seizures. One might speculate that the seizure provides some sort of substitute for the REM sleep the individual usually needs.

Sleep deprivation can occur either when the duration of sleep is inadequate or when the sleeping time is repeatedly interrupted, especially during Stage IV or the REM stages. Any individual who must work various shifts with intervening days off, such as a nurse, may experience sleep deprivation. Patients may be sleep-deprived due to pain or drugs, or to the requirements of constant nursing care.

Drugs and sleep

The work of Evans (1970) and others reveals that hypnotics decrease REM sleep, even though the sleeping time itself may be lengthened. Many sleeping medications, including the group called barbiturates, decrease REM sleep. None of the hypnotics induces natural sleep.

The amphetamines also greatly inhibit REM sleep. This class of drugs, known colloquially as "speed" or "uppers," has recently figured prominently in drug abuse. Much of the aberrant behavior of the "speed freak" may be attributable to long-term REM sleep deprivation.

Discontinuing any of these drugs causes REM sleep to become abnormally high, which is probably a "catch-up" mechanism. It is highly important for the nurse to know that the patient withdrawing from these drugs also frequently experiences vivid, frightening nightmares. If the person is made so uncomfortable by these episodes as to feel a need to return to the drug, a cycle of drug dependency can begin. Fortunately, this withdrawal period is relatively short. Talking with the patient about the feelings that accompany withdrawal and their cause may be a highly valuable service to the patient. Offering emotional support may prevent the patient from using drugs unnecessarily.

Nursing concerns with sleep

Basic knowledge about sleep is very important to nurses, who are themselves susceptible to sleep disturbances and sleep deprivation. Medication errors and deviations from aseptic technique can easily occur when the nurse is overly tired. Irritability may strain interpersonal relations. When sleep loss does occur—and it is sometimes unavoidable—the nurse must take special precautions in practice.

Most nursing history forms ask for no data on the patient's sleep patterns. One might append such information as the number of hours of sleep the patient normally needs, the usual bedtime, and factors conducive or disturbing to the patient's sleep. For example, a ticking clock soothes some and irritates others.

Awareness of medications being given or withdrawn enables the nurse to observe for signs of sleep problems and to offer reassurance if unpleasant dreams or other side effects occur.

The recumbent position can increase bronchial and nasal secretions, causing a cough. Anticipating this outcome in the case of the respiratory patient, and securing an order for an appropriate cough medication before the patient's bedtime, may prevent hours of sleeplessness.

Many assessments nurses make are simple observations, such as of skin color or rate of respiration. Others are much more subtle. To assess sleep deprivation accurately, one must be familiar with the patient's situation during the previous few days. Has the patient been in intensive care for some time, experiencing numerous interruptions of sleep? Has the patient recently been placed on REM-inhibiting drugs? Does the chart indicate several nights of poor sleep due to pain or stress?

Such information enables you to consider signs and symptoms that indicate the patient is sleep-deprived. Irritability, intermittent dozing, frequent complaints of pain inconsistent with the degree of pain usually produced by the underlying condition, and complaints of fatigue are all noteworthy. If sleep is disturbed due to pain, it is much more sensible and helpful to administer the prescribed pain medication than the sleeping medication. It is advantageous not to give medication known to interfere with REM sleep, since the relief of pain often allows sleep to ensue naturally.

Repeated studies have shown that at least some of the confusion and disorientation displayed by patients in intensive care units is caused by sleep deprivation due to continual interruption of Stages III and IV and REM sleep. Careful planning of nursing care, which allows for nursing procedures to be performed in specified time blocks, enables patients to sleep for more extended periods.

The value of comfort-promoting measures cannot be underestimated. The nurse who spends time providing care before the patient's bedtime may considerably minimize the need for sleep medications. An unhurried backrub, the straightening or replacement of wrinkled or soiled linens, and perhaps a warm, noncaffeinated beverage all enhance the ability to sleep. Offering the bedpan or urinal at bedtime prevents sleep from being interrupted.

Nursing Actions That Promote Sleep

1 Gathering pertinent data on the patient's sleep patterns
2 Being aware of the patient's medications and their effects
3 Taking steps to prevent coughing
4 Planning care to provide sufficient time for sleeping
5 Encouraging daytime activity
6 Eliminating or minimizing disturbing factors in the environment
7 Repositioning the patient to prevent restlessness
8 Adjusting binders, dressings, and casts as needed
9 Giving emotional support to relieve stress and anxiety
10 When appropriate, administering pain-relievers rather than sleeping medications

Binders, dressings, and casts are also known to cause discomfort and restlessness. Rewrapping a binder, reinforcing or replacing dressings, and padding or repositioning casts can easily prevent such a problem. Repositioning the patient incapable of turning independently lessens muscle fatigue, which in turn encourages relaxation.

Eliminating or minimizing disturbing factors in the hospital environment is also helpful. Unpleasant odors, excessively warm or cool temperatures, and unnecessary lights and noises—including conversation within proximity of the patient—may all prove distracting and interfere with sleep.

As well as providing physical comfort, the nurse strives to provide for maximum peace of mind, remembering that stress and anxiety frequently cause restlessness and/or insomnia. The patient's anxiety could very well be related to tests just performed or about to be performed, apprehension over his or her condition, or the strangeness of the hospital environment. The nurse who listens and discusses such concerns with the patient is promoting sleep.

Lastly, boredom often causes the bedridden patient to sleep off and on throughout the day, becoming wakeful and demanding at night. You might contact the family or occupational therapy department or, on your own initiative, provide a stimulating daytime activity or exercise to help the patient sleep more soundly at night. See the list of nursing actions that promote sleep above.

Conclusion

Illness causes stress and places undue demands on both the physiological and psychological response systems of the individual. Thus sleep is even more important than usual to persons who are ill. To provide for adequate sleep when planning nursing care and to intervene appropriately when sleep problems arise are essential elements of good nursing practice.

CARE STUDY / A patient with sleep deprivation

Mrs. Julie Stafford is a fifty-seven-year-old patient with bronchitis and emphysema. A long-term heavy smoker, Mrs. Stafford has experienced increasing respiratory difficulty over the past few years. In recent weeks the infection has made breathing so difficult that Mrs. Stafford has become dependent on frequent use of an IPPB (Intermittent Positive Pressure Breathing) apparatus.

On admission Mrs. Stafford reported feeling anxious as well as "generally tired," and appeared pale. Her respirations were shallow and rapid. Mr. Stafford said his wife had been sleeping poorly for two to three weeks.

The physician's orders include bedrest, an antibiotic, a mild tranquilizer, pain medication, and IPPB treatments every two hours.

The staff nurse assigned to Mrs. Stafford begins her assessment by reading the data in the record, which notes the history of sleeping poorly and the feeling of tiredness and anxiety, and the physician's orders. A visit to Mrs. Stafford confirms the persistence of the same concerns. The nurse notes the patient's exhausted appearance. A menu order lies on the bedside table unmarked. When asked if she would like to complete the form or needs help to do so, Mrs. Stafford dismisses the subject by saying, in a mildly irritated manner, "I really don't care what I eat. I just want to be left alone." When asked if her husband has left the hospital, she replies, "I really can't remember." She requests pain medication every three hours. Her medical and nursing management is such that Mrs. Stafford's sleep is interrupted about once an hour. Mrs. Stafford appears to be experiencing the problem of sleep deprivation.

The staff nurse determines that nursing intervention is needed. Knowing that the normal sleep cycle lasts about ninety minutes, she thinks the patient needs an extended period of uninterrupted sleep. The nurse arranges to talk with the physician, to whom she describes the patient's sleep history and behavior. The physician and nurse examine the current blood gas reports and, noting improvement, decide that the 2:00 p.m. IPPB treatment might be omitted. The physician writes the order to omit the treatment, and the plan is explained to the patient. Mrs. Stafford seems to welcome the intervention. At 12:00 she receives her noon meal, medications, the IPPB treatment, and a relaxing backrub. The hospital telephone operator is instructed not to place calls to the patient for four hours. The room is darkened. A sign noting the time span during which the patient is not to be disturbed is placed on the closed door of the room. At 3:00, the plan is explained to the p.m. staff nurse.

Evaluation is termed positive by the staff nurse at the 4:00 p.m. report. Mrs. Stafford awakens from four hours of deep sleep stating that she feels "so much better." She appears to breathe more easily and requests a colorful gown in preparation for evening visiting hours.

Study terms

BMR (basal metabolic rate)
circadian rhythm
cortex
electroencephalogram
electroencephalograph
hallucination
hypnotic
insomnia
paradoxic sleep
REM (rapid eye movement)
sleep cycle

sleep deprivation
sleep stage
theories of sleep
   chemical
   feedback
   instinctual
   neurohormonal
   pituitary
   vascular
tonus

References

The Anatomy of Sleep. 1966. Nutley, N.J.: Roche Laboratories.

Evans, J. I., and Ogunremi, O. 1970. Sleep and Hypnotics: Further Experiments. *British Medical Journal* 8:310-312.

Kales, A., *et al.* 1970. Hypnotics and Altered Sleep-Dream Patterns. *Archives of General Psychiatry* 23:9:211-218.

Kleitman, N. 1963. *Sleep and Wakefulness*, rev. ed. Chicago: University of Chicago Press.

Lavie, P., *et al.* 1975. Ultradian Rhythms: The 90 Minute Clock Inside Us. Part 2, *Psychology Today* 8:5:54-56.

Long, B. 1969. Sleep. *American Journal of Nursing* 69:9:1896-1899.

Luce, G. G. 1975. Internal Tempos: To Live in Harmony with the Earth, Trust Your Body Rhythms. Part 1, *Psychology Today* 8:5:52-53.

O'Dell, M. L. 1975. Human Biorhythmology: Implications for Nursing Practice. *Nursing Forum* 14:1:43-47.

Oswald, I. 1969. Human Brain Protein, Drugs and Dreams. *Nature* 233:5209:893-897.

_____. 1971. The Biological Clock-Shift Work. *Nursing Times* 67:9:1207-1208.

Owen, M., and Bliss, E. 1970. Sleep Loss and Cerebral Excitability. *American Journal of Physiology* 18:1:171-179.

Wyeth, R. J. 1973. Treatment of Insomnia. National Institute of Mental Health. Washington D.C.: U.S. Government Printing Office.

18 Sexuality

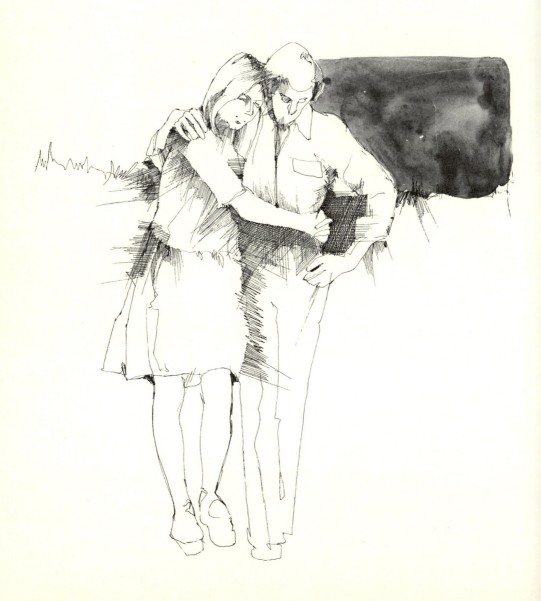

Objectives

After completing this chapter, you should be able to:

1 Differentiate between sexuality and sexual behavior.

2 Explore your own feelings about sexual variations and behavior with regard to caring for patients.

3 List three major classes of drugs that may cause sexual alterations.

4 List the factors that may decrease or increase libido during illness.

5 Specify surgical procedures that may precipitate sexual problems for the patient.

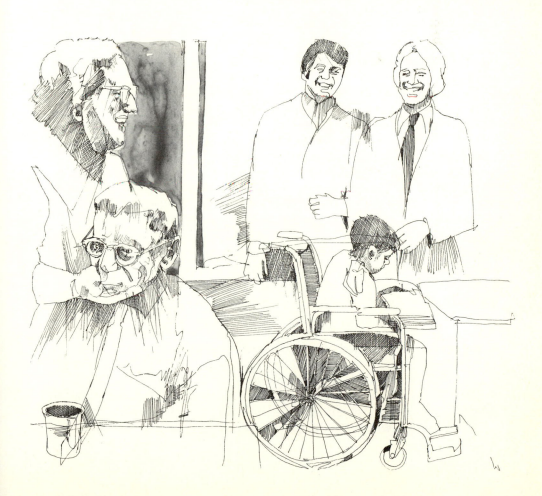

I T IS READILY EVIDENT that we in the United States are currently experiencing a sexual revolution. Although there is considerable controversy over the extent of this revolution, it is inescapably obvious that sexual attitudes are changing. Women are demanding and assuming sexual freedom enjoyed in the past only by men and a new openness with regard to sexuality is allowing individuals to explore their sexual feelings honestly and to seek help with sexual problems.

It is important for nurses to keep in mind the distinction between sexuality and sexual behavior. Sexuality, regardless of its expression, is an integral aspect of the total person. It is an awareness of one's femininity or masculinity, a vital component of one's body image and orientation toward life. Although we will in this chapter be focusing on sexual behavior, or the expression of sexuality, we must keep in mind the concept of sexuality itself as a feeling about oneself as a sexual being.

Variations in sexual behavior

Sexual behavior is the expression of sexuality. *Heterosexuality*—sexual relations between a man and a woman—is the norm in American society. Alfred Kinsey and his colleagues, after collecting a large volume of data, published two books (1948, 1953) on the sexual behavior of the American male and female. These books document a higher incidence of two variations from the norm than their authors had suspected: *homosexuality*, or sexual relations between two members of the same sex; and bisexuality, or sexual relations with members of both sexes. It is unclear whether more people are homosexual or bisexual now, or whether open communication has simply made sexual variations more apparent. Until very recently, both homosexuality and bisexuality have been considered "deviant" behavior, often punishable by law. In the last few years, homosexuals (most of whom prefer to be called *gay*) have formed groups protesting discriminatory practices against them. In 1973 and again in 1974, the American Psychiatric Association (APA) resolved at its annual convention that homosexuality, in and of itself, does not constitute mental illness.

Just as a certain proportion of the general population is homosexual, so may be some members of the health care team, including nurses. It is impossible, of course, entirely to suppress our emotional and sexual lives when practicing nursing. Our attitudes unavoidably influence our interactions with patients and with our peers. Remaining objective and nonjudgmental is not always easy, but patients should be regarded as persons who have problems and need care, regardless of their sexual life styles. Similarly, nurses should evaluate each other in terms only of nursing proficiency, not of sexual preference. It must be understood that nurses never impose their sexual views on their patients.

Stereotyping, unwise in any situation, is particularly futile when one tries to "guess" another person's sexual life style. The notion that males who are "limp-wristed" and females who are "mannish" are gay is simply false. Studies of gay persons reveal no overwhelming preponderance of particular traits. These findings lend support to the practice of accepting people as they are, on the basis of objective data.

Although, as we have said, homosexuals have become much more vocal and are in many cases speaking out honestly in defense of their chosen sexual style, gay patients rarely divulge such relationships. In light of generally negative staff attitudes toward homosexual patients, this reticence is understandable. The homosexual patient is often socially ostracized, even to the point of being placed in a single room or alone in a multiple-occupancy room. The usual light conversation and inquiries about job and family are noticeably absent. The patient's visitors are scrutinized by the staff, and attempts are occasionally made to limit them, which is not done with other patients. Some degree of relief is often evident when such a patient is discharged.

If we consider nurses as a sociological group, we can better understand the sources of the judgmental behavior nurses sometimes exhibit toward persons whose sexual life styles differ from the majority's. Nursing's roots are in religion; many schools of nursing were originally religious in nature. And even with the current prevalence of nonsectarian settings, nursing continues to be subject to dictates on moral and sexual conduct. Also, nurses come largely from the middle class; few are very wealthy or very poor. The middle class, like other social classes, has characteristic values, which have tended to be conservative, particularly in the realm of sexuality. Social changes are usually initiated at the fringes of society, and gradually make their way to the center. Nurses, as participants in the mainstream of the culture, may give way to change somewhat reluctantly. We need, however, to accept the new openness toward homosexuality and to respond to gay persons in a more objective, professional manner.

Sexuality in relation to nursing practice

Think back on the nursing process and evaluate the completeness of your assessment. Do you routinely assess for sexual problems? Are sexual problems not an appropriate subject for assessment? Sexual problems do arise as a result of illness and surgery, and yet we often ignore their existence. Because of the private nature of sexual matters, you might choose not to ask the patient direct questions about sex for purposes of assessment. Sometimes the nurse has only a "feeling" that a patient is facing sexual problems. At other times a patient or the patient's partner may feel a need to talk about such problems and approach the physician or nurse. A male patient may be more comfortable talking with a male physician or a male nurse; female patients might also prefer to speak to a doctor or nurse of their own sex.

One sensitive problem that may occasionally present itself to the nurse is a suggestive or seductive advance by a patient. Pretending such an incident did not occur is usually not helpful, for it can only encourage the same behavior to be repeated. It is usually more expedient to confront the situation, saying calmly but briefly that you care about the person professionally but that personal advances are inappropriate and may even interfere with care. Because you state your concern for the patient as a person and do not respond with rejection to such an incident, a working relationship and a friendly professional atmosphere can be reinstated.

You must closely examine your own dress and behavior to discern whether even unconsciously, you are "sending messages" that could be construed as sexually provocative. In general, women express sexuality more visually than do men; men do so more verbally. For example, a female nurse in a very short, tight, form-fitting uniform may convey a highly sexual image to the patient. The male nurse may exhibit his sexuality by making a lighthearted but sexually suggestive remark to the patient. Neither of these approaches is professional. Patients, frequently bored and isolated from their usual forms of sexual release, are especially vulnerable to both visual and verbal nuances. Any frank sexual remark or overture to any patient by any nurse, regardless of the sex of either, is extremely inappropriate and unprofessional.

On the other hand, it has been said that many nurses appear almost *asexual*, or sexless, and regard their patients the same way. Perhaps this apparent lack of sexual awareness is assumed as a defense in order to perform intimate tasks. Such nursing tasks as cleansing the areas of elimination and the genitals can make both the nurse and the patient uncomfortable. It is not uncommon for a penile *erection* to occur in the male during such care. This reflex should not be construed as a sexual overture. The erection mechanism is both voluntary, arising from the cerebral cortex, and involuntary, originating in the lumbar portion of the spinal cord. Even the very young infant has erections, and the adult male may experience them during the REM sleep stage. The adult male commonly awakens with an erection due to a distended bladder. An erection during care is usually simply a reaction to the stimulus of touch, and not an expression of erotic feelings. If the patient shows signs of embarrassment or makes an apologetic remark, you might say that you hope he will not feel uncomfortable, since such an occurrence is not uncommon and is due to a reflex that is not under his control.

Masturbation is the term for self-stimulation for the purpose of eliciting sexual pleasure, possibly terminating in sexual climax. Once thought harmful, masturbation is now increasingly accepted as a natural component of psychosexual development and a useful outlet for sexual tension in some individuals. Nevertheless, cultural taboos are still associated with masturbation, and it remains an emotionally charged subject. It may happen that you observe patients masturbating. Mental patients to whom cultural values are not for the moment important may masturbate openly. Only if such behavior becomes excessive and is preferred to normal relationships does it pose a problem. When the patient improves and re-establishes a sexual relationship, masturbation usually diminishes or disappears.

Retarded and brain-damaged persons may masturbate openly as do many children. Understanding that such a person's emotional and intellectual life may be at the child's level makes this behavior appear congruent or appropriate. The family and the staff can become upset, viewing such behavior as indelicate. An example is a nineteen-year-old boy with considerable brain damage due to a motorcycle accident. As his state of awareness improved, he engaged in masturbation. His mother, embarrassed and upset, asked the nurse to do something to stop him. When the nurse explained that such behavior is not unusual in patients with brain injury and, in fact, could be a sign that the patient was becoming aware of himself and progressing toward more complete consciousness, the mother became more accepting.

What if the nurse happens upon an adult patient in the act of masturbating? Leaving the patient in privacy is a reasonable response. Such behavior should be looked on as satisfying an immediate need, and no response should be made that would cause the patient to feel guilty or ashamed. The same suggestions apply in the case of the elderly patient, male or female, who engages in masturbation. We now know that sexual interest persists late in life, and outlets for it may be nonexistent for some elderly people. Because the elderly who are institutionalized may suffer sensory deprivation, sexual self-stimulation is perhaps therapeutic. Although encounters with masturbating patients will probably be very infrequent, you should prepare yourself to meet the situation in the most knowledgeable and understanding manner possible.

Aging and sexuality

It was once thought that sex between persons past child-bearing age was "not nice" and not necessary, but such attitudes no longer prevail. Current data show that sexual activity enjoyable for both partners may continue into the seventies and eighties, and beyond. It is incorrect to assume that every elderly patient in our care is no longer interested in sex and has no active sexual life. It is true that some elderly couples have, for health-related or psychological reasons, mutually decided to conclude their sexual activity. Unfortunately, such a decision is sometimes unilateral, causing friction between the partners. Physiologically, the aging process causes structural and hormonal changes in the sexual organs that may bring about a decline in libido and sexual frequency. However, this circumstance should not have a disruptive effect on sexual interest and performance. Aging persons need to know that sex in the later years is perfectly acceptable, enjoyable, and natural, and nurses too should abolish their preconceptions.

Drugs and sexuality

Few, if any, of the drugs used to treat patients have no side effects. Such side effects are at best distressing to the patient, and at worst dangerous. Physicians very often choose to prescribe a certain drug for a patient, regardless of its side effects, because it is the best agent for a specific condition. Drugs commonly cause skin rashes, blood disorders, nausea, respiratory depression, and a host of other reactions, and can cause changes and problems in every system of the body. Over 118 drugs may specifically cause changes in libido (sexual interest) or sexual performance (Journal of Drug Research, 1974). The three main classes of such drugs—*anorexic* (appetite-reducing), *antihypertensive* (blood-pressure-lowering), and *antidepressive*—are used very frequently and generally cause a decrease in libido.

There are many other drugs that may affect sexuality. Some hormones and the dopamine derivatives can greatly increase libido. This consequence can be frightening to the family, the staff, and the patient in that it dramatically alters the patient's self-image.

To retard malignant or abnormal cell growth, a hormone of the opposite sex may be prescribed in rather large dosage. Some degree of masculinizing effect on the female and feminizing effect on the male undergoing such therapy is almost unavoidable, and a supportive, empathetic attitude is essential on the part of the nurse.

Although many of the potential side effects of drugs are mentioned to the patient so that he or she will inform the physician if they occur, there is doubt in some minds that information about possible sexual alterations should be provided in all cases. The issue is whether this information might be suggestive enough to trigger problems not otherwise caused by the medication. On the other hand, patients on some of these drugs have been known to become very upset over decreased libido and difficulty in sexual performance, not realizing such changes are drug-induced.

The drug information circulated by the pharmaceutical companies citing sexual difficulties due to certain drugs usually focuses on the male response: lack of sexual desire, failure to attain or maintain an erection, and ejaculation of semen too early or not at all. Such deficiencies in males appear to be more readily measurable than are deficiencies of response in females, but lack of sexual desire and inability to attain climax may occur in the female to an equally distressing degree. A trusted nurse is often the one person to whom the patient confides sexual problems. He or she may express great relief when you explain that it is *possible* the problems may be drug-related. When the physician is consulted, the drug may or may not be discontinued, depending on its importance in the treatment of the underlying condition. If the drug is not withdrawn, the patient and his or her partner may need continuing support and counsel with regard to the sexual problem created.

You can do patients a service by keeping in mind the drugs a given patient is taking and by observing for side effects. It is a strong argument for on-going assessment that problems of a sexual nature are thus detected before they cause the patient undue emotional distress and anxiety.

Illness and sexuality

Illness causes both general and specific problems relative to sexuality. Illness generally causes major changes in the patterns of daily living, and the unfamiliar environment of the hospital exaggerates these disruptions. Not only is sexual activity interrupted; jobs, hobbies, and family and community responsibilities must also be abandoned.

Sexual activity is enhanced by rest and a state of well-being. Among the most common components of illness are *lassitude*, or fatigue, and general malaise, neither conducive to an interest in sex. All the body's resources are combating the illness, and the patient's mind is focused on his or her health, on missing work, and/or on the burden the illness represents for the family. Furthermore, illness is usually accompanied by some degree of mental depression, which is well known to reduce *libido*, or desire.

Let us look more closely at specific illnesses that may have a direct effect on sexuality. Sterility and impotence are higher in male diabetics than in the general population, and diabetic women tend to give birth to larger-than-normal infants. A rather special case is the patient who has suffered a heart attack. People occasionally do suffer heart attacks during sexual intercourse, due to the increased expenditure of energy. Thus fears about resuming such activity on recovery are not entirely unrealistic. Only the physician can determine what instructions are appropriate for a given patient, but sex need not be eliminated. Depending on their cardiac status, some persons resume sexual relations almost immediately while others must delay doing so. If there is risk for a male patient, the female partner can be instructed to assume the more active role in intercourse. Teaching records are available for the patient to listen to, if the physician chooses to use such aids. Sexual adaptations will be discussed in more detail later in the chapter. Participating in sexual activity can, in some instances, cause anxiety in epileptics who equate specific aspects of the sex act with components of the seizure. There is at this time no evidence to substantiate the notion that seizures are brought on by sexual activity. Living as normally as possible is desirable for the epileptic.

We have noted the decrease in libido caused by the distraction of illness, fatigue, and a change in the environment. However, the opposite may at times be true. A patient who has been in the hospital for a long time may exhibit a revived interest in sexuality. For example, the heart patient, under orders for bedrest, who feels rested and refreshed and no longer extremely anxious, as in the earlier acute phase of illness, may begin to joke or talk about sexual matters. The nurse can become upset and fail to realize that persistent talk about sex may indicate either sexual problems or accumulated sexual tensions. Assessment and evaluation are necessary in this situation. First, you should acknowledge the behavior by saying something to the effect that the patient "certainly has quite a repertoire of jokes" or "must be improving to be showing so much interest in sexual matters." You might then say that it is not unusual when patients are rested and beginning to feel like their old selves again to experience renewed interest in sexual matters. This remark can lead to discussion if the patient wishes to talk.

Surgery and sexualtiy

Some surgical procedures that involve the genitourinary system have an undeniable effect upon sexuality. However, *any* surgical procedure may alter body image substantially enough to alter the patient's feelings about his or her own sexuality. The male patient who undergoes a bilateral *orchidectomy* (removal of both

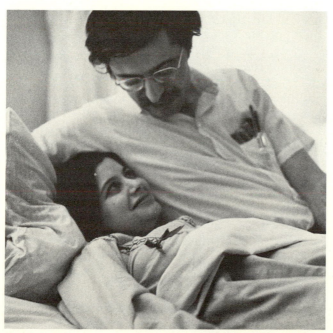

The hospitalized patient faces temporary disruption of his or her sex life.
Chris Maynard

testicles) suffers almost total loss of libido due to cessation of androgens and may or may not receive hormonal supplements, depending on the characteristics of his illness. The female who undergoes "surgical menopause" (removal of the uterus, fallopian tubes, and ovaries) may experience a decline but not total loss of libido, depending on her particular hormonal system. Again, hormonal supplements may or may not be administered. In any case in which libido is lost partly or completely, sexual counseling is in order to prevent feelings of failure, guilt, or inadequacy in the patient who simultaneously faces illness. You can be very helpful in encouraging the patient and the patient's sexual partner to undertake sexual counseling.

Other sexually related conditions requiring surgery, though they have no direct physiological effect on libido or performance, have vivid psychological components that can bring about sexual problems even in medically sophisticated patients. The impact of such psychological factors must never be minimized. For example, the man who chooses to have a *vasectomy*—an interruption of the tubes that deliver sperm—for purposes of contraception, may have problems with sexual performance following the procedure. In fact, this consequence is so common that physicians now recommend counseling before the procedure is performed. Women sometimes experience decreased libido after a hysterectomy, or removal of the uterus, which should not affect sexual interest. Particularly in a society that equates breasts with womanliness, the woman who must undergo a *mastectomy*, or removal of a breast, is subjected to sexual trauma. She may feel that she is no longer the woman she once was, and is therefore not the same sexually. The emotional support of the person to whom she relates sexually is essential. The nurse can often talk honestly and openly with both partners, together or separately, in order to help reinstate the patient's feelings of femininity.

The patient, male or female, who has had a *colostomy* needs very special attention from the nurse with regard to sexuality. A colostomy, which is performed for many medical conditions, is the surgical interruption of the intestines, a portion being brought through the lower abdominal wall to form a new opening for the excretion of feces. The intestinal opening or *stoma* appears moist and of normal pink hue, and varies in size from individual to individual. Your responsibility for helping the colostomy patient maintain sexual integrity begins when you perform the first dressing change. If your face reflects acceptance, without a flicker of aversion, a significant step toward acceptance on the part of the patient has been taken. The displacement of the intestine is no mi-

nor matter for the patient psychologically, and should be treated
by the nurse as a priority in the process of assessment. After discharge from the hospital, unexpected excretions, the wearing of
ostomy bags, and possible odor may totally eliminate sexual desire
on the part of both participants. It is hoped that such problems are
short-lived. A light dressing or attractive underclothing to cover
the stoma can minimize feelings of repugnance. Pamphlets on daily living after colostomies, which include information on sexual
activity, are available from several organizations.

In all cases of amputation, scarring, and incisions that violate
the body's integrity, the nurse must be aware of problems of body
image and, specifically, of sexuality. Each surgical patient warrants a
realistic assessment for potential sexual problems.

Handicaps and sexuality

Many persons suffer from chronic conditions and diseases of
the muscular, skeletal, cardiovascular, and nervous systems that render them medically handicapped. Their lives must, of necessity, consist of numerous adaptations and adjustments in order to function as
normally as possible. In planning and giving care to the handicapped, health care personnel have focused primarily on helping
such patients ambulate, dress and feed themselves, and perform basic hygiene. Only recently have those caring for the handicapped begun to take into consideration the sexual needs of the patient. It must
be remembered that the patient's sexual needs usually involve another person equally fully. The patient may, with therapy and walking devices, learn to walk again. But this may be only a hollow tri-
umph in the wake of a broken marriage or the loss of a meaningful
relationship.

Counseling for sexual problems

Some facilities require the agreement of the attending physician in a referral for sexual counseling. The sexual counselor uses
many techniques, but it has been found that, with paralyzed or totally incapacitated patients, the first step after separate interviews
with the partners is to provide a climate in which each can share
with the other fears about their sexual status. The male patient
might be thinking, "Am I really still a man at all?" "Will my wife

leave me if I can no longer sexually satisfy her?" or even "Is it fair to remain married?" His wife may be thinking, "Can he ever be the man to me he once was?" or "I feel it's wrong to have sexual longings when he cannot participate in sexual activity," or even "There is no way I can leave him now without unbearable guilt," or "I'm locked into a relationship no longer sexually alive." The airing of these otherwise forbidden thoughts allows the couple to begin to come to grips with the problem they share, and constructive therapy can begin. The problem is often less severe if it is the woman who is handicapped, since she is more often receptive than aggressive. When it is the man who is handicapped, the wife may be instructed to assume a more aggressive role and to take the superior position during intercourse. Social training sometimes makes it very difficult for the husband to be sexually passive and the wife aggressive without feelings of humiliation on both parts. Some universities have made excellent films illustrating the sexual act between a handicapped and a nonhandicapped person, using the female-dominant position. A trained counselor can often give such a couple long-term guidance leading to a reaffirmation of their relationship and mutual sexual satisfaction.

A word must be added about the assumption that handicapped persons do not have sexual interest or reach sexual climax. Each case is entirely individual, but studies indicate a more optimistic picture than once prevailed of the sexual-activity of the handicapped. Though new sexual techniques must often be taught and certain adaptations made, the joy of relating sexually need not end.

Until quite recently, little was written for the health professional on the treatment of sexual dysfunction. Now, however, there is a plenitude of articles on the subject in the health literature. This is welcome, since sexual dissatisfaction has played a prominent role in the dissolution of many marriages and has caused unhappiness for many single people. Patients are now more likely to discuss sexual problems with nurses or physicians in an effort to seek help.

Conjoint therapy, which is now in favor, is the treatment of a couple by a male and a female therapist, one or both of whom is a physician. Often the nonphysician is a nurse with special training. Each sees the patient of his or her own sex alone, after which the four interact to resolve problems.

You should know how to guide couples or individuals looking for a competent, reputable therapist or counselor. Most large hospitals and university medical centers now have sexual dysfunction clinics and there are many private clinics that treat sexual dysfunction and other mental health problems. In all probability, smaller communities too will have such resources in the not-too-distant future. A telephone call to the nearest university, large hospital, or medical society will furnish the caller with the names of one or more persons or groups trained in treatment of sexual dysfunction.

It is important to warn patients to avoid or carefully check up on sexual dysfunction clinics that advertise. Regulations establishing guidelines for this newest of therapies have not yet been implemented, and some disreputable therapists who use questionable techniques are practicing. Sound counseling, however, has enabled large numbers of people to find new satisfaction in their sexual lives.

Conclusion

Though our personalities are rooted in sexuality, the sexual aspects of our lives and feelings must not be overtly expressed in nursing practice or interfere with care. Except for those injurious to others, sexual variations have achieved some acceptability. It is time for nurses to broaden their vision to acknowledge sexuality as an integral part of the patient's total personality. Widespread changes are taking place in sexual attitudes, and nurses must adapt or lose many opportunities to care for people in a skillful and valuable way. Dealing with sexuality requires a high degree of trust between patient and nurse, since the subject is very private and continues to be fraught with taboos. Many patients, no matter how trustful of the nurse, are reticent about divulging their problems openly. And, buffeted by the psychological and physiological strains of illness, patients face a multitude of problems. It falls to the nurse to assess for problems and offer support and guidance.

CARE STUDY / A patient in need of sexual counseling

Ed Jefferson, a twenty-seven-year-old *quadriplegic* (a person all four of whose extremities are paralyzed) is in a rehabilitation unit. He has an attractive wife, who visits regularly, and a young daughter. During the seven weeks since his injury, he has been highly motivated in his sessions with the physiotherapist and has talked about regaining all function. A minimal degree of shoulder movement has returned, but the physician has told Ed that he will in all probability never regain the use of his legs.

Miss Stevenson, a registered nurse, has been caring for Ed. In the physician's statement and Ed's subsequent depression she perceives a potential problem. Miss Stevenson knows that, although many quadriplegics can maintain a penile erection, Ed's sexual function may be compromised.

While giving care, Miss Stevenson notices that Ed is becoming increasingly quiet. He develops a headache or nausea just before the physiotherapist's visits and pleads not to have therapy. He no longer initiates conversation, simply answering direct questions and making his immediate needs known. He watches less television than he once did, and spends long periods of time with his eyes closed but awake. Notably, just before his wife's usual daily visit, he complains about all sorts of minor matters. He appears edgy and apprehensive at these times, and his wife also appears unusually quiet. She shows concern for her husband and at times seems uncomfortable. They talk together primarily about their child.

The possibility that the patient's sexual function may be compromised appears to be affecting the psychological status of both husband and wife and the relationship between the two. Miss Stevenson decides that nursing intervention is needed. She recognizes that she cannot provide sexual counseling, but knows that a sexual counselor is available in the community.

While bathing Ed one day, Miss Stevenson says "You know, many persons who are paralyzed worry a great deal about whether or not they'll be able to function sexually in the future. It's certainly normal to have this concern, and if you have had some feelings about this, would you like to talk to someone trained in this area who can guide both you and your wife toward some solutions?" In the process of validating her conjecture, she has formulated an appropriate plan to refer the couple to someone equipped to offer counseling.

A look of relief comes over Ed's face as he admits that sexual functioning has been one of his primary concerns. After consulting with the physician, the nurse makes a referral to a therapist trained in sexual counseling.

Miss Stevenson feels satisfaction as she realizes that her goal has been reached: Ed and his wife will receive help. Evaluation of her nursing action is positive.

Study terms

androgens
anorexic
antidepressive
antihypertensive
asexual
bisexual
climax
colostomy
contraceptive
ejaculation
erection
fallopian tubes
gay
heterosexual
homosexual
lassitude

libido
mastectomy
masturbation
menopause
orchidectomy
ovaries
quadriplegic
sexual awareness
sexual behavior
sexual variations
sperm
stereotyping
stoma
testicles
uterus
vasectomy

References

Comarr, A. E., and Gunderson, B. B. 1975. Sexual Function in Traumatic Paraplegia and Quadriplegia. *American Journal of Nursing* 75:2:250-255.

Hanlon, K. 1975. Maintaining Sexuality After Spinal Cord Injury. *Nursing '75* 5:5:58-62.

Journal of Drug Research, 10:2 (May 1974). Published by the Society for the Study of Sex.

Keaveny, M. E.; Hader, L.; Massoni, M.; and Wade, G. 1973. Hysterectomy: Helping Patients Adjust. *Nursing '73* 3:2:8-12.

Kinsey, A. C.; Pomeroy, W. B.; and Martin, C. E. 1948. *Sexual Behavior in the Human Male,* 1953. *Sexual Behavior in the Human Female,* Philadelphia: W. B. Saunders.

Krizinofski, M. T. 1973. Human Sexuality and Nursing Practice. *Nursing Clinics of North America* 8:4:673-681.

Kroah, J. 1973. How to Deal With Patients Who Act Out Sexually. *Nursing '73* 3:12:38-39.

Lindl, K., *et al.* 1974. Spinal Cord Injury: You Can Make a Difference. *Nursing '74* 4:2:41-45.

McCary, J. L. 1973. *Human Sexuality,* 2nd ed. New York: D. Van Nostrand.

Pengelley, E. T. 1974. *Sex and Human Life.* Reading, Mass.: Addison-Wesley.

Smith, J., and Bullough, B. 1975. Sexuality and the Severely Disabled Person. *American Journal of Nursing* 75:12:2194-2197.

Wilson, R. 1973. Counseling Patients About Sex Problems. *Nursing '73* 3:11:44-46.

Winchester, A. M. 1973. *The Nature of Human Sexuality.* Columbus, Ohio: E. Merrill.

Part Four
Major Challenges in Patient Care

19 Pain

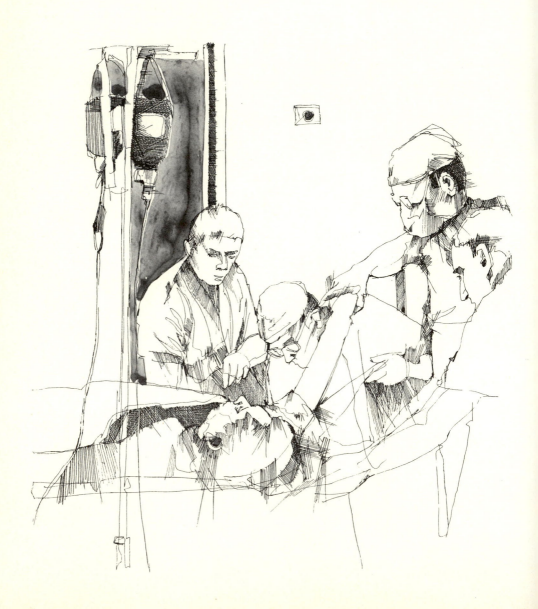

Objectives

After completing this chapter, you should be able to:

1 Explain, in your own words, the purpose of pain.

2 Discuss the three routes the pain impulse may travel after reaching the spinal cord.

3 List the physiologic responses to pain.

4 Discuss the various ways people respond to pain.

5 Assess a patient with regard to pain.

6 List five major categories of nursing intervention to relieve pain and give examples of specific actions in each category.

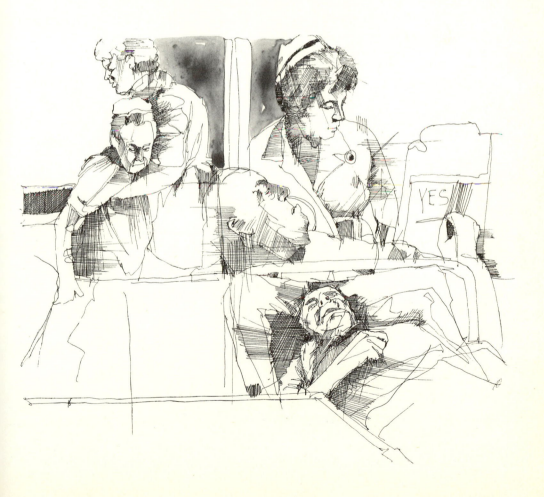

PAIN IS A PERSONAL and essentially lonely experience. It cannot be shared, and words are inadequate to explain the feeling to someone else. Pain can crowd out the rest of the world, making itself the center and focus of consciousness. Pain is frequently what prompts a person to seek medical care and often continues to be the person's primary concern during treatment. What is pain? What is its purpose? What causes it? What can be done to alleviate pain? Answers to these questions are highly important for nurses.

The nature of pain

Pain is a warning system. It lets us know when something is wrong, and thus enables us to protect ourselves from injury or care for an injury that has already occurred. Some individuals' pain perception is decreased or lacking due to disease or a congenital defect; thus unnoticed injuries, such as burns from an excessively hot heating pad, may occur to them. Lack of ability to perceive the pain might also lead to neglect of an injury, and thus to infection and further tissue damage.

Free nerve endings, which are pain receptors, pervade all tissue but are most prevalent in skin and surface tissues. Receptor nerve endings, for touch and temperature, also appear to be able to transmit pain impulses when they are excessively stimulated. Thus, pain may be caused by a variety of stimuli, including some that have chemical, mechanical, and thermal sources. *Ischemia* (lack of adequate blood supply to tissues) may, in some instances, cause

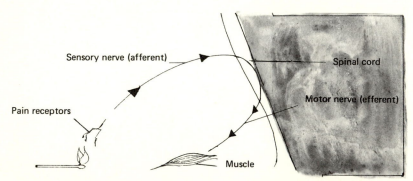

FIGURE 19.1   FIRST PATHWAY FOR PAIN IMPULSES: THE SIMPLE REFLEX ARC

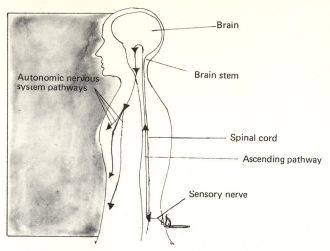

FIGURE 19.2   SECOND PATHWAY FOR PAIN IMPULSES

very severe pain in the affected part. Excessive stretching of tissues is a source of much visceral or internal pain. For example,
when the bowel is overstretched or the bladder excessively distended, such pain occurs.

When sensory nerves are aroused by a painful stimulus, three
processes occur. First, a reflex withdraws the body part from the
stimulus. The pain impulse travels along the sensory nerve to the spinal cord and is transmitted directly to a motor nerve (see Figure 19.1).

Second, the impulse travels up the spinal cord to the brain
stem, where the autonomic nervous system is activated. *Cutaneous
(superficial) pain* usually stimulates the sympathetic division of the
autonomic nervous system, which results in increased respiratory
rate, increased heart rate, and high blood pressure. *Visceral (internal)
pain* may cause the parasympathetic division of the autonomic nervous system to be stimulated, which increases blood flow to internal
organs and decreases respiratory rate, pulse, and blood pressure (see
Figure 19.2).

Other autonomic responses to pain are increased perspiration;
tearing of the eyes; dilation of the pupils; increased blood flow to
the brain, which increases alertness and causes restlessness; and
changes in gastrointestinal function, resulting in nausea and even
vomiting.

Third, the pain impulse, after reaching the brain, moves
through the thalamus, where the pain is perceived (recognized as

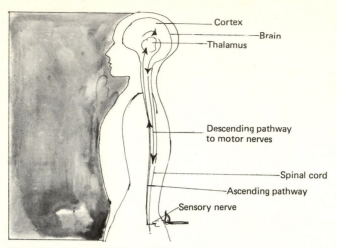

FIGURE 19.3   THIRD PATHWAY FOR PAIN IMPULSES

pain), to the cortex, where the perception is registered and interpreted and appropriate action is determined. It is in the cortex that
the location of the pain is identified (see Figure 19.3).

On occasion, pain may be identified by the patient as occurring elsewhere than its actual location. This phenomenon, called *referred pain*, occurs most frequently in the internal organs, where
there are fewer pain receptors because larger areas are served by the
same pathway. A familiar example is the heart attack that manifests
itself as pain radiating down the left arm.

Melzack and Wall (1965) have proposed that the spinal cord,
where the transmission of impulses from sensory fibers to ascending
fibers occurs, is characterized by a complex mechanism they call "gate
control." According to this theory, pain-inhibiting impulses travel
down the spinal cord constantly. Therefore, pain impulses must be
sufficient to overcome these pain-inhibiting impulses if they are to
travel upward to the brain to be perceived. Theorists suggest that disturbances in this mechanism may be responsible for cases of constant
pain with no observable cause. If the inhibiting impulses are lacking,
there may be a constant upward flow of minor impulses that are
perceived as pain. This theory has been neither proven nor dis-
proven, but has been valuable in enhancing our understanding of
chronic pain.

Phantom pain is pain perceived in a body part that is no
longer persent, such as an amputated leg. This phenomenon does
not seem to result from stimulation of the sensory nerves, since

surgery to sever nerves at the spinal level has not always relieved such pain. Phantom pain is not well understood, and research into its cause is continuing. The gate control theory has been applied to this problem, and it has been suggested that the pain impulses originate higher in the spinal pathways, at some point where the gate control mechanism has failed, or in the brain itself. It is important to recognize that phantom pain is not imaginary; the person truly experiences pain.

Responses to pain

Physiological reactions

The basic physiological reaction to pain initiated by the autonomic nervous system varies greatly in intensity, in response to the intensity of the pain. Reactions may range from mild, in which the heart rate and respirations increase only slightly, to massive, in which a state of shock ensues and the person loses consciousness. That people can learn to alter basic autonomic responses to pain is apparent in certain native American cultures, in which individuals were accorded recognition for their ability to endure great pain with no visible reaction, and in Hindu mystics who developed the same ability for religious reasons. It generally takes a long time and considerable effort to achieve such control.

The *pain threshold* is the amount of painful stimulation needed for pain to be perceived. Experiments have shown that the pain threshold is fairly uniform in all people. Pain reaction, however, varies dramatically.

Other reactions to pain are determined by interpretation by the cerebral cortex. The sensation of pain is compared with other experiences of pain, and is defined as "sharp," "aching," "cramping," or whatever. Its intensity is classified in light of prior experience as mild, moderate, or severe. It is important to remember that, since pain is a subjective experience, its intensity is rated subjectively. In other words, you cannot classify the intensity of someone else's pain. Although you may become highly knowledgeable about the levels of pain that usually accompany given conditions or procedures, the individual's pain is unique. Some researchers have developed external means of measuring pain, but they are still experimental.

The cortex also notes the location of pain, its original source, whether it *radiates* (appears to spread from its source), and whether position changes or movements ease or increase it.

Interpretations of the type, intensity, and location of the pain are then integrated with feelings about pain, prior experiences of pain, cultural and social attitudes toward pain, ideas about the origin or purpose of this particular pain, and current emotional and physiological status to produce a reaction to the pain.

Reaction to pain may be very different if it has been experienced before, and the person knows exactly what to do about it, than if the pain is entirely unfamiliar. For example, the person who suffers chronic sinus headaches may have a whole regimen of pain-relieving measures, including medications prescribed by a physician, and will thus react very differently to sinus pain than to unfamiliar pain of equal intensity in the abdomen.

Cultural responses

Different cultures are characterized by very different patterns of response to pain. The passive or nonresponsive attitude of members of certain native American tribes in the face of the most extreme pain has become legendary. This attitude, manifested in many cultures throughout history, has been named for the Stoics of ancient Greece. *Stoicism*, then, is one way of responding to pain.

Other cultures encourage *expressive responses*, or verbal and nonverbal expression of feelings of pain. Such expression may take the form of talking, moaning, praying, or cursing. Verbal and nonverbal expressions of pain are not necessarily congruent with the intensity of the pain stimulus. This is understood and accepted among persons of the same cultural background, and to keep one's feelings hidden is considered inappropriate.

The mainstream of American culture tends to lean toward the stoic attitude. It is considered good and brave not to express pain and, conversely, weak and bad to do so. Such acquired responses are not so potent that autonomic responses to pain are inhibited, however.

As a nurse, you must carefully examine your own attitudes toward pain in order to guard against making value judgments of another person's behavior in response to it. If you feel that pain should be expressed and encourage the characteristically stoic individual to do so, the patient may feel demeaned and lose some self-esteem. If, on the other hand, you try to induce an expressive person to withhold such feelings, you may be seen as rejecting his or her needs.

Recognizing the cultural values of the patient is also necessary when you are planning intervention. In the case of a patient who is stoic, you may need to base intervention on nonverbal cues, since pain may be greater than the patient's statements indicate. You also need to be very alert to nonverbal cues in the case of the expressive person, because intervention based only on verbal statements might be inappropriate to the actual degree of pain experienced.

Psychological responses

Pain arouses anxiety in many individuals, because it indicates that something is wrong and interrupts normal life patterns. Anxiety may be manifested in a variety of ways, depending on its severity (see Chapter 6). The severity of the anxiety may not be a function of the severity of the pain. Pre-existing anxiety often greatly accentuates reactions to pain.

Other emotions may also be evoked by pain. Some people feel guilt, having previously learned to equate pain with punishment. They perceive severe pain as punishment for some wrongdoing, and children in pain tend to do the same. For some people, pain may be a means of relating to others in such a way as to elicit their attention and concern. For them, pain is rewarding.

In some situations, pain may be seen as a means to an end. A woman in childbirth may see the pain of labor as worthwhile because it results in the birth of a much-desired child. Adherents of certain religious beliefs see pain as earning merit or favor from God.

When pain seems useless or undeserved, the reaction to it may be anger or increased tension and anxiety. This reaction may characterize the woman delivering an unwanted child or the person who has a body part removed. Such feelings tend generally to enhance both perception of intensity of pain, and reaction to pain.

Assessing the patient's pain

As is true of all other nursing situations, the first task is to assess the patient with regard to pain. Respiration, pulse, skin color, evidence of wincing, restlessness, and inability to sleep are important indications of the patient's physical response to pain. The patient may have tensed muscles, the brow may be furrowed, and a position that relieves stress on the painful part may be maintained. The person may move slowly and carefully in order to protect the painful site, or may resist moving at all. Such nonverbal cues may be the only evidence of pain in the child or the person unable to communicate.

Other patients can tell you about the location, severity, and type (sharp, dull, throbbing, or whatever) of their pain. (See the list of common terms used to describe pain on page 345.) Factors related to the pain, such as when it began, changes since it began (increasing, decreasing, radiating), and measures successful in combating it in the past may also be communicated. Factors that predate the pain but might have a bearing on its origin are also significant. Not all of these questions are, of course, appropriate to ask every patient.

Some individuals express themselves better than others with regard to pain. Because pain is a subjective sensation, words are often inadequate to describe it. For some, the effort of talking about the pain being experienced is too great for their physical and emotional strength; such individuals should not be pressed to do so. Children may not have large enough vocabularies to describe their pain, or may use words in their own ways. For example, one four-year-old repeatedly told the nurse she had a headache. This was duly noted on the chart. Only when a more perceptive nurse asked the child to "point to the hurt" was it discovered that the pain was in the abdomen. The child called any kind of pain a "headache."

Information gathered by means of observation and interview must be integrated with information on the patient's sociocultural background and current medical status. A complaint of severe, sharp abdominal pain is interpreted differently if the patient has just had abdominal surgery than if the patient is newly admitted to the hospital and has not previously complained of such pain.

Relieving the patient's pain

After a thorough assessment, plans for nursing intervention are formulated. Such intervention can take many forms, depending on such factors as the origin and severity of the pain, the patient's response to it, and medical orders regarding drugs, activity, and the like.

One of the most helpful ways to approach intervention is to consider the various aspects of the total pain experience and to decide at which point intervention is possible. Intervention may be aimed at (1) eliminating the source or stimulus of pain, (2) preventing the pain receptors from reacting, (3) interrupting the impulse somewhere along the pathway, (4) decreasing perception of pain, or (5) altering the patient's interpretation of and response to the pain.

Eliminating the source of pain

Eliminating its cause is certainly the most long-lasting and effective means of dealing with pain. Such actions as removing open safety pins, changing wet bedding, and smoothing wrinkled sheets are all

Terms Used to Describe Pain

aching	intractable
burning	knifelike
cramping	lancinating
crushing	pinching
cutting	pounding
dartlike	radiating
dull	tearing
electric-like	throbbing
gnawing	sharp
heavy	shocklike

aimed at eliminating the source of pain. For the postsurgical patient who has gas pains, helping expel the gas by administering return-flow enemas or encouraging movement to increase peristalsis is the most effective approach. The nurse who automatically thinks "medication" when a patient says "I hurt!" is doing that patient an injustice. More complex or inaccessible sources of pain are more problematic, and may not be subject to nursing intervention. The surgeon must remove painful calluses on the feet or a gall bladder filled with stones to provide long-term relief of pain.

Certain drugs may, by reducing inflammation and swelling of a body part, reduce or eliminate the pain caused by those conditions. When severe muscle spasms are the cause of pain, muscle relaxant drugs will help. Massage can also relieve muscle spasms, especially in the neck and back. When pain is caused by *ischemia* (lack of blood supply to a body part), measures to increase blood flow may reduce pain. Intervention to remove the source of the pain is the best long-term response to pain; however, it is not always possible. Whenever feasible, it is the preferred method of intervention.

Protecting the receptors for pain

It is sometimes possible to protect the receptors from the source of pain. Examples are putting petroleum jelly on excoriated buttocks to protect the skin from urine and putting a cloth over the eyes to protect them from light. The patient with trigeminal neuralgia, a disorder of the fifth cranial nerve, may use a silk scarf to protect the overly sensitive nerve from air movement that might stimulate it. There is evidence that aspirin may exert some of its effect by decreasing the sensitivity of pain receptors. Ointments containing topical anesthetic agents are also used to decrease the ability of pain receptors to function, notably in products for hemorrhoids and sunburn.

Interrupting the pathways for pain

Interruption of pathways for pain is usually a physician's responsibility, though nurses performing expanded roles are accepting some such responsibilities. A local anesthetic may be injected at a point along the nerve pathway to interrupt the transmission of pain impulses. Injections are most commonly done just proximal to the origin of the pain (as in dental work) or close to the spine. Spinal anesthesia, the injection of drug agents into the spinal canal to provide total blockage of the pathway, allows surgery to be performed.

Pain pathways in the spinal thalamic tracts may be interrupted surgically in certain cases of long-term intractable pain. This procedure, called a *chordotomy*, cannot be guaranteed successful because of anatomic variations in the spinal cord, but has been immeasurably helpful in certain cases.

The *dorsal column stimulator (D.C.S.)* is an electric stimulation device recently developed for use in the control of intractable pain. The device is surgically implanted along the spinal column. When activated, it provides an electrical stimulation, which is felt as a buzzing sensation and can interrupt a pain impulse and prevent pain perception. The person can activate the D.C.S. when pain begins, and thus stop the pain. It is expected that use of the dorsal column stimulator will increase as more information becomes available about its effectiveness.

A *transcutaneous nerve stimulator (T.N.S.)* functions in the same manner as a dorsal column stimulator through electrodes temporarily attached to the skin.

Decreasing the perception of pain

Pain is perceived in the thalamus and then transmitted to the cortex. Narcotics given before the pain occurs or before it becomes severe block pain perception. Thus more effective relief will be obtained by giving medication before pain becomes severe. When a painful experience is anticipated, a narcotic given beforehand can prevent the perception of severe pain.

Concern about addiction to narcotic analgesics sometimes prevents nurses from using these drugs effectively. Available evidence indicates that addiction is extremely rare among those who are experiencing severe pain. It also seems to show that the chance of addiction is reduced if the person in pain is not required to demonstrate excessive reaction to pain in order to receive such medication. Thus, the person with short-term acute pain (such as a new surgical patient) does not become addicted when given narcotics regularly during the acute postoperative period. The person with severe pain of a terminal nature, such as terminal cancer, is less likely to become addicted or to need increasing amounts of medication when pain medication is given on a regular schedule and can be depended on. Absence of anxiety about pain and absence of fear that relief will be withheld seem to be key factors in preventing addiction.

It appears that hypnosis, when effective, can also work to block pain perception. Though used in some health care settings, hypnosis is not yet a common method of pain relief. The person using hypnosis must have an education which provides a thorough understanding of all the various aspects of its use.

Acupuncture, which has been practiced as a medical art in the Orient for hundreds of years, is receiving increased attention from medical researchers. In acupuncture, long slender needles are inserted into specific points on the body. These needles may be twirled, heated, or attached to a mild electrical current. The effect is to provide anesthesia to a given body part. Interestingly, the part anesthetized is not necessarily in close proximity to the entry point of the needle. Many kinds of surgery are performed in China using only acupuncture for anesthesia, and the process has also been used to treat different types of long-term pain. Our understanding of acupuncture is still limited, and there are many theories about how it works. Its use is experimental in this country.

Distractions that preoccupy the attention and prevent pain from being perceived also function at the level of the brain. For example, if a person with a headache becomes engrossed in a hobby, the head pain may recede from awareness, only to return when the distraction ceases. Pain is not perceived because all cerebral cortex activity is focused elsewhere, and impulses from the thalamus are blocked. When concentration decreases, impulses will be transmitted to the cortex and pain will be noticed. This mechanism is most effective in cases of relatively mild pain. However, if concentration is extreme enough, even severe pain may not be perceived until the attention disperses. For example, a football player in a big game may not realize he is injured until after the play is completed. Thus you can sometimes assist a person in pain by helping him or her find an engrossing activity. This approach will not necessarily minimize perception of very severe pain that is already present, but may serve to increase such patient's comfort. Visitors, a television program, a book, or anything else the patient is interested in can be an effective distraction. You need to be careful not to convey the idea that pain from which a person can be distracted is trivial. The importance or strength of the distractor is the primary factor.

Modifying the interpretation of pain

Pain interpretation may be modified by many factors. In the hospital, the most common agents are again the narcotic analgesics. While the narcotic given before pain becomes severe may block perception of pain, the same narcotic given after pain has become severe acts to modify interpretation. The patient may even say that the pain is still present but no longer matters. The patient may appear less anxious and able to rest or relate to others, and the physiological response to pain may be gone.

Pain interpretation may be modified by an interpersonal process involving the nurse and the patient (see Chapter 7). A person who interprets pain as punishment can be helped to examine and deal with such feelings. This process may in turn decrease anxiety about pain, reduce physiologic response to pain, and change the patient's interpretation of the severity of pain. Other interpretations of pain may be dealt with in the same manner.

Interpretation of pain may also be modified by comforting measures to counteract the pain impulses. Bathing to remove excess perspiration, combing the hair, or providing a backrub that is soothing to the skin may help decrease the severity of the pain. It is important to find out what the individual regards as soothing, since people vary greatly in their choice of comforts.

A *placebo* is an inert substance given in place of a pharmacologically active drug. It is effective when it has the effect that might be expected from the drug for which it substitutes. Though the effectiveness of placebos is not clearly understood, we do know that *all* medication is subject to a *placebo effect*—that is, the effect is greater than the drug itself accounts for. This phenomenon appears to be related to the atmosphere of trust and confidence in which the drug is given. You will find that medications for pain are more effective if you accompany them with explanations of their effectiveness and an attitude of certainty that they will indeed help to relieve the patient's pain.

Helping the person with chronic pain

Some pain does not respond to measures taken to relieve it. The condition responsible for the pain may be one for which there is currently no means of correction, such as severe arthritis; or there may be no visible cause. Narcotic analgesics are not advisable in such cases, because they can become addicting. This kind of chronic pain may threaten one's occupation, undermine interpersonal relationships, and destroy the fabric of life.

To modify such persons' reactions to pain, a variety of methods have been used. Behavior modification techniques that reward non-pain-oriented behavior and ignore pain-oriented behavior are meeting with some success. This approach suggests not that the pain is not real, but that it is the person's response to pain that disrupts his or her life.

Such techniques are not to be used lightly, since they can change a person psychologically as surely as surgery does so physically. The patient must be knowledgeable about the situation and consulted as to the treatment plan, and must give informed consent just as would be required for surgery. Success with these techniques comes only with a total health team approach.

Evaluating pain relief measures

At each point, the result of nursing intervention must be evaluated. Additional measures may need to be undertaken to make the patient more comfortable. If medication is given, information about the expected effect and the time elapsed before it takes effect will be needed to judge its effectiveness. The physician may need to be consulted if you determine that the medication is not effective. In any situation, the patient will benefit from the knowledge that you care about his or her pain and are actively working to alleviate it.

Conclusion

Pain is a complex phenomenon. In planning intervention for the relief of pain, you will find it useful to consider the various aspects of the total pain experience and to try to intervene as early as possible. Intervention is often more effective if it is multifaceted and aimed at more than one component of the pain.

Although medications to relieve pain are an important tool, they are by no means the only way of dealing with pain. The effective nurse carefully assesses the patient and then brings to bear measures aimed at a particular individual and problem.

CARE STUDY / A patient in pain

On Friday, Jeff Brown, a student nurse, is assigned to care for Mr. Ralph Jarvis, who had a cholecystectomy on Tuesday morning. Jeff is standing at the nursing station, checking the Kardex, when the orderly walks up and says, "Mr. Jarvis needs a shot for pain."

Jeff goes to Mr. Jarvis' room to make an assessment before planning intervention. He enters the room, introduces himself and describes his role, and then asks Mr. Jarvis to describe his pain. Mr. Jarvis says, "It's sharp and all across here," indicating his lower abdomen. Jeff thinks about the surgery, the length of time since the surgery, and the patient's description of the pain, and then says, "Mr. Jarvis, it sounds to me as if you may be having gas pains. This is usual this length of time after surgery, and the location indicates the same thing. Your doctor has ordered a 'return-flow enema' to relieve gas." Jeff then explains the procedure. "I'll give you one right now and we'll see if it helps."

Jeff performs the enema, and a large amount of gas is returned. After the procedure is over, Jeff asks Mr. Jarvis how he feels. Mr. Jarvis replies, "Wow, that did the trick—I feel pretty good. I don't think I need that shot now."

Jeff then returns to the nursing station to record the entire process on Mr. Jarvis' chart.

Study terms

acupuncture
addiction
analgesia
anesthesia
ascending fibers
autonomic responses
behavior modification
chordotomy
cutaneous (superficial) pain
dorsal column stimulator (D.C.S.)
expressive responses
"gate control" theory
hypnosis
ischemia

pain impulse
pain interpretation
pain perception
pain reaction
pain receptor
pain response
pain threshold
phantom pain
placebo effect
referred pain
radiating pain
spinal anesthesia
stoicism
visceral (internal) pain

References

Armstrong, M. E. 1972. Acupuncture. *American Journal of Nursing* 72:1582-1588.

Bellars, K. 1970. You Have Pain? I Think This Will Help. *American Journal of Nursing* 70:2143-2145.

Janzen, E. 1974. Relief of Pain: Prerequisite to the Care and Comfort of the Dying. *Nursing Forum* 13:1:48-51.

McCaffrey, M. 1973. Intelligent Approach to Intractable Pain. *Nursing '73* 3:11:26-32. Care study.

_____. 1973. Patients in Pain. *Nursing '73* 3:6:41-50. Pictorial.

_____, and Moss, F. 1967. Nursing Intervention for Bodily Pain. *American Journal of Nursing* 67:1224-1227.

Melzack, R., and Wall, P. 1965. Pain Mechanisms: A New Theory. *Science* 150:11:970-979.

Pain and Suffering. 1974. *American Journal of Nursing* 74:3:489-519 (special section). Part I: The Spectrum of Suffering. Part II: Recognizing Pain. Part III: The Gate Control Theory. Part IV: Acupuncture. Part V: Electrical Stimulation in Chronic Pain. Part VI: Use of the Dorsal Column Stimulator. Part VII: Drugs to Treat Pain. Part VIII: Psychogenic Pain.

Pain. 1966. Part 1, Basic Concepts and Assessment. *American Journal of Nursing* 66 (May 1966): 1085-1108. Part 2, Rationale for Intervention. *American Journal of Nursing* 66 (June 1966): 1345-1368.

Schultz, N. V. 1971. How Children Perceive Pain. *Nursing Outlook* 19:670-673.

Turnbull, F. 1971. Pain and Suffering in Cancer. *Canadian Nurse* 67:8:28-30.

Weiner, C. L. 1975. Pain Assessment on an Orthopedic Ward. *Nursing Outlook* 23:508-516.

Wiley, L., ed. 1974. Intractable Pain: How Nursing Care Can Help. *Nursing '74* 4:9:54-59.

20 Death: The Problem of Loss

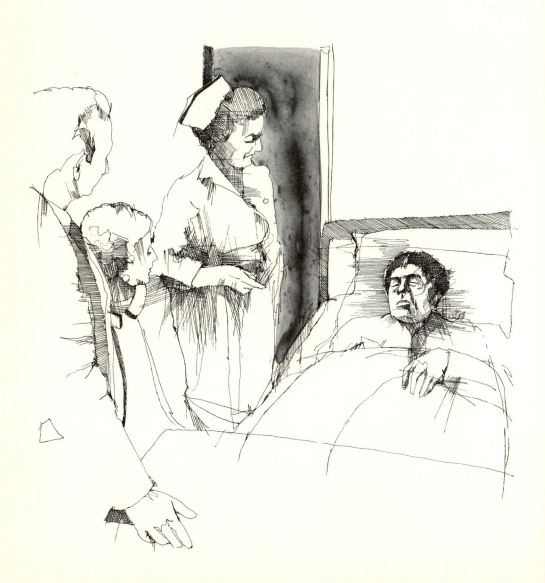

Objectives

After completing this chapter, you should be able to:

    1 Discuss American attitudes toward death.

    2 Name and briefly discuss the five stages of dying identified by Dr. Elisabeth Kübler-Ross.

    3 Identify the two major concerns of the dying patient and the three major concerns of nurses caring for the terminally ill.

    4 Discuss measures that can be used when interacting with the dying patient and his or her family.

    5 Name and briefly discuss the four stages of grief identified by Engel.

    6 Define the role of the nurse in helping the grieving.

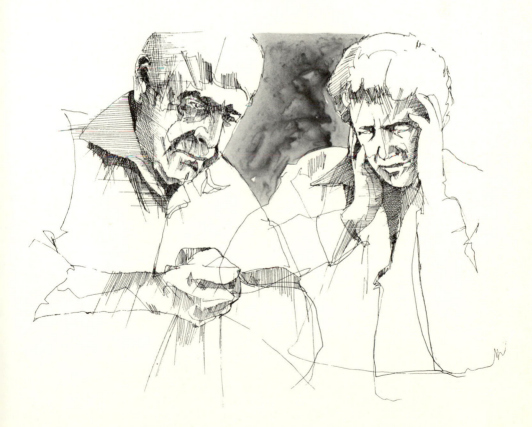

D EATH IS THE ULTIMATE and loneliest experience all human beings
face. We are the only species aware of our own mortality, and
this knowledge may bring not only loneliness and helpless-
ness but also outright fear of annihilation. However, even these feelings can be accompanied by growth—a growth in perceptiveness
leading to a feeling of relative contentment and acceptance. It is to
these ends that we as nurses must direct our actions.

When asked why they have chosen nursing as a profession,
most student nurses quickly and understandably reply that they
wish to help people get well. We are a recovery-oriented society.
Medicine is designed to cure, or at least to prolong life. Only recently
has this stance begun to become less rigid. The subject of death and
dying is being explored honestly, with the result that some guidelines are being developed for those who interact with dying people
and their families.

Society and death

In primitive societies, death was accepted as the natural
conclusion to life. Death occurred daily in the life of the village, to
animals and humans alike, usually within full view of members of
the community. Observance of the loss was in direct proportion to
the value of the deceased to the tribe: a young hunter or presti-
gious leader elicited an outpouring of grief not paralleled by that
felt for elderly persons or even children. Except for those wounded
on hunting expeditions or in accidents and worthy of salvage, dying persons who could no longer feed themselves were rarely
helped to eat; instead they were allowed to die.

In contemporary society, death is no longer visible, except on
television and in the movies. Though it is not unusual to read about
the death of thousands in a natural disaster as we sit comfortably in
our living rooms, many people live their entire lives without viewing
a dead person. Thus death in our culture is often depersonalized.
That is, death is perceived as something abstract that happens only
to others, and even thinking about it can be largely avoided.

Who is dying?

The capacity of modern technology to prolong life far beyond
the natural course of disease makes the classification of patients as
dying less clear-cut than heretofore. One of the frequent dilemmas
facing the nurse is preparing psychologically for the impending loss

of the patient and then watching that individual live on indefinitely, sometimes in pain and hopelessness, with the help of life-sustaining devices. Families face the same painful situations. Equally disturbing are patients who might be expected to respond to life-saving medical measures, but who die suddenly when such measures are not forthcoming. And there are those with life-threatening conditions whom the nurse does not classify as dying, but who are experiencing the same feelings and reactions as those close to death. In summary, the nurse must interact with each seriously ill patient by sharing his or her fears and cares and simultaneously living with uncertainty as to the patient's prognosis. This is a difficult task.

The stages of dying

In *On Death and Dying* (1969) Dr. Elisabeth Kübler-Ross has described five *stages of dying*. Dr. Kübler-Ross and students of theology at the University of Chicago observed and interviewed several hundred dying persons, and it gradually became obvious to

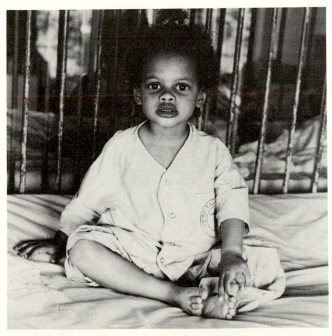

Preparing psychologically for the possibility of losing a patient is a difficult and often painful task.
Anna Kaufman Moon / Stock, Boston

them that persons facing death appeared to pass through five stages: denial, anger, bargaining, depression, and acceptance. Let us take a brief look at each of these stages.

Denial

The stage of denial is a period of coping, during which the individual is at least consciously denying that something of serious consequence is occurring. Dr. Kübler-Ross refers to this stage as that of "No, not me!" Denial usually lasts a relatively short time, primarily because events make the truth apparent and denial no longer possible. During this stage the patient may "doctor shop," request the repeat of certain tests, or flatly state that the test results are someone else's. Within certain limits, denial should not be contradicted, but allowed to subside slowly as the patient gradually adjusts to the upsetting news.

Anger

Perhaps no other stage is as difficult for nurses to deal with as anger. Dr. Kübler-Ross calls this the "Why me?" stage. It seems blatantly unfair to the patient that he or she has been "chosen" to die while so many others remain healthy. The feeling of anger becomes almost intolerable at times, and the health care team may bear the brunt of it. The family is sometimes reprieved because the family's love makes

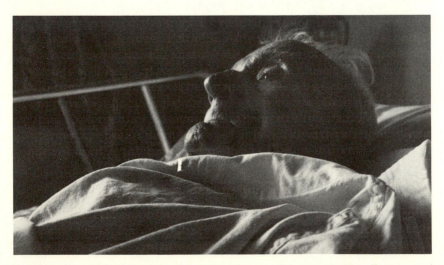

Death is the ultimate and loneliest experience all human beings face.
Frank Siteman / Stock, Boston

such outpourings unacceptable to the patient. The physician may also escape anger, as the one person who may be able to help and whom the patient thus does not dare to alienate.

It is often the nurse on whom anger focuses, in the form of excessive demands or complaints about care. The nurse may be made very uncomfortable by feeling anger in return and regretting that the person will not recover so that an appropriate response can be made. Using the skills of communication, firmness, and kindness, you can tell the patient you understand that he or she is seriously ill and angry about the consequent restrictions and that you would like to provide the very best care. However, you can say, some limitations must be set so both your goals can be accomplished. Such a confrontation is not disconcerting to the patient, and at times a patient will express relief at being treated as a person who can still elicit feelings in others. "Clearing the air," in such instances, is very therapeutic.

Bargaining

The third stage described by Dr. Kübler-Ross, bargaining, may be quite short, intermittent, or not apparent to the nurse. Often the patient bargains for time: "If I can only make it until my son's graduation . . ." Occasionally a patient will say, "If I were only a better person . . ." Dr. Kübler-Ross says that bargaining is an attempt to postpone and is helpful to the patient.

Depression

When bargaining fails to delay the course of the illness or bring about a cure, impending death becomes a reality that can no longer be avoided psychologically. The sense of losing one's life, family, and total earthly environment is often accompanied by feelings of deep depression and profound sadness. To do your own "grief work" but remain close to the patient is a notable nursing achievement. Crying during this stage denotes awareness, and it is therefore inappropriate for the nurse and/or family to admonish the patient not to cry. The stage of depression may be lengthy, and in some patients does not lift. Ideally, the patient will move through this stage to that of acceptance.

Acceptance

Dr. Kübler-Ross cautions nurses not to confuse acceptance with resignation. It is not usually a happy experience, but the pain is gone and the struggle is over. The circle of interest diminishes. The family may need support during this stage, for they may be less accepting than the patient.

Disengagement

The period of acceptance, the final stage described by Dr. Kübler-Ross, is sometimes followed by a sixth stage that might be called disengagement. One frequently sees this phenomenon shortly before the death occurs. The dying person may become very quiet, even withdrawn, but not necessarily sad. He or she wants to see only intimates or no one at all, is apathetic, and appears aware that the end is very near. A dying teenager said to his father, "Take the radio home, Dad, I won't be needing it anymore," and died within a few hours. The dying person has, in fact, passed beyond acceptance and said his or her goodbyes.

Nurses—as observers, sharers, helpers, and supporters in the dying experience—must understand that not all patients pass sequentially through the various stages. It is not uncommon for a dying person to revert from a period of apparent acceptance back into a state of depression. Bargaining may punctuate the dying process, only to be replaced by depression or anger. The family and members of the health team may in a sense accompany the patient through the stages of dying, sharing many of the patient's feelings.

Patients' responses to dying

Just as almost everything one has experienced affects one's life, almost everything that has occurred in one's life affects one's response to dying. One's ethnic, religious, and cultural background influences one's feelings about death, as do age and stage in life. An adolescent on the threshold of adulthood, a young mother with a family, and an aged grandfather with grown children may see their deaths in very different lights. The diagnosis and degree of deterioration or surgical mutilation have profound effects. The nurse must attempt to understand the patient's reactions to death within *the patient's* frame of reference.

Concerns of the dying

The primary concerns of dying patients differ quite strikingly from the major concerns of nurses caring for the dying. The dying are in a dependent role, much of their well-being and comfort subject to those around them. Nurses, however, play an independent role, assuming control of the care situation.

What are the major concerns of dying persons? Let us look closely at the two concerns most evident in interviews with the dying: fear of pain and fear of abandonment.

Fear of pain

Pain, as we have seen, has different meanings for different individuals. To the dying, pain may mean several things. It may mean that the disease is progressing, that "things are getting worse." That death is impending is an understandable interpretation, and occasionally a welcome one, if the illness has been long and painful. But pain is ordinarily unwelcome to the dying, destroying hope and draining the individual of energy that could be used to relate to family and friends. About 40 percent of dying patients experience severe pain during the course of their illnesses. One study shows that the pain can be adequately controlled in 95 percent of these patients (Lamberton, 1973).

Just as one's previous experiences with death affect one's dying, past experiences with pain affect the response to pain. For example, a patient who has had only infrequent experience of moderate pain, which has been satisfactorily controlled, is unlikely to be very fearful that pain will get out of control. On the other hand, the patient who has had severe uncontrolled pain fears it and lacks trust that it can be coped with.

Managing the pain of the terminally ill is a very important component of care planning. Drug addiction is uncommon in the terminal patient suffering severe pain, and large dosages of drugs are tolerated without bringing about psychological or physiological dependence. The patient should be given liberal amounts of pain medications so as to be as comfortable as possible until death. Tranquilizers are often prescribed in conjunction with narcotics, primarily to relieve anxiety.

Medication should be administered before the pain becomes intense and more difficult to control. British hospitals do not wait for the terminal patient to ask for medication and have no p.r.n. (whenever needed) orders; instead, oral pain medications are given to terminal patients routinely, "by the clock." They report that almost all their patients remain on oral preparations until twenty-four to forty-eight hours before death and are relatively pain-free. The pain of dying is very real, directly related to the pathology of its cause, and aggravated by anxiety. It must never be treated lightly. Pain management also involves finding time to listen and to allow the patient to talk freely about his or her fears.

Fear of abandonment

Losing a loved one is a heart-wrenching experience for a family, and can be nearly unbearable in cases of extended terminal illness when the goodbyes seem never-ending. Thus the abandonment the patient fears may be not physical—although this sometimes happens—but psychological. In short, not being "in touch" with the dying person is a form of abandonment. Long after the patient accepts and wants to talk about dying, the family may simply deny it. Family members may talk endlessly about the patient coming home. Or they may keep all conversation superficial, saying nothing that is meaningful to the patient. Visits become shorter. One young mother always brought her young children, who naturally became bored and rambunctious, necessitating her early departure from the bedside of her dying mother. An even more extreme example was the mother of an eight-year-old boy dying of leukemia. The boy was asking for his mother and several phone calls were made, all unsuccessful. Finally she said sadly, "Don't you understand? I simply *can't* come." With the support of the nurse, many families are able to maintain contact with their loved one, finding out for themselves that patients do not talk about dying at great length but only want to communicate their feelings on occasion to those who mean the most to them.

Concerns of the nurse

Nurses have three primary concerns. The first is "to tell or not to tell"—that is, how much should the patient be told that he or she does not already know? The second, closely related to the first, is communicating with the dying. And the third is euthanasia, which is now being widely debated.

Should the patient be told?

Whether or not a patient should be told the extent and prognosis of the illness is the responsibility of the physician. Dr. Kübler-Ross' interviews with dying persons reveal that most know that they are dying. It is reasonable and kind of the physician to reveal only what the patient wants and is willing to know, which varies greatly with different patients. Nurses often find themselves in the uncomfortable position of not knowing exactly what the patient and family have been told. The nurse might tactfully ask the attending physician what information has been shared with the patient and the family.

Experience in interacting with dying persons will enable you in a very short time to determine how much the patient knows or is willing to know about the diagnosis, mostly by listening.

Communication with the dying

Nurses often express the fear that, if the patient asks a direct question, they "won't know what to say." Such direct questions are fairly infrequent. Although each case is unique, certain guidelines for communicating with the dying can be offered.

Perhaps the most valuable thing the nurse can do is to plan sufficient time to sit with the patient and listen undisturbed. Studies show that nurses spend far less time in the rooms of the dying than they do with recovering patients. They tend to enter the room only to perform a task and to leave immediately after completing the task, fearful that the patient will confront them about the illness. Keep in mind that, even with very critical patients, you do not know whether they will die. Thus it is very risky, for your own peace of mind as well as the patient's, to make rigid predictions. It is far better, if the occasion arises, to let the patient know you understand that he or she is seriously ill. Nurses are often so concerned about *giving* information that they fail to simply *listen* to the patient, which is the essence of therapeutic interaction with the dying.

Euthanasia

No current issue appears to be of more concern to nurses than *euthanasia*, which means "peaceful death." Perhaps this is the case because euthanasia is a philosophical and ethical question that may intimately involve the nurse. There are two kinds of euthanasia: active (positive), which is the use of toxic substances or other methods to end life; and passive (negative), which is the withdrawal of or the decision not to use extraordinary means to prolong life. Active euthanasia is legally murder. Several test cases have come before the courts, all ending in acquittal. Public sentiment, as well as that of the medical community, appears to be growing in support of negative euthanasia, which is, in fact, practiced. Local medical societies and the Catholic Church have spoken out against the dehumanization brought about by the use of extraordinary means when there is no reasonable hope of recovery. This issue relates directly to that of "death with dignity." In our recovery-oriented zeal, do we on occasion deprive dying patients of their dignity? This is a searching question for nurses, and far too complicated an issue for absolute answers to suffice. Among the questions that must be answered are: What are extraordinary means? What do the physician, family, and patient see as appropriate? Nurses must be true to themselves. No nurse should participate in any decision or practice he or she considers ethically unacceptable.

Nursing the dying

It is up to the nurse to examine his or her own feelings about and attitudes toward death, which are highly personal in nature. Determining one's position on an imaginary continuum from total fear and denial of death to acceptance of it as the natural end to life can enable one to be more honest in a relationship with a dying patient.

In addition to the comfort measures afforded all patients, there are many other things you can do, including providing as cheerful an environment as possible, welcoming and making the family as comfortable as you can, and responding to the patient's pain. Respecting the patient as a person and maintaining his or her dignity is essential.

Hope should never be completely withdrawn. The will to live is a powerful force in most human beings. One author tells us that it is unacceptable to say, "There is nothing more I can do," since this depends on one's definition of "doing." Relationship, caring, and comfort can always be offered.

Death care

Death care, the cleansing and preparation of the body after death, may be as simple or as detailed as the hospital requires. It is best to check the procedure of the facility where you practice. After the patient is pronounced dead by the physician, usual practice is that all equipment is discontinued, clean dressings are applied, teeth and eyeglasses are sent with the body, and valuables are signed for and given to the nearest relative. It is a nursing responsibility to see that the body leaves the unit properly and with dignity.

The grief of the survivors

Life is, among other things, a series of losses: loss of a prize in school, loss of a desired position in one's working life, loss of a relationship due to divorce, and so on. Again, how one has coped with previous losses largely determines how one copes with the loss of a loved one or of one's own life. The stages of grief, as described by Engel (1964), are not very different from the stages of dying we have outlined.

The stages of grief

Shock and disbelief

The survivors feel that the death simply cannot have happened. Even if the illness has been prolonged, some degree of disbelief is present. Though perhaps only momentary, it recurs for a time to those close to the patient.

Developing awareness

As the shock subsides, even days later, awareness begins to dawn that the death has actually taken place. Crying at this time denotes such awareness, and should never be discouraged.

Restitution

Restitution is the observance of the death in the form of services or the gathering of family and friends. Formal, traditional funeral services are becoming less common, particularly in large urban areas.

Resolution of the loss

This stage involves realignment of one's relationships with others, a new relationship, or a new focus in life. The latter may take the form of a new career or job.

Leininger and Hofling (1960) compare the experience of grief to a ship that has lost its anchor in a heavy sea. The grieving person must put aside other things for a time and attempt to right the floundering ship. A substitute anchor is found and the sea also calms. It is not unusual for much of the grieving process to occur even before the patient is biologically dead. The end of the relationship, due to coma or disengagement, triggers the grief mechanism. During the period of bereavement, the nurse may note the survivor acting more dependent, taking on symptoms or mannerisms of the deceased, needing to talk about the deceased, and gradually refocusing attention on reality. Saying such things as "the way he would have wanted me to be" or "carrying on for her" is commonplace. All these are normal reactions to grief.

Because the nurse often sees people experiencing grief, it is important to recognize incomplete or abnormal coping in order to be able to provide help or support. Extreme exaggerations of the normal grief process, such as dependency to the point of nonfunctioning, persistent symptoms or mannerisms of the deceased, and constant dreams or even hallucinations of the deceased, all constitute unsuccessful coping and may indicate a need for help. Disturbances of the digestive tract, insomnia, heavy sighing, pacing, and unresponsiveness to others are other signs to watch for.

It may be said that grieving has taken place satisfactorily when the survivor can remember the deceased comfortably, recalling both the pleasures and the disappointments of the relationship.

Caring for the grief-stricken

Nurses can be of great help, both at the time of the death and later—since some families turn to the nurse for continued guidance. There is much that can be done to give support to the grieving person. The first thing to recognize is that nurses also grieve, feeling a personal loss along with the family. Such grief should never be construed as weakness.

The religious and cultural background of the family must be taken into consideration: different religions and cultures grieve in different ways, and what is comforting to the family should be foremost in the mind of the nurse as well. If the news of the death has not yet been given by the physician, the nurse can try to bring the family members together, knowing that they can often give needed support to one another. If one family member has appeared "strongest" to the nurse during the illness, this person might be best able to undertake arrangements and support of the grief-stricken.

The environment in which news of the death is received is important. If possible, it ought to be away from the general confusion of the hospital. Places for all the members of the family to sit are essential. The nurse might offer coffee to relieve the initial tension. Crying, as we have said, should not be discouraged. It is no longer unacceptable for nurses to cry, but control must be maintained if the nurse is to remain effective in helping. Viewing the body, if requested by the family and if the body appears peaceful, can be helpful in bringing home the reality of the death.

During the grieving period, the survivor may make unwise decisions, such as to sell a beloved home. In such a situation the

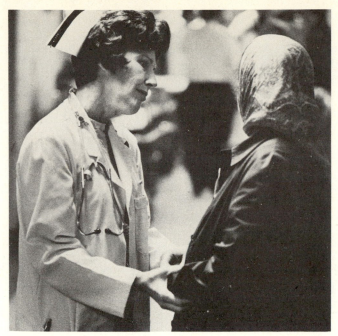

Family members need nursing support at the time of death.
C. Wolinsky / Stock, Boston

nurse can attempt to refocus attention on the death and encourage
the delay of major decisions. The nurse should support realistic and
constructive adaptive changes in the lives of the survivors, but it is
not up to the nurse to suggest such changes.

Anger at the nursing staff and physician is occasionally expressed by grieving family members at this time. The nurse should
recognize that such accusations are usually expressions of guilt and
grief, and should be treated as such.

Perhaps the most important support the nurse can offer the
family is touch. At a time when words are inadequate, the steady
arm or gentle hand of a nurse expresses care and shared feelings.

Conclusion

Nursing the dying, while certainly sad, is not without its sat-
isfactions. A long-term relationship with a dying person can be
deeply meaningful for the nurse. Each patient dies in his or her own

way, and some dying patients are examples of human beings at their finest. The dying person who talks less about dying than about living can be a rare and treasured experience for the nurse.

Care of the dying and the management of grief have rightfully come into prominence during the last few years. If we could choose, children and adults would never die in our care, but death is a sober fact of nursing practice. No one needs our skills, caring, and gentleness more than those whose lives are about to end.

Study terms

abandonment
acceptance
anger
bargaining
communication
death
death care
dehumanization
denial
depersonalization
depression
deterioration
disbelief
disengagement
dying
euthanasia
   active (positive)
   passive (negative)
extraordinary means
grief
hope
mutilation
realignment
resignation
restitution
shock
stage of dying
terminal

References

Drummond, E. E. 1970. Communication and Comfort for the Dying Patient. *Nursing Clinics of North America* 5:1 (March 1970).

Engel, G. L. 1964. Grief and Grieving. *American Journal of Nursing* 64:9:93-98.

Glaser, B., and Strauss, A. L. 1965. *Awareness of Dying*. Chicago: Aldine.

Gray, R. V. 1973. Dealing With Dying. *Nursing '73* 3:6:26-28.

Griffin, J. G. 1975. Family Decision: A Crucial Factor in Terminating Life. *American Journal of Nursing* 75:5:794-796.

Hofling, C. K., and Leininger, M. M. 1960. *Basic Psychiatric Concepts of Nursing*. Philadelphia: J. B. Lippincott.

Kavanaugh, R. E. 1974. Helping Patients Who Are Facing Death. *Nursing '74* 4.5:35-42.

Kobrzycki, P. 1975. Dying with Dignity at Home. *American Journal of Nursing* 75:8:1212-1213.

Kübler-Ross, E. 1969. *On Death and Dying*. New York: Macmillan.

––––––. 1974. *Questions and Answers on Death and Dying*. New York: Macmillan.

LaCasse, C. M. 1975. A Dying Adolescent. *American Journal of Nursing* 75:3:433-434.

Lamberton, R. 1973. *Care of the Dying*. London: Priory Press.

Lester, D., et al. 1974. Attitudes of Nursing Students and Nursing Faculty Toward Death. *Nursing Research* 23:1:50-53.

Lewis, C. S. 1973. *A Grief Observed*. New York: Seabury Press.

Reiner, E. E. 1975. Helping the Survivors of Expected Death. *Nursing '75* 5:3:60-65.

Ufema, J. K. 1976. Dare to Care for the Dying. *American Journal of Nursing* 76:1:88-90.

Wertenbaker, L. T. 1957. *Death of a Man*. New York: Random House.

Whitman, H. H., and Lukes, S. J. 1975. Behavior Modification for Terminally Ill Patients. *American Journal of Nursing* 75:1:98-101.

Williams, J. G. 1976. Understanding the Feelings of the Dying. *Nursing '76* 6:3:52-56.

Zopf, D. 1975. The Dying Patient: Meeting His Needs Could Be Easier Than You Think. *Nursing '75* 5:3:16-18.

21 Sensory Disturbance

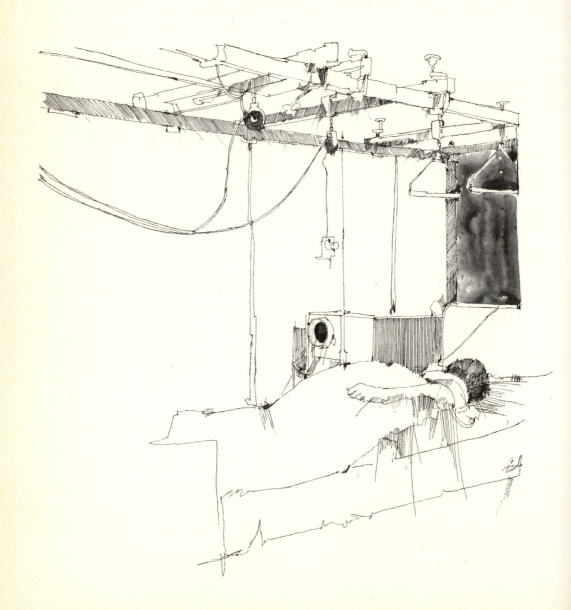

Objectives

After completing this chapter, you should be able to:

    1 Define sensory deprivation and sensory overload.

    2 Identify situations that might predispose to sensory disturbance.

    3 Assess for sensory deprivation or sensory overload, taking into consideration the condition, environment, and symptoms of the patient.

    4 Describe nursing intervention for both sensory deprivation and sensory overload.

    5 Evaluate the effectiveness of prevention or intervention in cases of sensory disturbance.

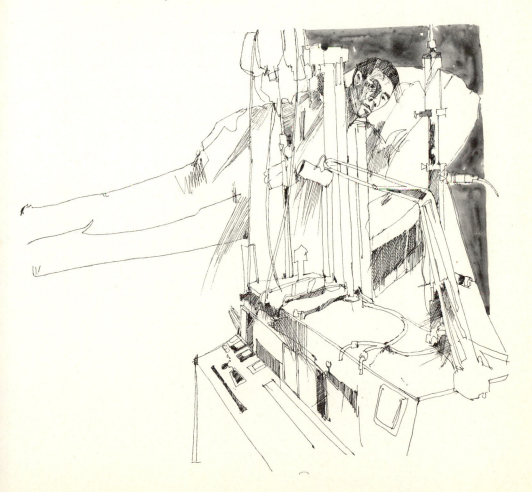

FOR MANY YEARS, the assessment of patients' problems by nurses focused virtually exclusively on physical needs. It has gradually become apparent that psychological needs must be assessed as well. Only very recently, however, have nurses seen the necessity of assessing for disturbances related to sensory input.

Normal sensory input

When we speak of *sensory input*, we are talking about all the messages and impressions that are transmitted to the brain by any of the five senses. Sights, sounds, tastes, odors, and the sensations of temperature and texture all make up what we call *input*. During our waking hours, thousands of these stimuli are registered in one's consciousness, where they are not only received but also interpreted and sometimes acted on. These messages are received in repetitive, "rapid-fire" manner, though we perceive them in a smooth-flowing pattern. For example, a symphony is actually a series of sounds—high and low, short and prolonged—all bombarding the ear.

At any given point in time for each individual there is an optimal level of input, or a specific number of stimuli that can be received with comfort. This level is very changeable. Suppose you are spending the evening studying. The input you are receiving is mostly visual, from books and papers, accompanied by some tactile input from the texture of the paper and the shape of the pencil. This is a time of relatively low input; higher input would make you uncomfortable and interfere with your concentration. The next day you attend a football game, where you experience very high sensory input; the colorful uniforms, the roar of the crowd, a marching band, and the smells of popcorn and hotdogs, all combine to make for a multitude of stimuli. Human beings both enjoy and need variations in sensory input. We tend to cope better with input if high-input periods are followed by lower levels of input.

Sensory disturbance

Sensory disturbances do not happen exclusively to patients in the hospital. However, the person who is not in the hospital can, by changing the environment or moving elsewhere, adjust sensory input to meet his or her needs. If while studying you want to increase input, you need only turn on the phonograph and continue to work. If the phone begins to ring repeatedly, the family returns home, or street noises become obtrusive, you may gather up books and papers and take refuge in the local library, where the environment is more subdued and input is decreased. Some people whose professions do not allow them to adjust their environments may suffer from sensory disturbance. Night-duty nurses, astronauts in spaceships, miners, and people who work in windowless rooms have all been reported to suffer from the effects of sensory deprivation due to monotony and lack of sensory stimuli. Control-tower operators in busy airports have experienced sensory overload due to the input produced by incoming and outgoing aircraft, monitoring equipment, and radio interchange with pilots. Thus there are two potential sensory disturbances: sensory deprivation and sensory overload.

Sensory deprivation

Sensory deprivation results from a lower level of sensory input than the individual needs for optimal functioning. Studies show that normal persons in experimental settings where sensory input is as low as possible experience irritability, inability to think clearly, perceptual distortion, and changes in brain wave pattern (Bexton, Heron, and Scott, 1954). That such symptoms occurred even though the subjects were aware of participating in an experiment on sensory deprivation suggests that sensorially deprived persons have little control over their reactions.

After less than three hours of lying in the recumbent position, patients can begin to exhibit signs of sensory deprivation (Downs, 1974). The recumbent position distorts visual images and auditory perception and forces the patient to adapt to a new spatial environment.

Because of new understanding of sensory deprivation, hospital rooms are becoming more colorful and visually stimulating. However, many rooms in institutions remain plain and dull, painted white or tan and sparsely furnished. Such a setting offers the patient little visual input.

Sensory overload

Sensory overload occurs when the individual receives more sensory stimuli during a given period than can be tolerated. It is usually a combination of stimuli, such as auditory, visual, and tactile, that overtaxes the patient's sensory receiving mechanism. A persistent barrage of input produces symptoms similar to those of sensory deprivation.

Again, all patients in the hospital are susceptible to sensory overload. A hospital unit, which is quite different in routine and pace than a private home, can bombard the patient with unfamiliar input. The patient awakened for the measurement of vital signs, disturbed for morning care, and subject to many tests and procedures will commonly exhibit irritability. Patients who are quite ill fare worse. The insertion of tubes or catheters and frequent injections represent additional input, as well as causing discomfort. Touch, which is very valuable to the patient suffering from sensory deprivation, can arouse anxiety in the patient with an overload of stimuli. Constant touching, turning, and testing may raise anxiety to the level of panic.

Assessing for sensory disturbance

In assessing a patient for sensory deprivation or overload, you should know something about the sensory level the patient is most accustomed to and accommodates best. A busy, outgoing, aggressive businessman who is suddenly placed on strict bedrest in a private room may develop sensory deprivation fairly rapidly. Conversely, the nursing-home resident who is transferred to the hospital could develop sensory overload because of a sudden rise in the level of input.

Assessment for potential or existing problems of sensory disturbance consists of studying (1) the condition of the patient, (2) the environment in which the patient is placed, and (3) whether or not the patient is experiencing any of the symptoms we have mentioned. The nurse sees such symptoms manifested in the behavior of the patient. Assessment is especially important when the patient is immobilized or less responsive than usual psychologically.

Each patient must be assessed as an individual. Irritability and unclear thought do not necessarily mean that a patient is sensorially disturbed. The same symptoms may be caused by such other conditions as generalized infection, electrolyte imbalance, drug intoxication, or illness itself. Thus, keeping in mind the patient's diagnosis will make your assessment more accurate and complete.

Common signs and symptoms

It has been observed, with normal persons in the laboratory and with institutionalized patients, that sensory deprivation and sensory overload produce similar symptoms.

The first symptoms may be irritability and childish responses. If sensory disturbance becomes severe enough, lack of clarity in thought and illusions can occur. *Illusions* are false interpretations of visible objects. An example is a rounded vase of fluffy pussywillows that the patient thinks is a bird with a tail of large feathers. If sensory disturbance becomes extreme, actual *hallucinations* can develop. A patient who hallucinates sees sights and/or hears sounds that are not actually there. A thorough assessment of the patient and the situation is necessary to determine whether sensory deprivation or sensory overload is responsible.

Patients in hospitals are in a "captive" environment in the sense that most have little control over the quantity of input they receive. Because the study of sensory input and its importance is relatively new, many patients and health care workers are unaware that certain feelings and symptoms are attributable to sensory disturbances, and not directly to the disease process.

Identifying sensory deprivation

Some patients are more susceptible than others to sensory deprivation. Using one or more of the three parameters—condition, environment, and symptoms (behavior)—consider several categories of patients for whom you might care. Patients who reside in chronic-care facilities, where they are in bed much of the time and may have roommates who are unable to communicate, infrequent visitors, and contacts with the staff only when care is given, commonly suffer sensory deprivation. Private rooms, intended to provide for rest in an undisturbed environment, may unwittingly promote deprivation of the senses.

Particularly susceptible to sensory deprivation are patients in isolation. Patients may be isolated for various medical reasons and with different degrees of stringency (see Chapter 11). It appears that sensory deprivation is directly related to the degree of isolation imposed. As a case in point, when you care for a patient in protective isolation for leukemia or burns, you usually wear a gown, a cap over your hair, a mask, gloves, and cloth boots over your shoes. The room is often sparsely furnished in order to diminish the chances of the spread of bacteria. We rely greatly on visual impressions of the people with whom we interact, and to see only people's eyes can be very disconcerting.

Patients who have suffered heart attacks often experience sensory deprivation because coronary care units are designed to provide low sensory input in order to allow for complete rest. Sensory deprivation can also occur to any patient who has suffered the partial or total loss of any of the senses, and to patients who have undergone eye surgery or are immobilized.

Patients with mild sensory deprivation often simply tell you that they are bored. At this early point you can prevent further disturbance by supplying additional input.

Identifying sensory overload

Assessment for sensory overload employs the same parameters as does assessment for sensory deprivation: condition, environment, and symptoms. Is the patient's condition such that he or she needs constant surveillance by sophisticated medical equipment and personnel? This situation makes for a multiplicity of stimuli within a small area. The presence of any psychological disturbance can also be a clue to sensory overload.

Intervening in sensory disturbance

Nursing actions in response to sensory disturbance are two-fold: prevention and intervention. Preventing problems from arising is a primary aim of all nursing action, and it is far preferable to prevent sensory disturbance than to intervene once it has occurred. If the patient's condition and/or environment seem to be potential causes of sensory disturbance, the nurse may be able to modify one or the other. It is usually easier to change the environment than the patient's condition. For example, you might be able to push the immobilized patient, bed and all, to an environment that provides a more satisfactory level of input, if only for a brief time. The bedridden patient with low sensory input could be transferred in bed to an occupational therapy session. And the patient who is experiencing too much input might be moved to a quiet area. Intervention to alleviate an existing disturbance uses similar tactics. The physician may allow the patient on strict bedrest to get up once a day, which would increase input. If the sensorily overloaded patient's condition permits, the physician might order the discontinuation of monitoring equipment.

Intervening in sensory deprivation

Studies show that the input provided to relieve sensory deprivation must be meaningful to the patient. Thus music the patient enjoys stimulates the senses, while incidental noise in the hallway has no

meaning for the patient and may be not only annoying but also ineffective in relieving symptoms. Only stimuli that are received and interpreted, and that serve some purpose for the individual, represent
effective input.

It may be that the hallucinations experienced by some persons
suffering extreme deprivation are functional in that they provide input. That is, the creation of hallucinatory images compensates for
lack of real input in the environment. When input is increased, hallucinations usually disappear.

The most meaningful input experienced by human beings is
personal contact with others. The few people who have dared lone
voyages across the ocean have reported severe sensory deprivation
and hallucinations, despite the abundance of sensory input provided
by the sea, changing weather, and wildlife. They attributed this phenomenon to loss of human contact, a hypothesis that has important
implications for nurses. Every member of the health care team has
meaning for the patient in that each helps plan and provide care. It is
frequently the nurse who spends the most time with the patient, and
thus has the best opportunities to offer the patient meaningful input.
Family and friends are equally important. Personal contact has the
advantage of providing input in various modalities. The nurse presents a visual image, provides auditory input by speaking, and may
touch the patient as well.

The significance of touch cannot be overemphasized. The
earliest meaningful input in our lives is touch: long before the infant can focus on objects or interpret sounds, stroking and fondling quiet his or her cries and produce a sense of contentment.
Touch continues to be an important part of our lives. For the patient in the hospital, touch is a means of orientation to the environment, reassurance in stressful situations, and an expression of
caring. In adulthood, some people use touch more expressively
and more spontaneously than others. Though you may initially
have to make a conscious effort to use touch, it soon becomes
automatic to touch a patient's hand or shoulder while speaking. It
is unusual for a patient to show any objection to this practice. In
fact, most find touch a warm, pleasant experience.

Another effective source of input is the radio or television.
Television has the advantage of being visual as well as auditory. If
the patient is unable to do so, you should choose music or a program
suitable for the patient. The family may be of help here. For example,
a soul-rock radio station is inappropriate for a seventy-six-year-old
patient but suitable for a teenager.

Taste is another source of input. If you are selecting a menu for
a patient who is unable to do so, you might choose foods character-

ized by a variety of tastes and consistencies. Taste can be particularly meaningful if a special treat is prepared and brought from home by a family member. An example is a teenager of Italian descent who had been badly injured. After several weeks in a coma, he regained consciousness and was beginning to feed himself. His sister brought in a small hot dish of homemade spaghetti, and with the initial spoonful he grinned broadly for the first time since his accident.

Olfactory stimulation should not be overlooked. A friend brought a teenage patient a small box of incense—an odor the patient associated with home. You might apply mildly scented skin lotions, deodorants, after-shave lotions, or colognes to the patient after a bath. And you might yourself wear a very light fragrance.

Intervening in sensory overload

After making an assessment, you can devise a plan for preventing or relieving sensory overload. It is a sound first step to make a careful nursing care plan, taking into consideration sources and levels of sensory input. Some of these sources might be eliminated, and input might be timed more satisfactorily. For example, you could plan to carry out several procedures at one time, allowing the patient periods of low input between periods of care. Input simultaneous with but unrelated to medical procedures can be therapeutic, relieving anxiety. Soft music for limited periods of time has proven effective.

Evaluating intervention in sensory disturbance

Evaluation involves checking for the presence and intensity of symptoms. If symptoms have diminished or disappeared, intervention is successful. What is effective with one patient, however, may not work with another. Individualization is a necessity.

Conclusion

Sensory disturbance in patients has been recognized as a problem only a relatively short time. The irritability and confusion it elicits is upsetting not only to the patient, but to the family and staff as well. With basic knowledge of sensory disturbance, assessment is not difficult. And once the problem is properly identified, nursing intervention is remarkably effective. Because sensory disturbance is a problem that calls for creativity and imagination, formulating a solution can offer a high degree of satisfaction.

CARE STUDY / A patient with sensory deprivation

Tim is a twenty-one-year-old college student who suffered extensive injury to the right side of his head in an explosion. After several weeks in a coma, he gradually regained awareness but remained confused much of the time. More time has passed and the confusion continues. An assessment is undertaken.

Though the surgical site is healing well, Tim has a large defect on the right side of his head—an area where part of the skull has been removed, leaving only the skin as a covering for the brain tissue. The physician has ordered the patient turned only to his left side and back to protect the area from pressure. Tim's left arm and leg are paralyzed, and he cannot turn himself. Because of the injury to the brain, he cannot see to his left with either eye. This, then, is the condition of the patient. As for his environment, the head of his bed is against the left wall of the room as the nurse enters, so that he faces a wall. The combination of this arrangement and the limitations of Tim's vision means that Tim can see only the ceiling and a part of the upper wall. The room itself is sparsely furnished. Symptoms of confusion are present: Tim thinks he is in his dormitory room and carries on long conversations with friends who are not present.

It is decided to offer Tim a variety of stimuli. A friend brings in a radio and tells the nurse the kind of music Tim likes. The radio is left on for measured periods of time and then turned off, in order to avoid monotony of input. Extension cords for electrical equipment allow for the bed to be moved to the right wall, and Tim to face the open doorway to the hall. His body position is changed frequently. Brightly colored travel posters, obtained free-of-charge from a local travel agency, are taped to the wall within Tim's line of vision. (Tim travelled all over the world with his widowed father, who was in the military, before his accident.) The posters recall to Tim many of the places he has visited, and he tells the nurse some of his experiences. Initially placed high on the wall near the ceiling, the posters are gradually lowered as Tim becomes able to view objects at a more normal level. Since Tim has always been interested in aquatic diving, a friend buys him *Diving* magazine, and friends and staff take turns reading passages to him when time permits. A small amount of his favorite shaving lotion is applied after morning care.

Tim's mental status gradually clears as input is increased. He begins to talk more, and soon becomes active in his own care and enthusiastic about recovering and continuing his college studies. He states later that he remembers the silence of his room and the blankness of its white walls. He talks about the frightening images he saw and his relief when familiar sights and sounds were introduced into his environment.

CARE STUDY / A patient with sensory overload

Maria Palmucci, a thirty-eight-year-old woman of Italian descent, is admitted to the acute care unit of the hospital with severe cardiopulmonary problems. Her room is designed for intensive care, the glass on the upper half of the wall contiguous to the hallway permitting close observation by the nursing staff. The room itself is a clutter of equipment, mostly electrical. Lights blink and sounds emanate from the appliances constantly. Oxygen and suction equipment bubble and gurgle. The ceiling lights are left on night and day to allow the nursing and medical staffs to perform tests, treatments, and procedures. Vital signs are taken hourly, oxygen and intravenous fluids are under constant scrutiny, and the patient is turned frequently. Mrs. Palmucci is becoming increasingly apprehensive.

The condition of the patient is such that almost constant attention and touching are required. Tubes and catheters add to the general confusion experienced by the patient. The environment inflicts a high level of visual, auditory, and tactile input on a continuing basis. A heart-monitoring machine is equipped with an alarm that rings loudly in response to even moderate movement on the part of the patient, as well as to heart irregularity. Mrs. Palmucci's symptoms are apparent in her behavior. Apprehension is fast escalating into panic. Mrs. Palmucci grasps the sheets until her knuckles are white. She *hyperventilates* (takes rapid, deep breaths) and her eyes appear frightened. At times she pulls at her gown and violently shakes her head. Though it is believed that the loss of REM sleep (see Chapter 17) exaggerates her state of mind, the primary problem is sensory overload.

The physician is consulted about Mrs. Palmucci's condition and environment. All unnecessary equipment is removed from the room. The ceiling lights are dimmed for long periods of time, leaving only a small, dim wall light. When the nurse is in the room, the shade on the large hallway window is pulled to shut out the sight of busy traffic up and down the hall. The door is kept closed to diminish sound. The heart-monitoring alarm is moved by the mechanical department of the hospital, so that it rings only at the nurse's station and does not continue to distress the patient. Suction equipment is turned off when not in use. The nurse plans for care to be provided at a few set times, so that the patient will not receive constant stimuli. Soft music is played in the unit for short periods of time. The nurse sets aside time to hold Mrs. Palmucci's hand in silence.

Within a very short time, Mrs. Palmucci grows quieter and her breathing becomes more regular and efficient. With the improvement in breathing, her cardiac status also improves. The look of fear on her face disappears and her body muscles relax.

Study terms

auditory	perception
electrolyte imbalance	recumbent
hallucinations	sensory deprivation
hyperventilation	sensory input
illusions	sensory overload
intervention	stimuli
olfactory	tactile

References

Bexton, W. H.; Heron, W.; and Scott, T. H. 1954. Effects of Decreased Variation in the Sensory Environment. *Canadian Journal of Psychology* 8:6:70.

Bolin, R. H. 1974. Sensory Deprivation: An Overview. *Nursing Forum* 13:3:240-258.

Cameron, C.; Kessler, J.; Kramer, W.; and Warren, K. 1972. When Sensory Deprivation Occurs. *The Canadian Nurse* 68:11:32-34.

Chodil, J., and Williams, W. 1970. The Concept of Sensory Deprivation. *Nursing Clinics of North America* 5:3:544-548.

Downs, F. S. 1974. Bed Rest and Sensory Disturbance. *American Journal of Nursing* 74:3:434-438.

Ellis, R. 1972. Unusual Sensory and Thought Disturbances After Cardiac Surgery. *American Journal of Nursing* 72:11:2021-2024.

Evans, F. M. C. 1971. *Psychosocial Nursing*. New York: Macmillan.

Hahn, J., and Burns, K. R. 1973. Mrs. Richards, A Rabbit and Remotivation. *American Journal of Nursing* 73:2:302-305.

Heron, W. 1971. The Pathology of Boredom. In *Altered States of Awareness*, pp. 60-64. San Francisco: W. H. Freeman.

Thomson, L. R. 1973. Sensory Deprivation: A Personal Experience. *American Journal of Nursing* 73:2:266-268.

22 Disturbances of Body Image Integrity

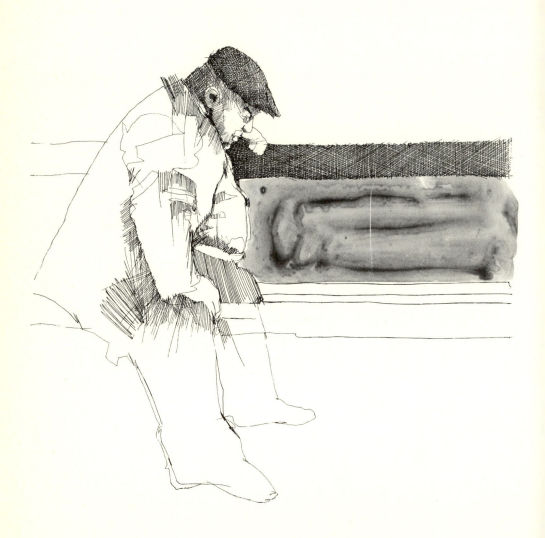

Objectives

After completing this chapter, you should be able to:

    1 Discuss the meaning of disturbance of body image integrity.

    2 Identify situations in which body image integrity may be disturbed.

    3 List the four stages in a response to disturbance of body image integrity.

    4 Assess an individual patient's response to his or her own situation with regard to body image integrity.

    5 List ways to prevent disturbances of body image integrity and to restore integrity if a disturbance is present.

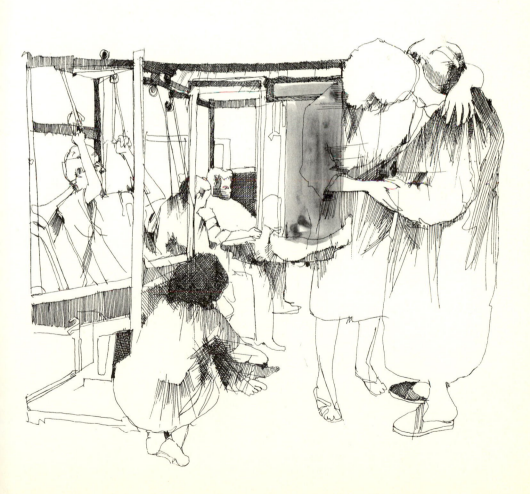

IN CHAPTER FOUR, on the life cycle, *body image* was defined as a multidimensional view of one's body that takes into account its appearance, kinesthetic feedback, sensory feedback, and internal feelings.

An individual who has an accurate body image that changes as the individual changes, and with which he or she feels comfortable, has *body image integrity*. This integrity can be disturbed if the individual fails to develop an accurate body image or persists in viewing his or her body in a way that is no longer realistic.

Illness frequently causes changes in the body. Because these changes are usually undesirable and often happen suddenly, disturbances in body image integrity occur commonly among ill persons. As a nurse, you will need skill in (1) identifying situations in which body image integrity may be threatened, (2) assessing the patient's response to such a situation, and (3) intervening to prevent a disturbance or help restore a body image integrity if a disturbance is present.

Common problems with body image integrity

In order to identify situations that may threaten body image integrity, you must consider both the situation and the individual.

Failure of normal development

Children are prone to failure of normal body image development while ill. The child may emerge from the illness having made no gains in psychological development. For example, an infant needs appropriate tactile input if he or she is to learn to distinguish the body from the environment. Touch is provided by cuddling, feeding, bathing, and playing with the infant. Even if the infant is fed and kept clean and dry, insufficient touch will retard development. The infant also needs to learn to identify feelings, such as hunger, that occur in the body. To do so, the infant must feel the discomfort, express it, be fed, and feel satisfaction. If fed on a time schedule without regard to the body's responses, the infant will not learn about them.

The toddler needs from others an accepting attitude toward touching various body parts, without labeling some body parts good and and others bad. Such simple procedures as shaving a body part before surgery can upset a toddler, who considers hair part of the body and does not necessarily recognize it as expendable. The toddler may view an intravenous tube infused to the arm as part of the body and need help in understanding both its placement and its removal.

School-age children need contact with peers and reassurance that they are "normal" and acceptable. Lacking such support, they can be expected to suffer self-doubt and become withdrawn.

The individual needs appropriate input at each stage of development in order to develop body image integrity.

Changes in external body appearance

A second category of situations that often cause disturbances in body image integrity involve changes in external body appearance. The person who experiences formation of a scar, head-shaving for surgery, loss of a limb, or a colostomy (surgery to open the colon through the abdominal wall) will probably need some support and assistance to maintain body image integrity. In order to participate fully in life, one must accept such changes and incorporate them into one's self-image.

The difficulty of doing so is a function of the individual's de-

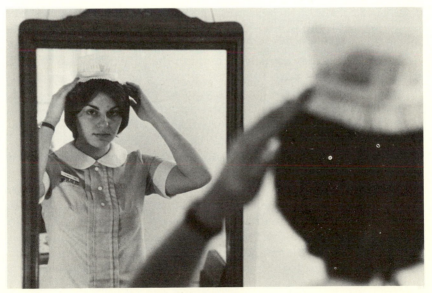

Lynn McLaren, courtesy of Newton-Wellesley Hospital

velopmental level, previous life experiences, and previous body image. For example, a facial scar may be readily incorporated into the body image, and even worn as a badge of pride, by a young man who fences as a hobby. The same scar on a teenage girl might elicit severe depression and cause her to withdraw from normal social life.

Changes in body function

Another group of conditions that often affect body image integrity involve changes in the body's functioning. Examples are a lung disease that limits physical activity, a stomach problem that requires dietary changes, and medications whose side effects include lessened alertness. The body does not respond as it has, and may be less acceptable. Some individuals deny such changes and jeopardize their future health by failing to follow prescriptions for activity and diet. Others find the change so overwhelming that they feel life is no longer meaningful.

Patients' responses to problems with body image integrity

The following pattern is common in patients suffering from disturbances in body image integrity. At first the patient may exhibit *disbelief and denial*, which must be allowed; but if denial persists for a long time and interferes with the patient's ability to participate in his or her own care, skilled psychiatric help may be needed. For a while, however, denial may actually be helpful: the patient whose energy is invested in coping with the physical problems of healing may not have adequate resources for simultaneous psychological changes.

As the reality of the change is acknowledged, the patient may express *anger*, not at anyone in particular but at the world in general. Such anger is characterized by a "Why me?" attitude. On occasion, it may be directed at the most accessible targets, the nurse and the family. Although such anger is not really personal, it is often difficult to make this distinction, and families may need to talk to someone who understands what they are feeling. If you are the target of anger, you too may need someone with whom to discuss your feelings if you are to continue to function effectively with the patient. It is important that you not reject the patient at this time. Though rejecting of others, the patient needs their acceptance in order to move toward self-acceptance.

Anger may be followed by severe *depression* as the patient grieves for what was and might have been. Attempts to cheer up the depressed patient are inappropriate. Instead, such a patient needs the constant concerned care and presence of others even when he or she is rejecting of others. Sitting with the patient in silence, with no expectation of response, may be especially helpful. Touch and other nonverbal communication is especially important.

Gradually, the person develops *acceptance* of the new body image. Integrity is restored, and energy can be focused on rehabilitation or returning to the mainstream of life. This process is gradual. Therapeutic interaction to help the patient think about the entire experience, verbalize it, and give it meaning, is most effective at this time.

Health care workers sometimes make the mistake of expecting this entire process to be accomplished very rapidly. Time is needed: time with others and time alone. Trying to hurry a person in the development of a new body image may only impede progress.

Assessing for problems of body image integrity

When you have identified a situation in which body image integrity may be disturbed, you will need to make a thorough assessment of the individual patient. First, consider the patient's *developmental level*. What might be his or her primary needs and concerns? How are those needs and concerns related to the current situation? Is the patient, for example, a young adult just beginning to develop interdependent relationships with the opposite sex? If so, changes perceived as diminishing sexual attractiveness or sexual ability may be especially upsetting. The removal of a uterus is likely to be less upsetting to a woman past childbearing age than to an eighteen-year-old who has never had a child.

Another area of concern is the person's occupation or usual *life role*. A singer's mouth is important to her, while a telephone lineman may consider his legs much more significant. The person whose occupation is sedentary will be less threatened by an illness that necessitates being sedentary than will someone whose previous job involved considerable physical activity. The woman who sees her position in life as dependent on her ability to entertain may be excessively upset by an ulcer that requires a special diet.

Cultural expectations may greatly affect a person's response to a body change. Because of Western society's definition of beauty in women, a woman who loses a great deal of weight might not be too upset; a man who associates being big with being masculine might find weight loss of greater concern.

As you assess the individual, consider his or her *strengths and weaknesses*. What assets will the person be able to bring to bear on the crisis? Some persons have developed strength by confronting previous crises successfully. Others have the support of strong religious beliefs. Always try to meet the family or significant other persons and to assess their strengths. Some family members may be very helpful, while others also need assistance in dealing with the crisis. Each individual has some strengths that can be built on.

Identifying the particular stage the person is experiencing in the process of reestablishing body image integrity will help you to respond in the most helpful way. In any event, your general assessments regarding developmental level and the like must be validated with the individual. What are the patient's behavior patterns? Observe for activity level, pacing the floor, chain-smoking, and other signs of anxiety. The person may refuse to discuss the change, or may become completely absorbed with it to the exclusion of all other topics. Neither is a healthy response. What are the patient's facial expressions? Muscles may be tense and the lips tightly drawn if the person is upset and anxious. The entire face may droop if depression is severe. Does the person's reaction seem appropriate to the situation? For example, laughing and joking about the loss of a leg indicate a serious problem. Such a loss is a major disability and requires considerable adaptation. Denial of the seriousness of the disability is a barrier to rehabilitation.

Always keep in mind that it is the person's own *perception* of the seriousness of the change that most profoundly affects his or her response.

Intervening in problems of body image integrity

There are many ways you can help the patient maintain body image integrity. Most are valuable in prevention as well as in dealing with an existing problem. Planning ahead for the maintenance of body image integrity may prevent the patient from experiencing severe difficulties.

A therapeutic environment that helps the person to accept the change can be provided by promoting cleanliness, enhancing the patient's personal appearance, and performing other tasks that demonstrate respect. Providing privacy and preserving modesty are also important. These considerations are sometimes overlooked in the case of children, but they too respond to recognition of their personal modesty.

Emphasizing unimpaired abilities and assets and putting no undue stress on the disability may help the person accept the change. Help the patient look for his or her own strengths.

By avoiding an exclusive focus on one part of the body, you may assist the patient to retain a broad perspective on the self. If, on the other hand, everyone who contacts the patient is interested only in his or her bowel function, the patient too will focus on that alone.

Such *perceptual feedback* as touching a scar or the stump of an amputated arm can provide valuable sensory input. Encouraging active movement of a changed part, such as an arm affected by a stroke, will provide for *kinesthetic feedback*. When active movement is not possible, passive movement (movement carried out by another person) is helpful.

Verbal feedback on the movements being performed is valuable in establishing understanding of the body's new feelings. For example, while exercising a leg, you may state, "Now I am bending your knee. Now I am straightening it out." *Visual feedback* by means of mirrors allows the patient to face reality and not to be overwhelmed by imaginings that exaggerate reality.

The patient, family, and friends may deal more effectively with a profound change if they are adequately prepared before actually confronting it. Thus it may be beneficial to describe the changes to the family in advance so they can maintain composure and provide support to the patient when they first view the change. With regard to the patient, there is a fine line between adequate preparation and frightening disclosures he or she is not ready for. The individual's response must be your guide in making such decisions. For example, a young woman refused to look at her colostomy for days after the surgery, and would not consider learning to care for it herself. A nurse, assessing the situation, learned that the patient was envisioning a "horrible black mess," and explained that the colostomy is a rosy pink mucous membrane approximately two inches in diameter. The patient then looked at her colostomy, decided it was not as bad as she had expected, and began learning self-care.

When changes in functioning occur, explanations at a level of sophistication appropriate to the patient are necessary. Such explanations should note possible changes in feeling and the effects that treatments and medications will have on functioning. Mistaken ideas often add greatly to the patient's fears and burdens. Finally, the nurse may be able to help the person understand what he or she is feeling. The techniques of interpersonal communication (see Chapter 7) are valuable in this endeavor.

Conclusion

Body image is a complex phenomenon encompassing all the ways a person perceives his or her own body. The development of body image is a lifelong process characterized by constant shift and change. Although patterns of body image development are identifiable, each person must be considered as an individual.

Body image integrity is essential to optimal functioning. Because illness causes myriad changes in the body and requires adaptation of the body image, the nurse must develop skill at identifying threats to body image, assessing individual situations with regard to the patient's body image, intervening to prevent problems, and helping resolve existing problems.

CARE STUDY / A patient with a disturbance of body image integrity

Eleanor Jacal, a student in a fundamentals of nursing course, is assigned Mrs. Katherine Meindl, age forty-eight, who had a left radical mastectomy three days ago. In preparing to care for this patient, Eleanor notes the following:

1 A radical mastectomy involves removal of a large amount of chest and axillary tissue, as well as the breast itself. The resulting scar is quite large. There may be some weakness and difficulty of movement in the arm on the operated side because of the role chest muscles play in arm movement.

2 A radical mastectomy is usually performed for a malignancy of the breast.

3 Although radical mastectomy is extensive surgery, by the fourth postoperative day it is usual for the patient to be ambulating and beginning self-care.

4 Movement of the arm on the operated side is usually ordered by the surgeon, and exercises are usually started in the postoperative period.

5 It is usual for the mastectomy patient to be upset about this change in body structure. She often feels a loss of femininity and concern over the response of significant family members, especially her sexual partner. Depression is common.

In making her plans, Eleanor anticipates spending a lot of time with Mrs. Meindl, who will probably be sad and need support.

The next morning, when Eleanor walks into Mrs. Meindl's room, she is surprised to see a woman in a beautiful bed-jacket, hair perfectly arranged, and make-up expertly applied, though it is only 7:30 a.m. Mrs. Meindl greets her with a smile and says, "I'm sure having a student will be fun. Of course, I'm not really a sick patient, so you won't have much to do." This is not at all the response Eleanor expected. She wonders if Mrs. Meindl is just an exceptionally well-adjusted woman.

When the surgeon arrives to change the dressings, Mrs. Meindl says "You do what you must—I'm really not interested. Eleanor and I will just continue our chat." Mrs. Meindl looks the other way and ignores the surgeon's comments throughout the dressing change.

Later, when Eleanor is discussing with Mrs. Meindl her plans after leaving the hospital, the patient states that she expects to begin her old activities immediately. "You see, my daughter will be coming home from college for vacation. She doesn't know I've had surgery. I don't want her to know that she has only half a mother."

The staff nurse visits during the morning to say, "Mrs. Meindl, often women who have had a mastectomy wonder about the various kinds of 'falsies' available. There is an organization called Reach for Recovery made up of women who have had mastectomies. A member of that group would be glad to visit and would be able to discuss this with you." "No!!" Mrs. Meindl almost shouts. "I—I mean, no, thank you. I'm not interested," she continues, in a calmer tone of voice.

As Eleanor is preparing to report off to the team leader at noon, she reviews her assessment data:

1 Mrs. M. appeared cheerful and outgoing on first contact.

2 She refused to look at the surgical incision or to listen to the surgeon's discussion of the surgery.

3 Mrs. M.'s plans are to take up her former activities without a recuperative period. This is not realistic.

4 She has kept the operation a secret from a college-age daughter.

5 She had called herself "half a mother."

6 Mrs. M. appeared upset when a "Reach for Recovery" visitor was suggested.

Eleanor decides that Mrs. M. has a problem of body image integrity because she is not discussing or showing evidence of facing the physical change in any way and because her emotional response to the problem appears to be interfering with her ability to be realistic about her care.

Since Eleanor will not be caring for Mrs. Meindl during the rest of her hospital stay, she decides to report her findings to the team leader. The team leader says, "I've been concerned about Mrs. Meindl. Her cheerfulness is too good to be true. After all, any surgery is serious and her attitude doesn't seem very realistic. I appreciate the specific information you've been able to give me. I do agree with your analysis of the problem. During our team conference this afternoon, we can bring this problem to the attention of the entire team and develop a plan for helping Mrs. Meindl."

The student nurse has researched background information, collected data on the patient, and analyzed the data, determining that a problem exists. In considering a plan of action she recognizes her own limitations, and reports her concerns to someone with the skill and opportunity to act. The process of assisting Mrs. Meindl with her problem is begun.

Study Terms

body image
body image integrity
developmental level
feedback
kinesthetic
life role
nursing assessment
nursing intervention

perceptual feedback
self-concept
stereotype
stimuli
  external
  internal
therapeutic environment
validation

References

Blaesing, S., and Brockhaus, J. 1972. The Development of Body Image in the Child. *Nursing Clinics of North America* 7:597-607.

Compton, C. Y. 1973. War Injury: Identity Crisis for Young Men. *Nursing Clinics of North America* 8:53-66 (March 1973).

Corbeil, M. 1971. The Nursing Process for a Patient with a Body Image Disturbance. *Nursing Clinics of North America* 6:155-163 (March 1971).

Dempsey, M. O. 1972. The Development of Body Image in the Adolescent. *Nursing Clinics of North America* 7:609-615.

Loxley, A. K. 1972. The Emotional Toll of Crippling Deformity. *American Journal of Nursing* 72:1839-1840.

Miles, M. S. 1969. Body Integrity Fears in the Toddler. *Nursing Clinics of North America* 4:39-51 (March 1969).

Murray, R. L. 1972. Body Image Development in Adulthood. *Nursing Clinics of North America* 7:651-660.

———. 1972. Principles of Nursing Intervention for the Adult Patient with Body Image Changes. *Nursing Clinics of North America* 7:697-707.

Neir, C. 1975. Coping with Newly Diagnosed Blindness. *American Journal of Nursing* 75:2161-2163.

Riddle, I. 1972. Nursing Intervention to Promote Body Image Integrity in Children. *Nursing Clinics of North America* 7:651-661.

Tierney, E. A. 1975. Accepting Disfigurement When Death Is the Alternative. *American Journal of Nursing* 75:2149-2150.

23 Aging

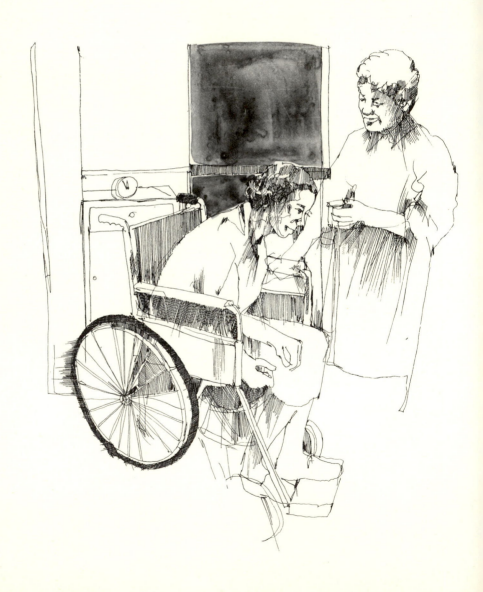

Objectives

After completing this chapter, you should be able to:

1 Discuss the major concerns of the elderly in society today.

2 Recognize the physical and mental changes and disturbances of the systems of the body brought about by the aging process.

3 Integrate this knowledge into the planning of care for the elderly patient.

4 Formulate specific adaptations and techniques for augmenting nursing care of the aging patient.

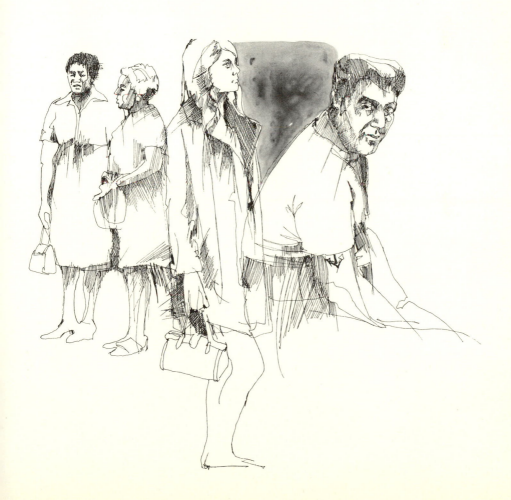

THERE ARE MORE elderly people in the United States today than ever before: one out of every ten Americans is over the age of sixty-five. This phenomenon is attributable to the dramatic increase in life expectancy. At the turn of the century, one could expect to live an average of forty-five years; at present, the average person lives into the late seventies. Many more persons are living into their eighties, nineties, and beyond. Since living longer increases one's chances of disease and illness, older persons are being admitted to acute and chronic care facilities with growing frequency. Also, Medicare, the federal health assistance program, and Medicaid, the general public assistance program, make entering a hospital or nursing home financially feasible for the older patient. As a result, the elderly may account for 60-70 percent of the patient population in an acute care hospital. In the chronic or nursing home setting, the elderly comprise 90 percent or more. *Geriatrics* is the health care specialty of old age. *Gerontology* is a broad field encompassing all that pertains to aging.

Precisely because of the rising numbers of elderly persons entering hospitals and nursing homes, schools of nursing are recognizing the importance of providing student nurses clinical experience in caring for geriatric patients. The skills of caring for the aging patient are essentially the same skills the nurse offers every patient, adapted to the physical changes and limitations that may accompany aging. However, special attention must be given to the psychological needs of the older person. Although the student nurse may not wish to pursue a career in geriatric nursing, knowledge of older patients and their needs is valuable. Contact with older persons is inescapable in nursing. Even in pediatrics, you may find that an older family member greatly influences the decisions and eventual recovery of a young patient.

What is aging?

There are many definitions of aging. In a sense, aging begins at the moment of birth, and each day is a part of the aging process. In another sense, aging is the biological maturation of mind and body. But at what point is one aged?

Aging, like all human experiences, is individual. Consider for a moment the eighty-three-year-old retired attorney, hospitalized for minor surgery, who sits up at night studying the new math, because, as he says, "It's so exciting. There's so much to know." At the other end of the spectrum is the sixty-eight-year-old woman lying impas-

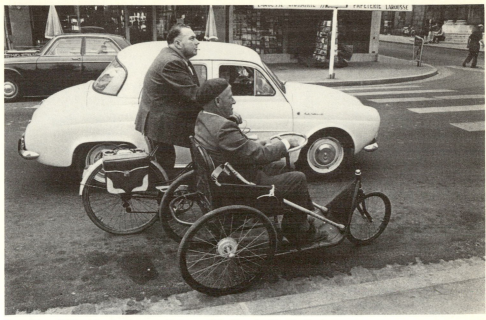

Top: *Harry Wilks / Stock, Boston*; Bottom: *Ellis Herwig / Stock, Boston*

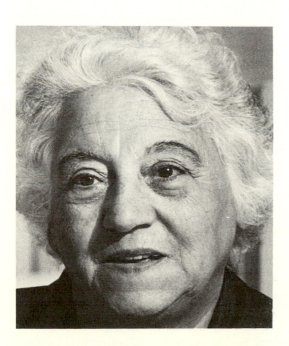

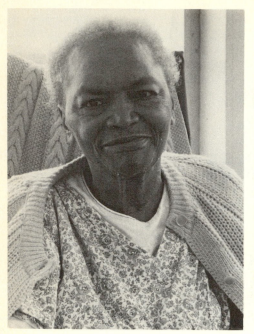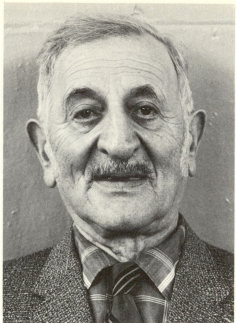

Left: *John Goodman*; Right: *Ira Gavrin*

sive in a nursing home bed, staring blankly at a rain-spattered window. Why do people age so differently? We can only speculate that variations depend on such factors as the patient's previous mental attitudes, health, and nutritional status, as well as the support of the family. Other factors, known and unknown, affect different individuals. Theories about the causes of aging are not germane here; it is important only that we remember that aging is a natural process.

Concerns of the elderly

In order to give comprehensive care to elderly patients, we need to know something about their concerns and problems. An unfortunate but all-important preoccupation of most elderly Americans is money, and how to make it cover the necessities of life. One out of every four older Americans is below the poverty level established by the U.S. Bureau of the Census in 1971. Another large segment of elderly people lives only slightly above the poverty level. To determine why this is so, several factors must be considered. First, though many have accumulated income for retirement through the federal Social Security program, this income alone has proven inadequate to meet the high cost of living today. Second, because employment savings plans were uncommon until relatively recently, the individual worker had to look ahead independently to secure his or her financial future. Third, money put aside years ago has been devalued by inflation. Furthermore, people are living longer, and any savings they have accumulated must thus last longer. And some elderly people who suffered illnesses or injuries before Medicare and Medicaid were established sustained financial losses they have never recovered.

Housing for the elderly is a national problem of considerable import. Many who have lived in the inner city for years no longer find their neighborhoods desirable—or even safe. Deteriorating neighborhoods, theft, and street violence have placed undue stress on older citizens and forced them to seek out less threatening environments. Finding adequate housing on a low fixed income is not easy. Large homes with high maintenance costs must often be traded for smaller, less expensive houses. Some elderly people purchase mobile homes and form their own retirement communities, while others must accommodate themselves to small furnished or unfurnished rooms with minimal cooking facilities. The U.S. Department of Housing and Urban Development (HUD) has subsidized a limited number of low and moderately priced public housing units, but the waiting lists are long for such accommodations.

Nutrition for the elderly is receiving increased attention. Because food costs have spiraled in the last few years, elderly people spend approximately one-third of their incomes on food. The older population has been found to have a high incidence of chronic malnutrition, due to food costs, the difficulties of shopping, long-standing poor eating habits, and poor meal planning. Attempts are being made to alleviate this situation through food stamps and community centers that provide one well-balanced meal a day.

Older persons also face the problems of obtaining mental health care services, securing adequate transportation, finding part-time employment, adjusting to the loss of a spouse or long-time friend, maintaining stable relationships with their children and grandchildren, and many others.

Organizations for the elderly

There are federal, state, and local organizations whose purpose is to provide for some of the needs of the aged. The Administration on Aging (AOA), a subdivision of the U.S. Department of Health, Education and Welfare (HEW), acts as a federal liaison to state and local agencies and publishes a monthly magazine, *Aging*. Many states and counties have their own councils on aging, and many communities are establishing senior citizen centers. The 1971 White House Conference on Aging defined the major problems of the elderly and pointed out the necessity for elderly people to join together to make their needs known and to exercise their political power.

In many localities, nurses are forming geriatric "special interest groups" to explore new knowledge, share concerns and techniques, and improve the quality of care for the older person. Geriatric nursing has come into its own as a specialty.

The nurse's attitudes toward the elderly

How quickly and how well the nurse relates to the older patient depends largely on past experiences with elderly persons. A nurse whose elderly aunt or grandparent has been cantankerous or disruptive to the family might find it harder to be empathetic and close to an elderly patient than would a nurse who has had a cherished relationship with an older relative.

Communication that is overly familiar can undermine a potentially good relationship with an elderly patient. Most older patients were raised with much more social formality than is usual now. First names were not used casually. It is best, then, for you to address the older patient by his or her last name until the patient requests that you do otherwise. Though hospitals are becoming increasingly informal, and many nurses and patients are on a first-name basis, it is prudent to show respect to the older person in this way. Another unfortunate commonplace practice is "talking down" to the elderly as if they were children. Terms such as "honey" and "dear" may be interpreted as degrading by the patient. The inclusive "let's do that" is also inappropriate, for it intrudes on the dignity of the patient and suggests dependency.

One must guard against stereotyping the aged. Often a patient's age elicits an unfortunate response before he or she even arrives, a response reflected in such remarks as, "Oh, but she's ninety-one. What are we supposed to do?" It sometimes appears that the limitations age imposes on good recovery make for lack of interest on the part of the nurse. As a professional, however, you must always strive for the maximal health and comfort of each patient, regardless of age.

The physiological effects of aging

The body of a young person makes the adaptations necessary to maintain homeostasis rather quickly. The elderly, due to cellular and tissue changes, respond or adapt more slowly to physiological and emotional stresses, and thus have more difficulty maintaining a state of balance. As nurses, we can help the older patient to make needed adaptations. This ought, in fact, to be the focus of care. For example, because the metabolism rate slows and body temperature lowers as one ages, the older person feels cold more acutely than the younger person. You can facilitate the patient's adaptation to a more comfortable body temperature by keeping the room temperature constant, guarding against drafts, and providing sufficient blankets and a sweater. Out of bed, the elderly patient may be more comfortable in shoes and stockings than in slippers.

Although individuals do not all experience the same bodily changes with aging, patterns can be discerned. The assessment process will be facilitated by familiarity with the potential effects of aging on the systems of the body.

Diminishment of the five senses

The five senses—seeing, hearing, smelling, tasting, and touching—diminish to some extent in the aging process. It is thought that these alterations occur because of degeneration of nerves, vascular irregularities, and/or local tissue changes. In some patients such diminishment is almost undiscernible; in others it is rather profound. While it may be obvious to you that a patient is partially blind or hard-of-hearing, you may overlook decreased sensitivity of taste, smell, and touch. When the patient has suffered a significant loss in one or more senses, a degree of sensory deprivation can result (see Chapter 21) and in turn can cause psychological depression. Patients are sometimes defensive about a loss of hearing or sight, and some frankly deny it. The nurse with ingenuity can frequently channel a patient's interest toward the use of a compensatory sense. For example, the elderly patient who was an avid reader and television viewer until loss of vision made both impossible could make use of "talking book" records available through a public library or an organization for the blind. Books with very large print are also available from the library, and some newspapers print large-type editions. The older patient with mental agility may want to learn a new skill, such as Braille.

The patient suffering from partial or total loss of vision has an added problem when entering the hospital. Accustomed to the arrangement of furniture at home, such a patient may find the hospital room confusing. Keeping furniture and personal items in the same places facilitates orientation. Patients who do not see well can distinguish objects better if they are painted bright colors. Beverage glasses should be only half-filled so as to spill less easily. Dishes arranged in the same position on the tray at each meal help the patient to eat independently. If the patient is totally blind, you should speak as you enter the room to allay the anxiety any of us would feel if we heard footsteps but could not see. It is also a kindness to touch the sightless patient as you speak, since touch provides warm contact with people the patient cannot see. When an older patient who has been using eye medication is admitted, be sure that the eye drops are available, that the physician writes an order for their use, and that they are given conscientiously. If contact lenses or glasses are needed, they should be cared for properly and the patient should be assisted in their use when necessary.

Loss of hearing is far more common among the elderly than is loss of sight. It has been estimated that one out of four persons over the age of sixty has a degree of hearing loss sufficient to be characterized "medically deaf." Among the several causes of deafness are disturbances of the auditory nerve or cerebral cortex and changes in the structure of the ear itself. A hearing aid is not helpful in all cases, and an examination by a specialist can determine whether or not such an aid would improve hearing. There are several things you can do, and instruct the family to do, to help the patient hear as well as possible. In assessing, it is not enough to observe that the patient has hearing loss. You should determine which ear is the least affected, so that when speaking you can stand facing the patient on the side where hearing is best. Sitting or standing at the patient's eye level is helpful because visual cues and lipreading help the patient understand what is said. Since hearing loss is often greater in the higher tones, lowering the voice slightly aids in communication. Speaking clearly and distinctly is helpful, because the elderly person may process information more slowly. One should never shout at the deaf, for shouting may be interpreted as a hostile outburst. You might guide the patient to a class on lipreading held in the community, if the patient shows interest.

Deafness is also a threat to the safety of the patient. The deaf person may not hear approaching cars that are out of the line of vision. A deaf apartment dweller may not hear a siren warning of a fire or emergency. It is often a good idea to offer the family guidance on care of the aged deaf.

Although it does not usually pose a serious problem, a loss of the sense of taste may cause the patient to become malnourished. Older patients frequently remark that food just doesn't taste as good as it once did. Dentures may interfere with both taste and texture perception. And food tastes appear to change with the aging process. One patient will crave sweets; another, who has always been fond of sweet foods, finds them no longer appealing. We know that color and consistency enhance taste, and diets planned with this in mind are no more expensive to prepare than bland, colorless diets.

The ability to smell also diminishes with age. Some older women use excessive perfumes due to a decreased olfactory sense. Because smell is a major factor in appetite, *anorexia* (loss of appetite) is in part attributable to olfactory impairment. Inability to smell smoke in time to flee from a fire could well affect the safety of the patient.

Although testing has shown that the sense of touch diminishes somewhat with age, this process rarely interferes with the individual's life. Men as well as women are taking up and enjoying such crafts as needlepoint, knitting, and weaving with increasing frequency. Difficulty working with fine yarns and patterns is often attributable to both visual loss and impairment of touch. The best solution is for the patient to use "bulky" knits and/or larger patterns. The primary problem posed by impairment of touch is the possibility of injury from sharp or hot objects. Such accidents might be prevented by avoiding hot water bottles and heating pads and by wearing shoes at all times to protect the feet. A deficit in touch could also cause a person not to note an injury, and thus to go without care. The older person should be encouraged to examine the extremities daily for signs of injury.

Changes in the skin

The integument, or skin, undergoes rather profound changes with aging. Wrinkling, though present to a degree even in children, is seen as an overt sign of aging. Research tells us that smoking, poor diet, and exposure to sun and weather hasten wrinkling. Prevention can be taught, but the person who already has extensive wrinkling has little recourse except cosmetic surgery, which is seldom undertaken by the elderly. Because older skin also becomes thin and dry, it is helpful to add oils directly to the tub or bedbath water or to apply palliative oils or lotions sparingly to the patient's skin immediately after the bath. The patient who is not soiled need not be bathed daily, since bathing is drying to the skin. Many older patients are used to bathing only once a week, and become upset at what they consider undue emphasis on cleanliness. Alcohol, often used in conjunction with rubs, should be avoided because of its drying effect on the skin. You should also be careful when placing an identification armband on the wrist of the elderly patient. An overly snug band can cause an abrasion, as can a tight watchband. Rubbing on sheets, lying on wrinkled bedding, and striking a siderail can all cause skin damage to the elderly. The slightest redness may be the forerunner of a difficult-to-heal decubitus ulcer, or bedsore.

Alopecia, the loss of hair, is another common result of aging. Not only scalp hair, but also hair in the axilla and genital area and general body hair are lost. Hair distribution becomes sparse. Baldness, though more common in the older male, also occurs in females. In women, baldness of the scalp is more "patchy" in appearance. It has been suggested that excessive shampooing, tight hats, and the practice of setting the hair tightly all promote balding, but evidence is not conclusive. Much male baldness is genetic and cannot be prevented. Baldness is important only if it affects the patient's body image. The use of a hairpiece should not be discouraged if it is beneficial to the patient's self-concept.

Musculo-skeletal degeneration

Musculo-skeletal changes due to aging affect the joints, long bones, and muscles, and can be very troublesome. The patient becomes more sedentary, and may even change position less frequently. It has been shown that the active, healthy person need not lose more than 30-40 percent of muscle tone and strength through aging. However, lack of exercise and improper diet often cause older people to lose a much greater proportion of their muscle tone. Weak muscles enhance the danger of broken bones, since they cannot provide adequate support. A moderate exercise program and a good diet adequate in protein will help the patient maintain muscle strength.

Bones often undergo degenerative changes with aging. The most common condition is *osteoporosis*, a metabolic failure to replace bone tissue, which leads to thin, porous bones that fracture easily. This condition occurs frequently in women over the age of sixty due to the reduction of estrogens. It also appears in men. Symptoms include low back pain, weakness, stooped posture, and a tendency to fracture bones. It is hoped that hormonal supplement therapy after menopause will greatly lessen the incidence of osteoporosis in older women, and early data appear to support this hope. In general, the diet should contain adequate calcium, protein, and vitamin D. Excess calcium in the diet will not prevent osteoporosis, which is a metabolic problem. The nurse must take extra precautions to guard such a patient agains accidents that could lead to the breakage of bones. If osteoporosis is severe, even grasping the long bones to turn the bed patient can result in a fracture. Ambulatory patients most often suffer fractures of the neck, the femur, and the trochanter. It has been speculated that, in many cases of hip fracture, the hip fractures spontaneously and causes the fall, rather than the reverse. Special care is needed for the patient with a fracture.

Most geriatric patients have some degree of osteoarthritis, which is assumed to be caused by the wearing of joint cartilage until the underlying bone is exposed. This situation in turn causes pain and immobility, and sometimes swelling, of the joint. Almost every person over the age of forty has some osteoarthritis in the cervical spine or neck, which may be asymptomatic until later in life when joints of the extremities also become involved. Treatment of arthritis consists of moderate exercise to maintain mobility, medications for inflammation and pain, and special therapies such as heat. When caring for the person with arthritis, a gentle touch is needed. The patient may be able to tell you how he or she moves most easily. Remember that the patient may be in constant pain.

Gout is a systemic illness whose most common symptom is swollen and inflamed joints. In addition to medication, the patient is often ordered to consume 3000-4000 cc. of fluid a day. Seeing to a fluid intake this high may take ingenuity on your part: a variety of juices and beverages and a schedule for intake made up with the patient's help are both beneficial.

Respiratory changes

The respiratory system is affected by changes in the musculo-skeletal system. Bone and muscle changes decrease actual chest size. There are also fewer alveoli, and those present become larger. The older person breathes slightly faster than the younger person in order to compensate for these changes. More important than actual chest size is decreased ability to cough. The collection of secretions that are not *expectorated* or spit out, is often a source of infection. Encouraging patients, especially those who are bedfast, to cough and deep-breathe can help ward off respiratory complications.

Cardiovascular complications

Changes within the cardiovascular system are complex. The most generalized complication that arises in the elderly is *arteriosclerosis*, a thickening of the middle wall of vessels that narrows the opening through which the blood flows. A more severe form of vascular compromise occurs with *atherosclerosis*, an additional thickening of the inner wall of arteries caused by the presence of deposits. This condition, which makes the vessels even more rigid and narrows the *lumen* (the interior of the vessels), affects every system of the body by diminishing the supply of blood to all organs.

The heart muscle itself is less efficient due to decreased blood supply, and a weaker beat often described as "thready" results. In conjunction with degenerative changes in the vessels supplying the heart muscle, the valves of the heart itself do not close as tightly as they once did. What are the consequences of all this for the patient? The blood pressure rises due to the increased force with which an unchanged volume of blood is pushed through a smaller lumen in the vessels. Because circulation is slow, the patient feels cold. Standing for a long period of time pools blood in the lower extremities and may cause dizziness. Lying on the extremities causes tingling and can disturb rest. The muscles stiffen, the muscles of respiration are no longer as vigorous, and overexertion can quickly exhaust the individual. The kidneys also receive less blood supply and are less productive than before. Drugs are excreted more slowly and can build up in the body, necessitating close observation for drug effects. The patient may be prescribed special drugs to facilitate functioning of the cardiovascular system, perhaps for the rest of his or her life.

Urinary problems

The genitourinary system is similarly affected by aging. As we have said, the vessels and renal arteries narrow. It is important to understand that, although the filtering process is less efficient, the volume of urine produced in a day remains normal; thus, in computing output for an elderly patient, the nurse should base findings on normal output. Studies show that bladder capacity lessens as one ages, necessitating that the bladder be emptied more frequently. Getting up at night to urinate is common, and interrupts the patient's rest. The sphincter, because it is muscular, loses some of its elasticity, and urine leakage can occur in both males and females. This is understandably disturbing to the patient, and a solution is not easy. The male can wear a device that consists of a penile covering much like a condom catheter, connected to a leg bag. Females may wear a light padding to protect against accidents. Muscular deterioration can also prevent the bladder from emptying completely, encouraging the growth of bacteria. Susceptibility to infections and the formation of stones (calculi) are the common results.

Gastrointestinal dysfunction

The gastrointestinal tract probably causes more patient distress than any other system of the body. Foods once easily digested can in the later years cause gastric or intestinal discomfort. Actually, the digestive system undergoes far less change than do other systems of the body. There is some decrease in the digestive juices and some reduction in the ability of the gall bladder to process fats. Much of the problem appears to be due to inadequate chewing of food because of ill-fitting dentures or poor teeth, inappropriate food choices, and emotional upset. Constipation in the elderly results largely, as we have said, from early and continued use of laxatives. Constipation is much more frequent than diarrhea. With old age and its accompanying muscular changes, the bowel becomes more unresponsive and laxatives less efficient. You may have considerable difficulty convincing the older patient of the need to increase fluid intake, include roughage in the diet, and exercise, though all contribute to healthy bowel functioning. It is often impossible to eliminate the use of laxatives once they have become firmly established.

Changes in the nervous system

Changes in the nervous system are of great concern to both the patient and the family. Neurons within the brain are lost from the age of twenty-five onward, and this loss increases with age. Also, arteriosclerosis affects vessels of the brain just as it does other vessels in the body. It is very important to note here, however, that a person's intelligence and emotional status are not directly affected by physiological vessel narrowing, as has been proven by autopsy examination of many older persons.

One of the most common maladies of the nervous system in the elderly is the *stroke* or *CVA*, meaning "cerebrovascular accident." Some five million people a year suffer strokes, the majority of them elderly. Strokes account for 12 percent of all deaths in the elderly. In general, a stroke is the obstruction or rupture of a vessel within the brain, causing blood to flow into the brain tissue. The manifestations of a stroke can be minimal or devastating. A patient may totally lose awareness. Loss of the ability to move or feel half of the body, loss of bladder and bowel control, and loss of speech are common. All or any of these complications may occur. The major goal of rehabilitative nursing is to restore function to the fullest degree possible.

Though the word *senile* means, in fact, the state of being old, it is commonly used with reference to mental deterioration, and thus has offensive connotations for many people. Lately, however, the term has come into use in diagnosis and appears on the charts of many older patients. In the context of diagnosis, senility means a state of physiological and psychological deterioration with age. At best, it is a broad and ill-defined term. Though no one knows whether the state of senility is reversible, a study undertaken several years ago sheds some light on the question. Five nursing-home patients who had been classified as senile were organized into a sharing group by the nurses. They met daily and talked about their past experiences and skills. At first, talk was minimal; but, as time went on, these patients renewed their interest in life, began caring for themselves again, and improved physically. One wonders, then, whether these people were truly senile. If so, can the state of senility be reversed? Far different, in any event, is the 107-year-old woman who exhibits little in the way of mental faculties and completely lacks reasoning power. Has her body outlived her brain? Unfortunately, less money was spent for medical research on aging in 1975 than on any other medical field. A vigorous investigation of the causes of senility does not appear to be in the offing.

Psychological concerns of the elderly

In considering psychological problems in the aging, we must look searchingly at our society. Undeniably, we tend not to look to older people with respect and recognition of their accomplishments and accumulated wisdom. The one word that best describes many elderly people today is "depressed." Chronic depression characterizes many people in their later years, and is caused in large part by loss: loss of home, friends, spouse, job, physical well-being, and of the significance of life. Because a depressed person is not pleasant company, further isolation results. Circularly, isolation causes even deeper depression.

Confusion is not uncommon in the geriatric patient. Often the patient recognizes such confusion and is frightened by it. Such a situation is not easily remedied, but there are things you can do to help. An older patient who is able to be of service in some manner will benefit from feeling needed. One older patient became much less confused and depressed when she was asked to help fold linen. Another patient wrote a letter for a fellow patient who could not write. Be creative! A replacement for a loss can be very therapeutic. A pet can, to a degree, replace human loss, and a volunteer job can replace past employment. What cannot be overemphasized is the importance of human contact—the feeling that people care. Calls and visits from friends and family and a caring attitude on your part are essential to the psychological well-being of the institutionalized patient.

In communicating with the elderly, it is beneficial to speak of the past, the present, and the future. The past is familiar, the present keeps thinking current, and the future—even the near future—suggests hope. Some nurses complain that care of the elderly is time-consuming because older patients seem to talk endlessly. "It's hard to get away," they complain. Remember that such patients are lonely and cherish the nurse's presence for even a short time. If you visit the patient frequently when care is not needed, communication will be improved.

Intervention is essential for the confused older patient, because confusion often increases if nothing is done about it. If the patient is confused about the time and place, informing the patient where he or she is and what time it is, including the day and month, is helpful. You might ask the family to bring a large-faced clock and a large-print calendar as aids to orientation. Sometimes confusion is only evident at night. A night light and siderails give the patient a feeling of security and enhance safety. Any necessary changes in routine should be undertaken slowly, since confused patients adapt poorly to sudden change. Another helpful technique is to make out a daily schedule, in large print, which allows the patient to keep track of the day's plan and to know what to expect at a given hour. Unrealistic plans and behavior should not be supported by the nurse. For example, if a patient tells you that he is going on a picnic and the snowy weather obviously makes such a plan impossible, it is not a kindness to agree. Simply point out that, although picnics are great fun on warm sunny days, the weather is poor and no plans for such a picnic have been made. Then, to minimize the patient's disappointment, offer an enjoyable substitute.

It is very poor practice to tell an elderly patient you will do something or be back at a specified time and not to follow through. Such a practice not only confuses the patient but also rapidly destroys trust. Specifying a time is good, but only if it is adhered to. Five minutes may seem like twenty to the inactive patient. Thus it is wise when you inform the patient that you will return in five minutes to suggest that he or she watch the clock. This practice calls on the patient's sense of time and enhances confidence that you will return as promised. These may seem like little things, but they are valuable to the aged.

Safety in caring for the elderly

Accidental injury or trauma sustained by the older patient is a particularly serious problem. The older patient heals slowly, and may develop pneumonia due to immobilization during recovery. Safety demands that you constantly observe the patient and the environment for potential hazards.

The patient, in a state of confusion, overzealous independence, or night disorientation, may try to get out of bed unaided. In many institutions it is mandatory for the siderails of every patient over sixty-five to be placed in the upright position at night, unless a waiver has been signed by the patient or the family. If the nurse describes this practice to the patient as a form of protection and not a punitive action, the patient will usually accept it. However, some patients will attempt to crawl over the rail, intensifying the danger. Soft wrist restraints or a vest restraint may then have to be applied. The call bell or button must always be placed so that even the restrained patient may call for help. The most restless patient becomes much quieter if he or she understands that you can be summoned at will.

Falls are of special concern to the elderly. Well-fitting hard-soled leather shoes are safest for older people. Bedroom slippers are often slippery and tend to fit poorly and give inadequate support; tennis shoes "catch" because of the rubber sole covering, and do not provide enough support. Spills are very dangerous, for both patient and nurse. If you see a spilled liquid, wipe it up immediately. Loose floor tiles, throw rugs, and such small items as bobby pins on the floor may all imperil the patient. Furniture should not obstruct passageways. Showers and tubs are very dangerous and a bath towel placed on the bottom of the tub provides for better footing. Handrails on bathroom walls offer support. And good lighting is essential for safety.

Another hazard is electrical appliances with worn cords or connections. Smoking is distinctly dangerous, and many hospitals have rules controlling it. Many chronic care facilities do not allow patients to have cigarettes or matches at their bedsides, which undermines patients' independence but may be necessary. Smoking in bed is dangerous for anyone, and particularly so for the older person whose reflexes may be impaired. The patient's safety is no minor matter, and perpetual vigilance by the nurse is indispensable.

Conclusion

Almost every specialty in nursing deals with elderly patients. Whatever your nursing interests, therefore, you must develop knowledge and skill in nursing geriatric patients. Moreover, you should examine carefully any preconceived ideas and feelings you hold about aging persons. It is highly unfortunate that some people consider the aged irrelevant or dispensable, forgetting that many leading artists, composers, and national leaders are well into the later years. It is important to remind ourselves that patients of all ages are unique individuals with specific problems. Let us give the elderly the kind of nursing care we ourselves would like to receive.

Study terms

alopecia
alveoli
anorexia
arteriosclerosis
atherosclerosis
empathy
expectorate
geriatric
gerontology

gout
lumen
osteoarthritis
osteoporosis
senile
sequence
stroke (CVA)
trauma

References

Birchenall, J., and Streight, M. E. 1973. *Care of the Older Adult*. Philadelphia: J. B. Lippincott.

Burnside, I. B. 1970. Clocks and Calendars. *American Journal of Nursing* 70:1:117-119.

Cahill, J. B., and Smith, D. 1975. Considerate Care of the Elderly: Little Things Mean a Lot. *Nursing '75* 5:9:38-39.

Costello, M. K. 1975. Sex, Intimacy and Aging. *American Journal of Nursing* 75:8:1330-1332.

de Beauvoir, Simone. 1972. *The Coming of Age*. New York: G. P. Putnam's Sons.

Evans, F. M. C. 1971. *Psychosocial Nursing*. New York: Macmillan.

Long, J. M., ed. *Caring for and Caring About Elderly People*. Philadelphia: J. B. Lippincott.

Markson, E. W. 1974. Readjustment to Time in Old Age. *Nursing Digest* 2:1:32-39.

"Nursing Care of the Elderly: Human Problems in Nursing," *Nursing '73* 3:4:18-22.

Patrick, M. 1973. Little Things Mean a Lot in Geriatric Rehabilitation. *Nursing '73* 3:8:7-9.

Pugsley, J. R., and Kolb, P. 1973. Jane and Sara Were Old and Helpless. *Nursing '75* 5:4:10-12.

Putnam, P. A. 1974. Orienting the Young to Old Age. *Nursing Outlook* 22:8:519-521.

Robinson, K. D. 1974. Therapeutic Interaction: A Means of Crisis Intervention with Newly Institutionalized Elderly Persons. *Nursing Clinics of North America* 9:1:89-96.

Stone, V. 1969. Give the Older Person Time. *American Journal of Nursing* 69:10:2124-2127.

Storlie, F. 1972. The Aged Poor. *Nursing '72* 2:5:19-34.

Thralow, J., and Watson, G. 1975. Remotivation for Geriatric Patients Using Elementary School Students. *Nursing Digest* 3:4:48-49.

Toussie, C. G. 1973. Mabel, You Don't Belong Here. *American Journal of Nursing* 73:12:2059.

Wilkiemeyer, D. S. 1972. Affection: Key to Care for the Elderly. *American Journal of Nursing* 72:12:2166-2168.

APPENDIX A Common Abbreviations

ABBREVIATION	LATIN MEANING	ENGLISH MEANING
@		at
abd.		abdomen
a.c.	ante cibum	before meals
A.D.L.		activities of daily living
ad lib.	ad libitum	at will
ax.		axillary
b.i.d.	bis in die	twice a day
B.M.		bowel movement
B.P.		blood pressure
B.R.P.		bathroom privileges
c̄	cum	with
cap.		capsule
c/o		complains of
D.O.A.		dead on arrival
et	et	and
Frax.		fractional, fracture
gtt.	gutta	drop
h.	hora	hour
H/P		history and physical
h.s.	hora somni	hour of sleep (bedtime)
I.M.		intramuscular
I.V.		intravenous
K.V.O.		keep vein open (with intravenous infusion)
L.L.Q.		left lower quadrant (of abdomen)
L.U.Q.		left upper quadrant (of abdomen)
N.P.O.	non per ora	nothing by mouth
n.r.	non repetatur	not to be repeated
"o"		orally
o.d.	omne die	every day
O.D.	oculo dexter	right eye
O.S.	oculo sinister	left eye
O.T.		occupational therapy
p.c.	post cibum	after meals
p.o.	per ora	by mouth

ABBREVIATION	LATIN MEANING	ENGLISH MEANING
p.r.n.	pro re nata	when needed
P.T.		physical therapy
q.s.	quantum sufficiat	sufficient quantity
q.d.	quaque die	each day
q.h.	quaque hora	every hour
q.2h.		every two hours
q.3h., etc.		every three hours, etc.
q.i.d.	quater in die	four times a day
q.o.d.	quaque alto die	every other day
R.L.Q.		right lower quadrant (of abdomen)
R.O.M.		range of motion
R.U.Q.		right upper quadrant (of abdomen)
s̄	sine	without
s.o.b.		short of breath
s.o.s.	si opus sit	if necessary
spec.		specimen
stat.	statin	immediately
sub q.		subcutaneous
tab.		tablet
t.i.d.	ter in dies	three times a day
T.K.O.		to keep open (intravenous infusion)
T.L.C.		tender loving care
T.P.R.		temperature, pulse, and respiration
U.A.		urine analysis
ung.	unguent	ointment

APPENDIX B   Abbreviations of Medical Conditions

A.R.D.S.	adult respiratory distress syndrome
A.K. Amp.	above-knee amputation
A.S.C.V.D.	arteriosclerotic cardiovascular disease
A.S.H.D.	arteriosclerotic heart disease
B.E.	bacterial endocarditis
B.K. Amp.	below-knee amputation
B.P.H.	benign prostatic hypertrophy
Ca.	cancer (carcinoma)
C.F.	cystic fibrosis
C.H.D.	coronary heart disease
C.H.F.	congestive heart failure
C.O.P.D.	chronic obstructive pulmonary disease
C.V.A.	cerebral vascular accident
D.&C.	dilation and curettage (of uterus)
D.I.C.	disseminated intravascular coagulation
D.T.'s	delerium tremens
F.U.O.	fever of undetermined origin
G.B.	gall bladder
G.C.	gonococcal infection
H.C.V.D.	hypertensive cardiovascular disease
L.T.B.	laryngo-tracheobronchitis
M.I.	myocardial infarction, mitral insufficiency
M.S.	multiple sclerosis
P.A.P.	primary atypical pneumonia
P.I.D.	pelvic inflammatory disease
P.V.D.	peripheral vascular disease
R.D.S.	respiratory distress syndrome
R.F.	rheumatic fever
R.H.D.	rheumatic heart disease
S.B.E.	subacute bacterial endocarditis
S.I.D.	sudden infant death
T.&A.	tonsillectomy and adenoidectomy
T.B. or T.B.C.	tuberculosis
T.I.A.	transient ischemia attack
T.U.R.	transurethral resection of the prostate
U.R.I.	upper respiratory infection
U.T.I.	urinary tract infection

413

Index

Abandonment, fear of, 360
Abbreviations, 110, 412-414
  of medical conditions, 414
Abdominal muscles, body mechanics
    and, 291-292
Abdominal paracentesis, 170-171
Abortion, 13
Absorption of drugs, 150
Acceptance
  of body image, 385
  dying and, 357
Activity, 282-301. *See also* Exercise(s);
    Immobility
  assessment of, 288-289
  benefits of, 284
  pain and, 347-348
  prescriptions for, 289
  in sleep, 305, 306-307
Acupuncture, pain and, 347
Addiction, narcotics, 347
Adolescence, 51-53, 61
  body image in, 52
  sexual development in, 52-53
Adulthood, 53-58, 61
  18 to 40 years, 53-55
  40 to 65 years, 55-57
  over 65 years, 57-58
Aesthetic needs, 38
Aggression, childhood, 51
Aging, 392-411. *See also* Elderly; Life
    cycle
  blood pressure and, 220
  cardiovascular complications of,
    403-404
  definition of, 394-396
  gastrointestinal dysfunction and,
    405
  hearing and, 400
  infection and, 177

  musculo-skeletal degeneration
    and, 402-403, 404
  nervous system and, 405-406
  physiological effects of, 399
  respiratory changes and, 403
  senses and, 399-401
  sexuality and, 324
  skin changes and, 401-402
  sleep and, 309-310
  smell and, 401
  taste and, 401
  touch and, 401
  urinary problems of, 404
  vision and, 399-400
Agnostics, 139
Air-borne pathogens, 179, 185, 186
Airway patency, 225-226
Albuminuria, 270
Alcohol
  backrubs and, 205
  fever reduction and, 230
  intravenous needle removal and,
    260
Allergies, drugs and, 149
Alopecia, 402
Alveoli, 223
  aging and, 403
Ambulation, 295-297
a.m. care, 198, 199
American Hospital Association, Pa-
    tients' Bill of Rights of, 12-13
American Nurses' Association Code
    for Nurses, 10, 11
Amphetamines, 311
Analgesics, 347, 348
Anesthesia, 346
Anger
  body image problems and, 384
  dying and, 356-357, 365

Laws, *See* Legal concerns
Laxatives, 275-276, 277, 278, 405
Learning, 120. *See also* Teaching,
    health
  anxiety and, 88-89, 124
  childhood and, 50-51
  definition of, 120
  environment and, 124-125
  external influences on, 124-128
  goals for, 121-122
  internal influences on, 123-124
  life experience and, 123
  motivation for, 124
  needs, assessment of, 120-121
  physiologic status and, 123
  previous education and, 123
  readiness for, 124
  vocabulary and, 123
Legal concerns, 8-10
  credentials and, 21
  dependent functioning and, 23
  drug administration and, 152
Liability insurance, 10
Libido, 326
  drugs and, 324-325
  surgery and, 328
Licensure, 21
Life cycle, 42-63
  adolescence (12 to 18 years), 51-53,
    61
  body image and, *see* Body image
  early childhood (3 to 6 years),
    49-50, 60
  infancy (birth to 1 year), 45-48, 59
  later years (over 65), 57-58, 61
  middle childhood (6 to 12 years),
    50-51, 60-61
  middle years (40 to 65), 55-57
  moving through, 58-59
  normal vs. usual in, 44
  nursing practice and, 59-61
  sexual development and, 45, 48,
    49, 50, 51, 52-53, 54-58
  stages of, 44-58
  tasks in, 47
  toddler (1 to 3 years), 48-49, 59
  young adulthood (18 to 40 years),
    53-55, 61

Life role, body image and, 385
Life style
  learning new, 120-121
  sexual, 320, 321
Life support, 224-226
  administering emergency, 225-
    226
  ethics of, 13
  recognizing need for, 225
Lifting, 290-292
Linens, care of, 181, 208
Lips
  care of, 207
  fever blisters of, 230
Listening, active, 105
Liver scan, 168-169
Long-term care, interdependent
    functioning and, 24-25
Loss
  aging and, 406
  grief and, 362-365
Lotions, backrub, 205
Love, need for, 34-36, 59
Lumbar puncture, 170-171
Lumen, blood vessel, 404
Lung scan, 168-169

Mandatory registration, 21
Masks, infection and, 186-187
Maslow's hierarchy of needs, 33-38
Massage, 205
Mastectomy, 328
  body image integrity and, 388-389
Masturbation, 323-324
Mattress, alternating pressure, 297-
    298
Meals, 250-252
  assisting patient with, 252
  environment for, 251
  patterns of, 246
  positioning for, 250-251
Meaningfulness
  of all behavior, 84-85
  of sensory input, 374-375
Meatus, urinary, 266, 267
Mechanics, body, 290-293
Medals, religious, 136, 142
Medication, *see* Drugs